Promoting the Health of the Community

Julie Ann St. John
Susan L. Mayfield-Johnson
Wandy D. Hernández-Gordon

Editors

Promoting the Health of the Community

Community Health Workers Describing
Their Roles, Competencies, and Practice

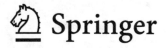 Springer

Editors
Julie Ann St. John
Department of Public Health
Texas Tech University Health
Sciences Center
Abilene, Texas, USA

Susan L. Mayfield-Johnson
Department of Public Health
University of Southern Mississippi
Hattiesburg, Mississippi, USA

Wandy D. Hernández-Gordon
HealthConnect One
Chicago, Illinois, USA

ISBN 978-3-030-56377-6   ISBN 978-3-030-56375-2   (eBook)
https://doi.org/10.1007/978-3-030-56375-2

This Springer imprint is published by the registered company Springer Nature Switzerland AG
The registered company address is: Gewerbestrasse 11, 6330 Cham, Switzerland

Foreword

Greetings from the Community Health Worker (CHW) team of Lisa Renee Holderby-Fox and Durrell Fox. We are pleased to welcome you to *Promoting the Health of the Community–CHWs: Describing Their Roles, Competencies and Practice!* Together we have approximately 58 years of experience as CHWs—28 and 30 years, respectively. Since the early 1990s, we have served our communities both in paid and volunteer CHW roles in community and clinical settings to promote health. In addition, we have served as CHWs for the CHW workforce—promoting a healthy workforce locally and nationally. We met two decades ago while organizing CHWs in Massachusetts to develop a statewide CHW network, which later became an association. This led us on the path to promote policy change to sustain and support the workforce, including successfully drafting legislation.

We are honored to serve as founding leadership of local, regional, and national CHW associations, coalitions, and networks. We have provided guidance to several national CHW projects and initiatives—often as a team. These initiatives have informed and progressed the local and national CHW movements. Our resumes include: providing leadership to the Center For Sustainable Health Outreach (CSHO) and the Unity Conference; the Community Health Worker National Educational Collaborative (CHW-NEC); the Health Resources and Services Administration (HRSA) 2007 Community Health Worker National Workforce Study; the Community Health Worker Core Consensus (C3) Project; the American Public Health Association (APHA) CHW Section; and the short-lived American Association of CHWs (AACHW). Most recently, we are founding board members of the National Association of CHWs (NACHW). Additionally, Lisa Renee served two terms as an appointed member to the National Healthcare Workforce Commission created by the Patient Protection and Affordable Care Act (ACA).

Over the years, we have proudly served our communities and contributed to achieving a vision where individuals, families, communities, and the CHW workforce are supported to thrive and to attain their optimal health and growth potential. We acknowledge that inequities and disparities continue to exist and have a profound impact on our communities and the CHW workforce. Hence, the struggle continues, and we shall overcome. We celebrate our advances and our continued work to address these inequities through utilizing currently available tools and by embracing the development of new resources, including the development of this book as a useful tool to apply in education and in practice. We believe the continued struggles for health equity have led to valuable lessons learned from each other, our family, communities, peers, and colleagues. We celebrate the dedication, role, and stories of CHWs. However, others have been telling the CHW story for too long. Over the past two decades, we have been encouraging our CHW peers to own and tell their stories and truths. Perhaps that is why the editors of this book, which tells the stories of CHW teams across the country, have asked us to contribute by writing this foreword.

We have known and worked with the editors of this book for many years. Although the number of years and projects we have worked together on varies, our relationships with the editors are all based on our shared desire to promote, sustain, and elevate the CHW workforce and profession. We have worked closely with our CHW peer and editor, Wandy D. Hernandez-Gordon, on numerous national CHW projects, policy efforts, and initiatives, including most recently serving as founding board members for NACHW. We have all served as past chairs of the APHA CHW Section. During our terms as chairs of the APHA CHW section, we assisted to lead efforts to develop a national CHW standard occupational code and APHA policies that support CHW self-determination and majority involvement on CHW workforce development task force and initiative teams. Susan Mayfield Johnson is a public health practitioner, researcher, and long-time CHW ally whom we have worked with and collaborated on many CHW professional and leadership development opportunities for two decades, including CSHO, the Unity Conference, APHA CHW section and other CHW meetings, conferences, and additional training opportunities. We have had the pleasure of working with Julie St. John and the many others as members of the National Community Health Worker Core Consensus (C3) Project team and the APHA CHW Section the past several years. Durrell has also worked with Julie on a statewide project in Massachusetts that utilized a curriculum that Julie developed to train CHWs in the areas of senior home visits to assess safety and prevent senior falls. In addition to calling these amazing women colleagues, they are also friends. We have met members of their families and have welcomed new members to all their families over the years. We consider them part of our family and valued members of our growing CHW family.

A rallying cry for CHW self-determination "Nothing about us, without us!" has increasingly been embraced by CHWs and allies nationally over the past few years. This book is an excellent example of an equitable partnership supporting CHW authors as members of 36 chapter teams made up of approximately 100 authors from across the country, providing a platform for CHWs to articulate and illustrate some of the day-to-day actions and activities that are essential to fulfilling CHW core roles. Teams of CHWs and allies across the country, consisting of voices from Alaska, Hawaii, east and west coasts, northern and southern states, and the middle of our country, have contributed their experience and wisdom to bring this book to life. Although CHWs are a diverse workforce who works in diverse communities, CHW core roles are foundational and common across the country.

Chapter 2 weaves the story of the C3 Project—a national project focused on engaging CHWs and stakeholders throughout the research process to build consensus around CHW scope of practice (roles) and CHW competencies, which include CHW core skills and qualities. The C3 story shares information about the project's methods and findings and also illuminates valuable information about how the journey of the project findings and recommendations were guided and navigated by CHW leadership on the project team and, even more powerful, were shaped by hundreds of CHWs through a rigorous CHW network/association review process.

This book includes several more illustrations of the critical importance of CHWs' role in the journey to advance the workforce. This journey truly models equity and CHW self-determination and leads to a destination that can have a positive impact on our communities, workforce, clinical and nonclinical providers, human services, and health and public health professionals. Part II of the book animates the C3 national list of CHW core roles by providing examples from the field representing the practical application of all ten national CHW core roles in action. To illustrate the core role of providing coaching and social support, there is a great story about "CHWs Extending Solutions to Violence." Overall, there are CHW models illustrating core roles from approximately 19 states and Tribal nations—which describe the national CHW scope of practice. There is some useful and practical information for readers interested in CHWs role in behavioral health, trauma informed care, oral health, cultural mediation, and systems navigation.

This book provides evidence that our CHW workforce makes a difference in people's lives, communities, and health outcomes. CHWs have been documented doing this work in the U.S. for decades and much longer internationally. Unfortunately, among policy makers and healthcare providers, there is still uncertainty of who we are as a workforce and the value we bring. We can think of no better resource to share the complete picture of the roles CHWs play, our contributions, impact on the communities we serve, and provide concrete examples, than the voices of CHWs. This is where the importance of this book lies. More than 20 teams of CHWs tell their stories. There is beauty in CHWs telling their own stories to provide examples of our nationally agreed upon core roles. The three editors, one of whom is a CHW, have over 60 years combined experience working with the CHW profession, and all were actively engaged with the C3 project. They are the right team to lead this project.

Over the course of our long careers, we have seen our workforce grow both numerically and professionally. We have seen opportunities for training and education expand and interdisciplinary collaboration and policies developed to support and sustain the workforce. Even with all the advances within the CHW workforce, there are still basic questions we are often asked like, "What do CHWs do?" and "How do we do it?" Until now, there has not been a comprehensive work to answer that question. *Promoting the Health of the Community: Community Health Workers Describing Their Roles, Competencies, and Practice* provides some long awaited answers.

CHWs occupy a special place in community health and wellness as well as in the lives we touch. We have shared our stories with each other, and this book provides a space to share our story with others in a meaningful way. Using the C3 framework of CHW core roles to share our stories is a unique method to give life to the roles of CHWs through practical, concrete examples. The editors understand the value of CHWs telling our stories and have honored, "Nothing about us without us." You are holding the next chapter in the collective CHW story. A collection of CHW stories in our own words, supporting the roles and skills of CHWs, is long overdue.

Roster Health   Lisa Renee Holderby-Fox
Stone Mountain, GA, USA

JSI Research and Training Institute, Inc.   Durrell Fox
Stone Mountain, GA, USA
March 2020

Preface

We are honored and elated to share this first edition of this Community Health Worker (CHW) book. CHWs are increasingly important members of the healthcare and public health professions. Yet, in spite of the exponential growth of CHWs interventions, CHW training programs, and CHW certification and credentialing by state agencies, a gap persists in the literature regarding current CHW roles and skills, scope of practice, CHW job settings, and national standards. Hence, the purpose of the book is to provide information about CHWs, the roles CHWs play as change agents in their communities, describe the integration of CHWs into healthcare teams, and support and recognize the CHW workforce. Specifically, the book highlights core roles and skills of CHWs that came from The Community Health Worker (CHW) Core Consensus (C3) Project. CHW teams across the United States share their stories about core roles they do in their respective communities, with an introduction to various roles and two examples from CHW teams who explain how they carry out the respective role, challenges, successes, and lessons learned.

The intended audience includes those interested in CHW scope of practice and/or certification/credentialing, CHWs, anyone interested in becoming a CHW, policy makers, CHW payer systems, CHW supervisors, CHW employers, CHW instructors/trainers, CHW advocates/supporters, and communities served by CHWs. The primary audience will find this book useful for numerous reasons. First, the book highlights nationally recognized standards for CHW roles, skills, and qualities, which were updated in 2016 from the National Community Health Advisor Study in 1998; the audience will receive information about these updated standards. This book also tells the story of how CHW teams are practically implementing these roles within a variety of settings and serving as change agents in their respective communities. Second, this book is written by CHW teams doing the work; each chapter includes a CHW author. Third, entities considering the CHW model and guidance on CHW scope of practice can utilize this book as a guideline developed by other successful CHW programs as defined by the chapter authors.

Abilene, TX, USA   Julie Ann St. John
Hattiesburg, MS, USA   Susan L. Mayfield-Johnson
Chicago, IL, USA   Wandy D. Hernández-Gordon

Acknowledgments

We could not have completed this book without the thousands of Community Health Workers, Community Health Representatives, Promotores, and others in this field who tirelessly serve our communities every single day to make a difference in the lives of its representatives, around our nation and globally. You provided the stories and the inspiration for this book. Thank you for sharing your thoughts, ideas, challenges, and success stories with us.

You contribute to making our community's health more equitable. You make a difference in the communities you serve; you have made a difference in our lives.

We also want to thank Springer staff for their guidance and support in the development of this book, especially Janet Kim. We also want to acknowledge and thank Miranda Rice and Brady St. John for their administrative support in compiling this book.

Lastly, we thank our family, friends, and colleagues who encouraged and supported us throughout this project.

Contents

12   Implementing Individual and Community Assessments   289

Jeffrey Tangonan Acido, Jermaine Agustin, Caitlin G. Allen,
Rebecca Anderson, Melanie Apodaca, Rachel Arasato,
Roshni Biswa, Gretchen Bondoc, J. Nell Brownstein,
Chasity Nohealani Cadaoas, Kristy Canionero, Ashley Corpuz,
Dennis Dunmyer, Selena Gaui, Leina'ala Kanana, Shawna Koahou,
Dominique Lucas, Sara S. Masoud, June Munoz,
Susan Oshiro-Taogoshi, Kelly Pilialoha-Cypriano, E. Lee Rosenthal,
Desiree Santana, Dalia Solia, R. Napualani Spock,
Julie Ann St. John, Malia Talbert, Nathan Tarvers, Lani Untalan,
Wes Warner, Shannon Watson, and Deborah White

Caitlin G. Allen, E. Lee Rosenthal, Sara S. Masoud,
          and J. Nell Brownstein
R. Napualani Spock, Julie Ann St. John, Leina'ala Kanana,
          Jeffrey Tangonan Acido, Jermaine Agustin, Kristy Canionero,
          Malia Talbert, Dalia Solia, Rachel Arasato,
          Kelly Pilialoha-Cypriano, Shawna Koahou, Shannon Watson,
          Gretchen Bondoc, Selena Gaui, Nathan Tarvers, Lani Untalan,
          Desiree Santana, Ashley Corpuz, Chasity Nohealani Cadaoas,
          June Munoz, and Susan Oshiro-Taogoshi
Dominique Lucas, Wes Warner, Melanie Apodaca, Roshni Biswa,
          Deborah White, Rebecca Anderson, and Dennis Dunmyer

13   Conducting Outreach   323

Caitlin G. Allen, Gabriela Boscan, Gregory J. Dent, Amy Elizondo,
Catherine Gray Haywood, Gail R. Hirsch, Teresa Mendez,
Laura McTighe, Katharine Nimmons, Janice Probst,
Floribella Redondo-Martinez, Carl H. Rush, David Secor,
Myriam Torres, and Ashley Wennerstrom

Editors and Contributors

About the Editors and Contributors

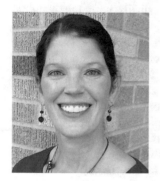 **Julie Ann St. John, DrPH, MPH, MA, CHW** is the Associate Professor, Department of Public Heath, Texas Tech University Health Sciences Center (TTUHSC), and the Associate Dean, Graduate School of Biomedical Sciences, TTUHSC, Abilene campus (Associate, tenured professor). She has her doctorate in public health from the University of Texas Health Science Center at Houston School of Public Health. She is a Texas-certified Community Health Worker Instructor, served on the Texas CHW Advisory Committee from 2011–2020, serves on the Interim Board of the Texas Association of Promotores and Community Health Workers, is a member of the American Public Health Association (APHA) CHW Section Council, and has worked with CHWs for 20 years. Her research interests include utilizing CHWs in community-based participatory research and community health development approaches, and she has served as the principal and co-investigator on numerous projects. She founded the National CHW Training Center at Texas A&M School of Public Health. Additionally, she teaches several undergraduate- and graduate-level public health courses.

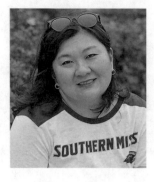

Susan L. Mayfield-Johnson, PhD, MPH, MCHES is an Associate Professor in the School of Health Professions, College of Nursing and Health Professions, at the University of Southern Mississippi in Hattiesburg. She has served as a CHW ally for over 20 years. Her research has focused on CHWs, vulnerable populations, health disparities, and qualitative research designs. Nationally, she is an advisory board member for the National Association of Community Health Workers (NACHW), section council member with the Community Health Worker (CHW) Section of the American Public Health Association (APHA), and a Master Trainer for the Women's Health Leadership Institute, Office of Women's Health, US Department of Health and Human Services. She also serves on the Southeastern Health Equity Council, as a part of the Regional Health Equity Councils with the National Partnership for Action to End Health Disparities for the Office of Minority Health. She also served as an International Outbound Fellow with the US State Department and Association of University Centers on Disabilities. In Mississippi, she serves on various statewide committees and advisory councils like the Health Equity Coalition, Mississippi Chronic Illness Coalition, Mississippi Food Policy Council, and the Mississippi Hypertension Coalition. Most recently, she was honored as a Health Care Hero by the *Mississippi Business Journal* and by the Mississippi Board of Trustees of the State Institutions of Higher Learning as the Diversity and Inclusion Educator of the Year.

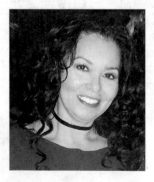

Wandy D. Hernández-Gordon, CD(DONA), BDT(DONA), CLC, CCE(ACBE), CHW has been involved with community health workers since she was a child as a consumer of services, to now as a community health worker national speaker and advocate for 28 years. Wandy has been a bilingual and bicultural specialized trainer at HealthConnect One (HC One) in Chicago, IL, since 1999 and is a Certified Lactation Counselor, DONA-Certified Doula Trainer, and Certified Childbirth Educator. Wandy served as President of the National Lay Health Workers/ Promotores Network from 2005 to 2007, and from 2012 to 2014 served as the Chair of the American Public Health Association's CHW Section. Wandy

served as an active member of the Illinois Statewide
Community Health Worker Advisory Board and in
2011 served as an advisory board member of The
Illinois AHEC Network and of the South Suburban
College Community Health Worker Technology
Advisory Community. Wandy is a co-founder of the
Chicago Community Health Workers Local Network,
formally known as Illinois Community Health Worker
Association, and is a coauthor on a peer-reviewed arti-
cle entitled "The Journal of Ambulatory Care
Management Community Health Workers Part 1."
Currently, Wandy chairs the Board of the National
Association of Community Health Workers, where she
brings vision and values to the table in support of unity
in the CHW workforce.

Contributors

Jeffrey Tangonan Acido, PhD Kokua Kalihi Valley Community Health Center, Kalilhi, HI, USA

Jermaine Agustin, CHW Wai'anae Coast Comprehensive Community Health Center, Wai'anae, HI, USA

Caitlin G. Allen, MPH CGA Consulting, Charleston, SC, USA

Alexandra Anderson, MPH New York City Department of Health and Mental Hygiene, New York City, NY, USA

Rebecca Anderson, MSW KC CARE Health Center, Kansas City, MO, USA

Melanie Apodaca, CHW KC CARE Health Center, Kansas City, MO, USA

Rachel Arasato, CHW Wai'anae Coast Comprehensive Community Health Center, Wai'anae, HI, USA

Diane Garzon Arbelaez Boston Medical Center, Boston, MA, USA

Cinthia Arechiga, CHW San Bernardino County, San Bernardino, CA, USA

Janae Ashford, CHW Detroit Health Department, Detroit, MI, USA

Melinda Banks, BA, CHWIII Sinai Urban Health Institute, Chicago, IL, USA

Mae-Gilene Begay, MSW, CHR/CHW Navajo Nation Community Health Representative (CHR)/Outreach Program, Window Rock, AZ, USA

Anastasia Belliard, DPT Loma Linda University Health, Loma Linda, CA, USA

Juan Carlos Belliard, PhD, MPH Loma Linda University Health, Loma Linda, CA, USA

Brook Bender, CHR Hualapai Tribe, Peach Springs, AZ, USA

Roshni Biswa, CHW KC CARE Health Center, Kansas City, MO, USA

Gretchen Bondoc, CHW Wai'anae Coast Comprehensive Community Health Center, Wai'anae, HI, USA

Tom Bornstein, DDS SEARHC Dental, Juneau, AK, USA

Gabriela Boscan, MPH National Rural Health Association, Washington, DC, USA

Arika Makena Bridgeman-Bunyoli, MPH, CHW Portland Children's Levy, Portland, OR, USA

J. Nell Brownstein, PhD Texas Tech University Health Sciences Center El Paso, El Paso, TX, USA

S. Kim Bush, MPA, CHWI, CHW, DrPH (candidate) The University of Texas Health Science Center at Tyler, Tyler, TX, USA

Gabriela Bustos, CHWII Sinai Urban Health Institute, Chicago, IL, USA

Chasity Nohealani Cadaoas, AA, CHW Maui Aids Foundation, Wailuku, HI, USA

Kristy Canionero, CHW Wai'anae Coast Comprehensive Community Health Center, Wai'anae, HI, USA

Olveen Carrasquillo, MD, MPH University of Miami, Miami, FL, USA

Heather Carter, EdD Arizona House of Representatives, Arizona Center for Rural Health, Mel and Enid Zuckerman College of Public Health, The University of Arizona, Phoenix, AZ, USA

Tamala Carter, CHW Penn Center for Community Health Workers, Penn Medicine, Philadelphia, PA, USA

Maria C. Cole, LMSW, MSW, MPH Baylor Scott & White Research Institute, Dallas, TX, USA

Ashley Corpuz, CHW Wai'anae Coast Comprehensive Community Health Center, Wai'anae, HI, USA

Naomi Cottoms, MA Tri County Rural Health Network, Inc., Helena, AR, USA

Megan Daly, MHA Loma Linda University Health, Loma Linda, CA, USA

Jill Guernsey de Zapien, BS University of Arizona Prevention Research Center, Mel and Enid Zuckerman College of Public Health, Tucson, AZ, USA

Gregory J. Dent Northwest Georgia Healthcare Partnership, Dalton, GA, USA

Yaminette Diaz-Linhart, MSW, MPH Brandeis University, Waltham, MA, USA

Ramona Dillard, BS, CHR/CHW Pueblo of Laguna Community Health, Albuquerque, NM, USA

Carolyn Dixon Where Do We Go from Here, Inc (formerly from Life Camp, Inc.), Queens, NY, USA

Cecil H. Doggette Health Services for Children with Special Needs, Washington, DC, USA

Teresa Campos Dominguez, CHW Multnomah County Health Department, Portland, OR, USA

Dennis Dunmyer, BBA, MSW, JD KC CARE Health Center, Kansas City, MO, USA

Amy Elizondo, MPH National Rural Health Association, Washington, DC, USA

Irene Estrada, CHW Penn Center for Community Health Workers, Penn Medicine, Philadelphia, PA, USA

Danielle Fastring, PhD, MS, MPH College of Osteopathic Medicine, William Carey University, Hattiesburg, MS, USA

Emily Feinberg, ScD, CPNP Boston University, Boston, MA, USA

Jill Feldstein, MPA Penn Center for Community Health Workers, Penn Medicine, Philadelphia, PA, USA

Maria Lourdes Fernandez, CHW Arizona Community Health Workers Association, Inc., Douglas, AZ, USA

Ivys Fernandez-Pastrana, JD Boston Medical Center, Lowell, MA, USA

Princess Fortin, MPH New York City Department of Health and Mental Hygiene, New York City, NY, USA

Durrell J. Fox, BS JSI Research and Training, Inc., Atlanta, GA, USA

Almitra Gasper New York City Department of Health and Mental Hygiene, New York City, NY, USA

Selena Gaui, CHW Wai'anae Coast Comprehensive Community Health Center, Wai'anae, HI, USA

Rebeca Guzmán, LMSW Detroit Health Department, Detroit, MI, USA

Catherine Gray Haywood, BSW Louisiana Community Health Outreach Network, New Orleans, LA, USA

Ilda Hernández Enlace Chicago, Chicago, IL, USA

Wandy D. Hernández-Gordon, AA, CHW HealthConnect One, Chicago, IL, USA

Gail R. Hirsch, MEd Massachusetts Department of Public Health, Boston, MA, USA

Lisa Renee Holderby-Fox, AS, CHW Roster Health, Stone Mountain, GA, USA

Dana Hughes, DrPH Philip R. Lee Institute for Health Policy Studies, University of California, San Francisco, San Francisco, CA, USA

Alexander Ross Hurley, MPH University of North Carolina, Chapel Hill, NC, USA

Jorge M. Ibarra, MD, MPH, FACE Texas A&M University, El Paso, TX, USA

Maia Ingram, MPH University of Arizona Prevention Research Center, Mel and Enid Zuckerman College of Public Health, Tucson, AZ, USA

Kim Jay, BA Sinai Urban Health Institute, Chicago, IL, USA

Stephanie Jordan, CHWII Sinai Urban Health Institute, Munster, IN, USA

Leina'ala Kanana, MSW Wai'anae Coast Comprehensive Community Health Center, Wai'anae, HI, USA

Shreya Kangovi, MD, MSPH University of Pennsylvania, Philadelphia, PA, USA

Francis Kham, CHW Immigrant and Refugee Community Organization, Portland, OR, USA

Shawna Koahou, CHW Wai'anae Coast Comprehensive Community Health Center, Wai'anae, HI, USA

Rhonda M. Lay, CHWIII Sinai Urban Health Institute, Chicago, IL, USA

Dane Lenaker, DMD, MPH SEARHC Dental, Juneau, AK, USA

Carmen Linarte, BA, MPH, CCHW University of Miami, Miami, FL, USA

Javier Lopez, MPA Red Hook Initiative, Brooklyn, NY, USA

Dominique Lucas, CHW, LMSW KC CARE Health Center, Kansas City, MO, USA

Elizabeth Mallott, RDH SEARHC Dental, Juneau, AK, USA

Helen Margellos-Anast, MPH Sinai Urban Health Institute, Chicago, IL, USA

Maria Martin, CHW, BSW PASOs, Columbia, SC, USA

Sahida Martínez, CHW Enlace Chicago, Chicago, IL, USA

Sara S. Masoud, MPH UT Health San Antonio, San Antonio, TX, USA

Susan L. Mayfield-Johnson, PhD, MPH, MCHES Department of Public Health, School of Health Professions, The University of Southern Mississippi, Hattiesburg, MS, USA

Laura McTighe, PhD Department of Religion, Florida State University, Tallahassee, FL, USA

Teresa Mendez, CHW Northwest Georgia Healthcare Partnership, Dalton, GA, USA

Paige Menking, MPA University of New Mexico Health Science Center, Albuquerque, NM, USA

Ella Miller Center for Appalachia Research in Cancer Education, Whipple, OH, USA

Katie Miller Center for Appalachia Research in Cancer Education, Whipple, OH, USA

Sue Miller, C-CHW Center for Appalachia Research in Cancer Education, Whipple, OH, USA

Kimberly Moler, PDHA II SEARHC Dental, Kake, AK, USA

Alejandra Morales, CHW Loma Linda University Health, Loma Linda, CA, USA

June Munoz, CHW Ho'ola Lahui Hawai'i Kauai Community Health Center, Lihue, HI, USA

Niem Nay-Kret Lowell Community Health Center, Lowell, MA, USA

Katharine Nimmons, MPH, MSc, CHWI Public Health Sciences Department, Texas A&M College of Dentistry, Dallas, TX, USA

Linda J. Nisley, C-CHW Center for Appalachia Research in Cancer Education, Whipple, OH, USA

Silvia Ortega, CHW Jurupa Unified School District, Jurupa Valley, CA, USA

Susan Oshiro-Taogoshi, BA, CHW Ho'ola Lahui Hawai'i Kauai Community Health Center, Lihue, HI, USA

Fatima Padron, BA, CHW Sinai Urban Health Institute, Chicago, IL, USA

Judith Palfrey, MD Harvard Medical School and Boston Children's Hospital, Boston, MA, USA

Colton Lee Palmer, MD Upstate Medical University, Syracuse, NY, USA

Michael Perry True 2 Life, Central Family Life Center, Stapleton, Staten Island, NY, USA

Kelly Pilialoha-Cypriano, CHW Wai'anae Coast Comprehensive Community Health Center, Wai'anae, HI, USA

Nadereh Pourat, PhD Fielding School of Public Health, UCLA Center for Health Policy Research, Los Angeles, CA, USA

Janice Probst, PhD University of South Carolina, Columbia, SC, USA

Floribella Redondo-Martinez, CHW, BS Arizona Community Health Workers Association, Inc., Douglas, AZ, USA

Keara Rodela, MPH, CHW Immigrant and Refugee Community Organization, Portland, OR, USA

Brendaly Rodríguez University of Miami, Miami, FL, USA

E. Lee Rosenthal, PhD, MS, MPH Texas Tech University Health Sciences Center El Paso, El Paso, TX, USA

Carl H. Rush, MRP Community Resources, LLC, San Antonio, TX, USA

Samantha Sabo, DrPH, MPH Department of Health Sciences, Center for Health Equity Research, Flagstaff, AZ, USA

Alix Sanchez, BA Multnomah County Department of Human Services, Portland, OR, USA

Desiree Santana, CHW Wai'anae Coast Comprehensive Community Health Center, Wai'anae, HI, USA

David Secor National Rural Health Association, Washington, DC, USA

Julie Smithwick, CHW, MSW University of South Carolina Center for Community Health Alignment, Columbia, SC, USA

Dalia Solia, CHW Wai'anae Coast Comprehensive Community Health Center, Wai'anae, HI, USA

Yanitza Soto, CHW, MPH Arizona Department of Health Services, Phoenix, AZ, USA

Joanne Spetz, PhD, FAAN Philip R. Lee Institute for Health Policy Studies, University of California, San Francisco, San Francisco, CA, USA

R. Napualani Spock, MA, MBA-PHA, MSW Hawaiian Community Capacity Building Resources, Makawao, HI, USA

Julie Ann St. John, DrPH, MPH, MA, CHWI Department of Public Health, Texas Tech University Health Sciences Center, Abilene, TX, USA

Kate Philley Starnes, JD, Med The University of Texas Health Science Center at Tyler, Tyler, TX, USA

Jessica Sunshine, MPH, MSW New York City Department of Health and Mental Hygiene, New York City, NY, USA

Katherine Sutkowi, MSW Consultant, Queens, NY, USA

Malia Talbert, CHW Wai'anae Coast Comprehensive Community Health Center, Wai'anae, HI, USA

Nathan Tarvers, CHW Wai'anae Coast Comprehensive Community Health Center, Wai'anae, HI, USA

Claireta Thomas, CHW Detroit Health Department, Detroit, MI, USA

Doretta Thomas, C-CHW Center for Appalachia Research in Cancer Education, Whipple, OH, USA

Melissa K. Thomas, PhD, MSPH, MSA, MCHES, C-CHW Ohio University Heritage College of Osteopathic Medicine, Athens, OH, USA

Aubry D. Threlkeld, EdD, MS Endicott College, Beverly, MA, USA

Lizdaly Cancel Tirado, MPH, CHW Benton County Health Services, Corvallis, OR, USA

Myriam Torres, PhD, MSPH University of South Carolina, Columbia, SC, USA

Kathryn Tucker, MPH University of Arizona Prevention Research Center, Mel and Enid Zuckerman College of Public Health, Tucson, AZ, USA

Lani Untalan, CHW Wai'anae Coast Comprehensive Community Health Center, Wai'anae, HI, USA

Virginia Vedilago, CHW, MA The Fenway Institute at Fenway Health, Boston, MA, USA

Maria M. Velazco, CHW El Pueblo Clinic, El Rio Community Health Center, Tucson, AZ, USA

Lorena Verdugo, CHW El Rio Community Health Center, Ventanilla de Salud Consulado de Mexico, Tucson, AZ, USA

Kelly Volkmann, MPH Benton County Health Services, Corvallis, OR, USA

Wes Warner, CHW KC CARE Health Center, Kansas City, MO, USA

Shannon Watson, CHW Wai'anae Coast Comprehensive Community Health Center, Wai'anae, HI, USA

Ashley Wennerstrom, PhD, MPH LSU Health Science Center—New Orleans, New Orleans, LA, USA

Behavioral and Community Health Sciences, School of Public Health, New Orleans, LA, USA

Center for Healthcare Value and Equity, School of Medicine, New Orleans, LA, USA

Deborah White, CHW KC CARE Health Center, Kansas City, MO, USA

Noelle Wiggins, EdD, MSPH Wiggins Health Consulting LLC, Portland, OR, USA

Geoffrey W. Wilkinson, MSW Center for Innovation in Social Work and Health, Boston University School of Social Work, Boston, MA, USA

Madeline Woodberry, BA, CHWIII Sinai Urban Health Institute, Chicago, IL, USA

Jessica Uriarte Wright, DrPH Houston Methodist Hospital System, Houston, TX, USA

Mike Young, MA PASOs, Columbia, SC, USA

DelAnne Zeller, RN The University of Texas Health Science Center at Tyler, Tyler, TX, USA

Part I
The Story Behind the Book

Chapter 1
Introduction: Why Community Health Workers (CHWs)?

Julie Ann St. John, Susan L. Mayfield-Johnson, and Wandy D. Hernández-Gordon

1.1 Why Community Health Workers?

Every individual who knows, has worked with, or has been supported by a Community Health Worker has a reason why they value Community Health Workers (CHWs). When asked to provide an answer quickly to the following question, "Why Community Health Workers?", we said the following:

> Community Health Workers (CHWs) see people. They make people feel valued and meet their needs. They make people matter. When you feel vulnerable, when you feel like you do not have support, CHWs help you to know that you are worthy of getting help.
>
> —Julie St. John

> CHWs need to be valued and respected for the authentic voice they represent—the under-served, undervalued, and overlooked community member whose human spirit has been invisible. CHWs will echo these voices until they are heard.
>
> —Susan Mayfield-Johnson

> Due to the equalities that a lot of minority and communities of color face, we need CHWs—knowing that the majority of CHWs are from the marginalized communities that they serve—to become that buffer, the mediator, the in-between, the bridge between the care professionals

J. A. St. John (✉)
Department of Public Health, Texas Tech University Health Sciences Center, Abilene, TX, USA
e-mail: julie.st-john@ttuhsc.edu

S. L. Mayfield-Johnson
Department of Public Health, School of Health Professions, The University of Southern Mississippi, Hattiesburg, MS, USA
e-mail: Susan.Johnson@usm.edu

W. D. Hernández-Gordon
HealthConnect One, Chicago, IL, USA
e-mail: wandyhdz@healthconnectone.org

© Springer Nature Switzerland AG 2021
J. A. St. John et al. (eds.), *Promoting the Health of the Community*,
https://doi.org/10.1007/978-3-030-56375-2_1

and the community. Inequalities, segregation, and systemic racism, all of these areas, CHWs
are there and continue to advocate, educate, compromise, and work on these issues.

—Wandy D. Hernandez-Gordon

As editors of this text, we are familiar with colleagues, coworkers, and friends who we call Community Health Worker (CHWs). We have also had incidents where we wished we had a CHW who walked with us through an experience—someone who had been through similar situations and could have told us what to expect, to communicate, to empathize, to listen, and to share. Even though we may have had knowledge or resources, having that individual to hold our hand, listen when we hurt, and advocate for our needs is important. In our opinion, everyone needs a CHW—they are that good at what they do, and they fill important, vital roles in the health, public health, and social services systems.

This chapter explains who CHWs are and what they do and answers the "why" for engaging the CHW model. Subsequently, the remainder of the book provides concrete examples of CHW teams across the nation sharing how they helped people going through those experiences where they wished they had someone there. Chapter teams from across the nation have contributed and shared their CHW stories to help us document the need for Community Health Workers.

1.2 Who Are Community Health Workers (CHWs)?

Community Health Workers (CHWs) are valuable, key members of the healthcare and public health professions. The Community Health Worker (CHW) Section of the American Public Health Association (APHA) defines a CHW as:

A frontline public health worker who is a trusted member of and/or has an unusually close understanding of the community served. This trusting relationship enables the worker to serve as a liaison/link/intermediary between health/social services and the community to facilitate access to services and improve the quality and cultural competence of service delivery. A community health worker also builds individual and community capacity by increasing health knowledge and self-sufficiency through a range of activities such as outreach, community education, informal counseling, social support and advocacy

A more informal definition is:

Indigenous members from a community who love their community and want to see people's health and lives improve—so they give unselfishly of their time and energy (often with no or little pay) not because it's a "job" but because it's a work of love for them. CHWs do everything from holding hands when someone is sick to calling thirty agencies to assist a resident with a particular need

CHWs have unique knowledge and experience of individual, family, and community needs, including cultural characteristics, behaviors, and attitudes. Further, CHWs fill an intermediary or bridge function by explaining the complexities of the health, social service, and public health systems to help their community members better understand and access services more readily. Likewise, CHWs also educate and communicate with providers, organizations, and systems about individual and community cultures and needs in order to help the service delivery system improve access to and provide higher-quality, culturally appropriate services to clients and patients. As mentioned previously, CHWs build individual and community capacity by increasing individual, family, and community self-sufficiency and health knowledge; improving collaboration between service delivery agencies and the community; and influencing attitudes and practices through a variety of activities, roles, and skills. To strengthen this point, The Patient Protection and Affordable Care Act (ACA) formally recognized CHWs as important members of the healthcare workforce who provide direct outreach services and build individual and community capacity.

CHWs have numerous titles, including some of the following:

- Case work aide
- Community care coordinator
- Community health aide (CHA)
- Community health advisor
- Community health advocate
- Community health educator
- Community health promotor
- Community health representative (CHR)
- Community outreach workers
- Consejera/animadora (counselor/organizer)
- Environmental health aide
- Family service worker
- Health coach
- HIV peer counselor
- Lactation consultant/specialist
- Lay health advisor
- Lay health advocate
- Lay health worker
- Lead abatement education specialist
- Maternal/infant health outreach specialist
- Neighborhood health advisor
- Outreach educator
- Outreach worker
- Patient navigator
- Promotor(a) de salud (peer health promoter)
- Peer counselor
- Primary dental health aide (PDHA)
- Public health aide

We use the term Community Health Worker as an overall umbrella term, and it captures the essence of the various types of individuals serving in this capacity. In 2009, the US Department of Labor and Statistics recognized CHWs as their own occupational class, defining CHWs as individuals who:

> Assist individuals and communities to adopt healthy behaviors. Conduct outreach for medical personnel or health organizations to implement programs in the community that promote, maintain, and improve individual and community health. May provide information

on available resources, provide social support and informal counseling, advocate for individuals and community health needs, and provide services such as first aid and blood pressure screening. May collect data to help identify community health needs. Excludes "Health Educators" (21-1091)

Although there are numerous positions and titles that fall under the continuum of the CHW umbrella, we recognize the distinctions in funding, specified training, and needed certifications associated with certain titles and positions, for example, community health aides (CHAs), community health representatives (CHRs), and primary dental health aides (PDHAs).

Figure 1.1 depicts some key events in CHWs' rich history in the United States. Globally, the presence of CHWs dates back centuries, with models in European, Asian, and African countries. By the 1960s, countries, including the United States, began to implement more CHW-led programs. In 1968, the Indian Health Service (IHS) established the Community Health Aide Program (CHAP) in Alaska. In 1970, the American Public Health Association (APHA) established the New Professionals Special Primary Interest Group (SPIG), which became the CHW SPIG in 2000 and then the CHW Section in 2009. In the 1980s, the US Department of Health and Human Services funded a council comprised of the National Migrant Worker Council, Inc., an association of Catholic sisters, religious leaders, and volunteers to conduct a community assessment with Midwest farmworkers. This council became MHP Salud (Migrant Health Promotion) and launched its first Camp Health Aide Program using a community-centered CHW model, which led to other CHW programs in the Midwest, Texas, and Florida.

In 1998, the National Community Health Advisor Study final report identified core roles, competencies, and qualities of CHWs—providing recommendations to practitioners and policymakers regarding CHWs' scope of practice. In 1999 and the early 2000s, states like Ohio and Texas began to seek certification of Community Health Workers/promotores; certification has since followed in several other states. Then in 2007, the Health Resources and Services Administration provided a comprehensive, national report on the CHW workforce—highlighting CHWs as a cost-effective model to address health concerns in underserved communities. In 2009, the US Bureau of Labor Statistics adopted an occupational code for CHWs. Then, in March of 2010, the US Congress passed the Patient Protection and Affordable Care Act, which recognized CHWs as an important component in the "health care workforce." As the CHW movement and model grew stronger and gained national recognition, in 2013, the Centers for Medicare and Medicaid Services created a rule allowing state Medicaid agencies to potentially reimburse for preventive services provided by CHWs—diversifying CHW funding streams. In 2014–2018, The C3 Community Health Worker Core Consensus Project revisited CHW core roles and skills from the 1998 National Community Health Advisor Study and released an updated set of core roles and skills in 2016 and additional tools such as a CHW assessment toolkit and Roles and Competencies Implementation Checklist in 2018.

The most recent major accomplishment to advance the CHW field began in 2014 with the development of a National Coordinating Committee (NCC), with 20 CHW leaders and allies from around the country meeting regularly to develop plans for building a sustainable membership organization for CHWs—broadly defined to

Fig. 1.1 History of CHWs
in the United States

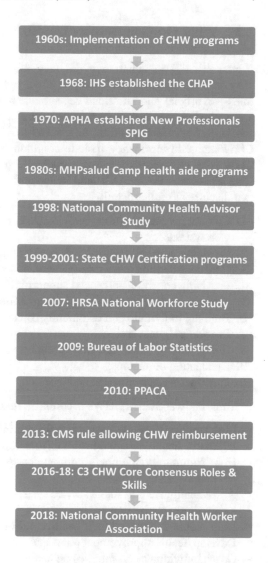

include CHWs, CHRs, promotores, and other workforce members—and allies. Formal strategic planning began in May of 2017 to draft recommendations about structure, governance, member services, and policy and program priorities. The NCC conducted a national survey of state, regional, and local CHW associations to assess the current capacity of workforce networks and to enable broader participation in planning for a sustainable membership organization for CHWs. In April 2019, the National Association of Community Health Workers was established. NACHW's mission is: "To unify the voices of the Community Health Workers and strengthen the profession's capacity to promote healthy communities." Clearly, there is a strong presence and record of CHWs nationally and globally, which brings us to what they do.

1.3   What Do Community Health Workers (CHWs) Do?

If you ask CHWs what they do, they might respond (and probably should), "Everything," and that would be just about right. Seemingly, CHWs fill numerous roles—in official and unofficial capacities, on the clock and off the clock. CHWs are integral change agents in their communities, which require multiple roles and activities. Regardless of all of the names of CHW-like positions that fall under the CHW umbrella term, they include common roles and skills. The framework of CHW roles utilized for this book was based from the Community Health Worker Core Consensus Project (C3) and includes the following ten roles, which chapter two discusses in fuller detail:

1. Cultural mediation among individuals, communities, and health and social service systems
2. Providing culturally appropriate health education and information
3. Care coordination, case management, and system navigation
4. Providing coaching and social support
5. Advocating for individuals and communities
6. Building individual and community capacity
7. Providing direct service
8. Implementing individual and community assessments
9. Conducting outreach
10. Participating in evaluation and research

Some daily activities CHWs accomplish that align with core roles include:

- Link families to needed resources (health insurance; food; housing; quality and affordable health care and health information; social services; transportation).
- Help community members communicate with healthcare and social service providers.
- Assist healthcare and social service systems to become culturally competent and responsive to their clients.
- Help people understand their health condition(s).
- Develop health improvement plans and strategies.
- Coach individuals and families on healthier behaviors and lifestyle choices.
- Deliver health information using culturally appropriate terms and concepts.
- Follow up with community members who have received services.
- Provide informal counseling and support.
- Advocate for local health needs at the local, state, and national levels.
- Provide some health services, such as blood pressure checks.
- Make home visits.
- Provide translation and interpretation for clients and providers.
- Conduct eligibility and enrollment.
- Organize health fairs and health education events.
- Conduct activities related to research studies (surveys, interviews, focus groups, data collection, etc.).

This is not an exhaustive list of CHW roles or the activities they do. CHWs' scope of work on a day-to-day basis varies based on their communities, their employers or volunteer agencies, the needs of their communities, their own unique skill sets and training, and a multitude of other factors. What is consistent about the CHW workforce are the general core roles and competencies, which CHWs will share throughout this book. Having answered who CHWs are and what they do, we will conclude with "Why CHWs?"

1.4   Why Engage the CHW Model?

Why do we need CHWs? Because everyone deserves to have a champion in their corner—and that is who CHWs are and what they do. CHWs present a compelling case for their engagement and integration in health and social service systems. Numerous studies demonstrated positive outcomes for participants receiving CHW services. Some of these outcomes include:

- Improved access to health and social services
- Increased health screenings
- Improved health outcomes
- Better understanding between community members and the health and social service systems
- Enhanced communication between community members and health providers
- Increased access to and utilization of healthcare services
- Improved adherence to health recommendations
- Reduced need for emergency services
- Reduced utilization of emergency departments for primary care needs

The evidence base continues to build the support for why CHW models improve health outcomes and reduce health disparities. CHW teams represented in this book describe how they carry out one of the core CHW roles in their respective community, institutional, academic, or clinical settings, and they share their personal stories of their impact in their communities, with clients, patients, and community members, in the entities they serve. Their stories answer, "Why CHWs?"

References

American Public Health Association. (2020). *Community Health Workers*. Retrieved from American Public Health Association: https://www.apha.org/apha-communities/member-sections/community-health-workers.
Centers for Disease Control and Prevention. (2016, January). *CHW job titles*. Retrieved from Division for Heart Disease and Stroke Prevention, Centers for Disease Control and Prevention: https://www.cdc.gov/dhdsp/chw_elearning/s1_p6.html.

Centers for Medicare & Medicaid Services. (2013, July 15). *Medicaid and children's health insurance programs: Essential health benefits in alternative benefit plans, eligibility notices, fair hearing and appeal processes, and premiums and cost sharing; exchanges: eligibility and enrollment.* Retrieved from Federal Register: The Daily Journal of the United State Government: https://www.federalregister.gov/documents/2013/07/15/2013-16271/medicaid-and-childrens-health-insurance-programs-essential-health-benefits-in-alternative-benefit.

ExploreHealthCareers.org. (2020). *Community Health Worker.* Retrieved from ExploreHealthCareers.org: https://explorehealthcareers.org/career/allied-health-professions/community-health-worker/#:~:text=The%20community%20health%20worker%20serves,health%20worker's%20responsibilities%20may%20include%3A&text=Advocating%20for%20local%20health%20needs,pressure%2.

Indian Health Service, U.S. Department of Health and Human Services. (n.d.). *Education and training.* Retrieved from Indian Health Service: https://www.ihs.gov/chr/education/.

LAWriter Ohio Laws and Rules. (2020, February 2). *Chapter 4723-26 Community Health Workers.* Retrieved from LAWriter Ohio Laws and Rules: http://codes.ohio.gov/oac/4723-26.

Lehmann, U., & Sanders, D. (2007). *Community Health Workers: What do we know about them? The state of the evidence on programmes, activities, costs and impact on health outcomes of using Community Health Workers.* Geneva: World Health Organization.

MHP Salud. (2014). *History of Community Health Workers (CHWs) in America.* Retrieved from mphsalud.org: https://mhpsalud.org/programs/who-are-promotoresas-chws/the-chw-landscape/.

National Association of Community Health Workers. (2020). *What we do.* Retrieved from National Association of Community Health Workers: https://nachw.org/about/.

Perry, H., Zulliger, R., & Rogers, M. M. (2014). Community Health Workers in low-, middle-, and high-income countries: An overview of their history, recent evolution, and current effectiveness. *Annual Review of Public Health, 35*, 399–421.

Rosenthal, E., Menking, P., & St. John, J. (2018). *The Community Health Worker core consensus (C3) project: A report of the C3 project phase 1 and 2, together leaning toward the sky, a national project to inform CHW policy and practice.* El Paso: Texas Tech University Health Sciences Center El Paso.

Rosenthal, E. L. (1998). *Final report of the National Community Health Advisor Study.* Tucson: The University of Arizona. Retrieved from https://crh.arizona.edu/publications/studies-reports/cha.

St. John, J. (2003). *Informal CHW definition.* Personal communication, TX, United States.

Texas Health and Human Services. (2019, December 6). *Legislation rules.* Retrieved from Texas Department of State Health Services CHW Program: https://www.astho.org/Maternal-and-Child-Health/Texas-CHW-State-Story/.

U.S. Bureau of Labor Statistics. (2018, March 30). *Occupational employment statistics.* Retrieved from U.S. Bureau of Labor Statistics: https://www.bls.gov/oes/2017/may/oes211094.htm.

U.S. Congress. (2010, March 31). *Patient protection and affordable care act.* Public Law 111–148, 42 USC 256a-1, § 5301, United States of America.

U.S. Department of Health and Human Services, Health Resources and Services Administration, Bureau of Health Professions. (2007). *HRSA national workforce study.* Bethesda, MD: U.S. Department of Health and Human Services, Health Resources and Services Administration, Bureau of Health Professions.

Viswanathan, M. K. (2009). *Evidence report/technology assessment number 181: Outcomes of Community Health Worker interventions.* Research Triangle Park: RTI International–University of North Carolina Evidence-Based Practice Center.

Chapter 2
The Community Health Worker Core Consensus (C3) Project Story: Confirming the Core Roles and Skills of Community Health Workers

E. Lee Rosenthal, Durrell J. Fox, Julie Ann St. John, Caitlin G. Allen, Paige Menking, J. Nell Brownstein, Gail R. Hirsch, Floribella Redondo-Martinez, Lisa Renee Holderby-Fox, Jorge M. Ibarra, Colton Lee Palmer, Alexander Ross Hurley, Maria C. Cole, Sara S. Masoud, Jessica Uriarte Wright, and Carl H. Rush

As a Community Health Worker (CHW), I feel confident that the Community Health Worker Core Consensus (C3) Project findings provide an opportunity for our workforce to be more fully understood as a professional workforce. Prior to this endeavor, we have been working in communities without defining our roles. We were trying to tell the story of what we do individually, not cohesively as a profession. Because of the efforts of the C3 Project, we now are equipped with tools that define and share our CHW roles and core competencies.

Floribella Redondo-Martinez—C3 Project Advisory Committee Co-Chair.
C3 Project Phase 2, 2016–2018.

E. L. Rosenthal (✉) · J. N. Brownstein
Texas Tech University Health Sciences Center El Paso, El Paso, TX, USA
e-mail: Lee.Rosenthal@ttuhsc.edu

D. J. Fox
JSI Research and Training, Inc., Atlanta, GA, USA
e-mail: Durrell_Fox@jsi.com

J. A. St. John
Department of Public Health, Texas Tech University Health Sciences Center, Abilene, TX, USA
e-mail: julie.st-john@ttuhsc.edu

C. G. Allen
CGA Consulting, Charleston, SC, USA
e-mail: caitlin.gloeckner.allen@emory.edu

© Springer Nature Switzerland AG 2021
J. A. St. John et al. (eds.), *Promoting the Health of the Community*,
https://doi.org/10.1007/978-3-030-56375-2_2

2.1 Introduction to the Community Health Worker Core Consensus (C3) Project

The Community Health Worker (CHWs) Core Consensus (C3) Project is a national project focused on engaging CHWs and stakeholders throughout the research process to build consensus around CHW scope of practice (roles) and CHW competencies, which include CHW core skills and qualities. The intent of the C3 Project is to support action through information, based on this research, to advance the CHW profession. The Project, which began in 2014, includes two phases each with several components. Phase 1 consisted of an analysis of CHW roles and skills and a consensus-building process; Phase 2 provided a deeper look at the influence of CHWs' work setting on the roles and skills they need and examined CHW skill assessment best practices. Additional work on stakeholder engagement and consensus building was also prominent in the second phase. Throughout both phases of the Project, the research team, which included CHWs, was committed to the

---

P. Menking
University of New Mexico Health Science Center, Albuquerque, NM, USA
e-mail: PMenking@salud.unm.edu

G. R. Hirsch
Massachusetts Department of Public Health, Boston, MA, USA
e-mail: gail.hirsch@state.ma.us

F. Redondo-Martinez
Arizona Community Health Workers Association, Yuma, AZ, USA
e-mail: floribella@azchow.org

L. R. Holderby-Fox
Roster Health, Stone Mountain, GA, USA
e-mail: lisarenee@rosterhealth.com

J. M. Ibarra
Texas A&M University, El Paso, TX, USA

C. L. Palmer
Upstate Medical University, Syracuse, NY, USA

A. R. Hurley
University of North Carolina, Chapel Hill, NC, USA

M. C. Cole
Baylor Scott & White Research Institute, Dallas, TX, USA

S. S. Masoud
UT Health San Antonio, San Antonio, TX, USA
e-mail: masoud@uthscsa.edu

J. U. Wright
Houston Methodist Hospital System, Houston, TX, USA

C. H. Rush
Community Resources, LLC, San Antonio, TX, USA
e-mail: carl@chrllc.net

integration of CHW leadership to create alignment and develop CHW ownership of Project findings, including the recommended lists of roles and competencies.

This chapter provides an overview of the history of and the rationale for the C3 Project, describes the Project's methods, and discusses findings and recommendations from each of the two phases. This chapter positions the work of the C3 Project into the broader context of workforce development efforts and examines C3 Project recommendations for the future. *This textbook provides a unique opportunity to look at contemporary CHW roles, as they are carried out by CHWs across the nation from the CHW's own point of view-role by role.* The C3 Project team is honored to have provided our identified CHW roles and competencies—based on recommendations from the CHW workforce—as an organizing framework for this groundbreaking and innovative book.

2.2   Factors Impacting Growth and Development of Community Health Workers in the United States

2.2.1   Implications for the C3 Project

Even with a rich history of contribution in improving health and healthcare access (Rosenthal & Brownstein, 2016), there are still those who have not heard of CHWs. The elder who guides the extended family, neighbors helping neighbors, and community members who serve as leaders, each of these connects to the role of CHWs in society throughout history. CHWs serve in many settings throughout the United States, including rural and urban community health centers, local and state health departments, and in diverse communities including immigrant, homeless, and other marginalized populations. CHWs' value is increasingly recognized in promoting access to care (Albritton & Hernandez-Cancio, 2017; Verhagen, Steunenberg, de Wit, & Ros, 2014) and in the prevention and management of chronic and infectious diseases (Addressing Chronic Disease through Community Health Workers: A Policy and Systems-Level Approach, 2015) as well as in promoting community development (Cosgrove et al., 2014). In spite of this, to date, there is an uneven integration of CHWs into systems of care in the United States.

Some of the barriers to CHW integration are *external* to the field itself, such as the limited understanding of top-level management about CHWs and what they can do, in contrast with that of CHW supervisors who often see the value and capacity of CHWs through observing their day-to-day work. Beyond these leadership challenges, we also see a lack of appropriate training and educational assessment, a lack of clear scope of practice protocols (Islam et al., 2015; Rogers et al., 2018) and changing strategies for payment for health services leading to challenges in identifying ongoing funding options. Additionally, given that CHWs often serve at the interface between health systems and communities (Torres et al., 2017), they tend to fall outside the bounds of services routinely covered by healthcare funding.

Finally, in some cases, simple limited political will to address the needs of marginalized populations influences the support of and demand for CHWs.

Likewise, there are several factors *internal* to the field that affect its growth and development. Many CHWs are paid stipends, wages, and salaries, but there is also a portion of the CHW field that serves as volunteers. Views on how to strengthen the field are impacted by CHWs' different vantage points on CHW work and service, though there is no uniform opinion dividing paid and volunteer CHWs. In addition to differences in how or if CHWs are paid, CHWs focus on a wide array of health, public health, and social issues which means they to some degree lack a common agenda and even a vocabulary, making it difficult for them to come together around shared concerns. The two factors together—the presence of both volunteer and paid CHWs and CHWs working on varied issues—have made building consensus and unity among CHWs challenging. Even when unity may exist on practice approaches, as is the case for many professions, disagreement on how to best advance the field overall is not uncommon.

Still other hurdles lie in the tension between the *internal* and the *external* barriers described above, such as debate about the value of state-based CHW certification. There are concerns about what some may refer to as the over professionalization of the field. We continue to explore options to maintain the organic nature and integrity of the CHW workforce while advancing and sustaining the profession. This brings funders, potential payers, employers, and CHWs into conflict with other stakeholders, including some CHWs who see the CHW approach as so closely aligned with natural helping systems that they are skeptical of any imposed standards and workforce development efforts. In spite of hurdles, the CHW field has entered a time of unprecedented recognition that has led to progress in CHW integration into systems of care. CHW unity and self-determination, rather than division, have characterized these changes that are well timed to the dawning of a new national CHW-led organization established by and for CHWs, the National Association of CHWs (NACHW). (NACHW is featured at the end of this chapter and NACHW leaders are featured as authors in Chap. 15 of this book.) This independent CHW-governed professional organization at the national level can model CHW self-determination and lead the CHW workforce in areas related to guiding and defining the workforce scope of practice, education and training, and sustainability.

Given these varied challenges to growth and development, importantly, over the past several decades, the CHW field has enjoyed crucial support from many organizations, including local, state, regional, and national CHW networks, alliances, coalitions, and associations. CHW-driven and focused conferences, where CHWs serve as facilitators and faculty, have also been key to the field's growth and development. These conferences include national events like the Unity Conference, the *Vision y Compromiso* Conference, and in the past, *the Red de Promotores* meeting and the National Association of Community Health Representatives triennial conference. State and regional CHW conferences have also been key to CHW workforce development progress in the last two decades. CHWs and stakeholders in the field have also often convened under the auspices of the American Public Health Association's CHW Section (Rosenthal & Brownstein, 2016).

The field has enjoyed support over this same time frame from several efforts within the Centers for Disease Control and Prevention (CDC) to support CHWs including a CHW Working Group.

2.2.2   Integration of CHW Leadership and Other Stakeholder Input Is a Key Value of the C3 Project Research Team

As described in the introduction, during the implementation of the C3 Project, no single national leadership organization existed that could represent the field like NACHW can now do moving forward. Given this, the C3 Project team worked to ensure CHW engagement and leadership in multiple ways, including adopting a guiding principle of CHW self-determination, which aligned with the self-determination policy statement put forward by the American Public Health Association in 2014 (Support for Community Health Worker Leadership in Determining Workforce Standards for Training and Credentialing, 2014). As with other work by the same research team in the mid-1990s (Rosenthal, Wiggins, and Brownstein et al.,1998), the C3 Project team used a community-based participatory research (CBPR) approach integrating CHWs and other key stakeholders in the leadership for all aspects of the Project (Minkler & Wallerstein, 2008). This integration varied across the two phases of the project.

In Phase 1, two CHW fellows served as advisory group chairs and were invited to attend all staff meetings. The Project also had a CHW consultant and established two distinct majority-CHW advisory groups that guided the initial review of roles and competencies and then a third CHW fellow was engaged to help lead the network review process. The team implemented major outreach efforts to all known CHW networks and associations for the CHW Network Review of proposed roles and competencies. In this effort, all known US CHW networks were invited to review proposed updates to the national list of CHW core roles and skills. Networks were asked to involve at least five members in the review process, with at least four of these being CHWs. This CHW-centered method was proposed by C3 Project CHW fellow Catherine Gray Haywood.

In the C3 Project's Phase 2, two CHWs served on the team as Project staff members, supported as other team members as project consultants. As in Phase 1, the Project team was guided by several majority-CHW advisory groups established to work on different aspects of the Project. In Phase 2, senior advising partners, including CHWs and others working to organize the field at the state and national levels, were invited to interpret and refine the findings and aid in the presentation of the Project's various final products.

In both phases, CHWs and other stakeholders engaged with the CHW workforce, assisted in the development of research strategies, aided in data interpretation, and guided the formation of recommendations. As intended, this leadership and these activities align with CBPR principles and practices, where members of the community of interest serve as equal partners in the development and conduct of the research as well as influence its application in practice and policy.

To put the work of the C3 Project in context, we now look briefly at other health disciplines and groups addressing public health to better understand the process of role and competency delineation overall.

2.3   A Look at Scope of Practice and Competency Development in the Health Sector

The Institute for Health Metrics and Evaluation reports that each of the recognized health professions of the modern healthcare team has achieved recognition through a process of defining their professional boundaries and occupational standards. Looking at other fields sheds light on the importance of and common features found in the development of core roles or competency guidelines or standards. Looking at competency development processes reveals that in almost all cases, multiple phases and stakeholder engagement are key. A closer look also reveals the need to routinely revisit consensus in a field to develop contemporary guidelines.

As reported in the *Journal of Public Health Dentistry* (Altman & Mascarenhas, 2016), in the late 1990s, US dentists with an interest in public health identified core competencies needed to practice and promote oral health. As in our C3 Project, a few decades later in the 2010s, a similar review of the 1990 dental public health competencies was undertaken. To renew earlier findings, the American Association of Public Health Dentistry, established in 1937, came together to undertake a renewed competency revision process. The review was multifaceted and engaged many stakeholders in the field at different stages in order to identify and promote a contemporary set of core competencies. Examining core competencies for preventive medicine residents provides another opportunity to understand the multifaceted approach to the development of guidelines for a workforce. In the *Journal of Preventive Medicine*, Lane, Ross, Chen, and O'Neill (1999) discuss the original preventive medicine competencies developed in the early 1990s; changes in the healthcare system by the end of that decade led to a revision. In the case of the 2.0 revision, a workgroup comprised of practitioners and academics developed the list of medical management competencies and updated the original competencies. The final version was submitted by the workgroup for dissemination as a component of the residency training manual for preventive medicine throughout the United States.

Looking beyond these broad public health-focused health professionals' competencies, we see numerous competency efforts within various fields undertaken to further refine practice. Several examples reveal a similarly deliberate engagement process with several phases that are as diverse as each specialty area. According to Dean et al. (2014), healthcare workers proposed evidence-based core competencies in health assessment and lifestyle behavior change to support their work in preventing the growing prevalence of noncommunicable diseases. The authors proposed an algorithm to assess patients and the appropriate behavior change interventions or referrals. This more technical process of consensus building was distinct from building competencies of a single workforce in that it aimed to address the health needs of the population across various workforce groups. In their article "Development of a competency framework for nutrition in emergency sectors," Meeker et al. (2014) discussed their review of literature for humanitarian competency frameworks, followed by their interview of experts, leading to the development of a framework for nutrition in emergencies. Once again, in this process, the agreement of the workforce with the proposed framework emerged as key, although this group likely encompassed an array of individuals from varied health professions. Finally, in the social work field, a scoping review of social work core practice roles in the provision of primary mental health care was proposed as the first step to developing practice guidelines for social workers providing mental health services in primary healthcare settings (Ashcroft, Kourgiantakis, & Brown, 2017). Sharing this step in the literature before conception, these authors kept the workforce informed, potentially serving to forge longer-term consensus to advance competency adoption and adherence.

With so many models to examine the competency development process, we can look back on the organic process that defined the NCHAS and the C3 Project (2014–2018) and recognize several elements that contributed to producing consensus-based recommendations for CHWs for use in education, practice, and policymaking in the field.

2.4   C3 Project Methods and Implementation

The C3 Project began in 2014 as an effort to develop contemporary roles and competencies (Phase 1). Following that work, the C3 Project team began the examination of the impact of workplace setting on CHW core roles and skills along with approaches to assessing skills (Phase 2). We now look at the methods used to implement these two phases of the Project; following that, Project findings, including recommended roles and competencies (again meaning to skills and qualities), will be presented.

2.4.1   Phase 1

In 2014, Phase 1 of the C3 Project began, which focused on answering the following questions:

1. Roles and competency changes: How have CHW roles and skills changed over time in the United States, particularly since the release of the NCHAS in 1998?
2. Today's roles: What contemporary roles (scope of practice) best capture the work of CHWs today in any setting?

3. Today's competencies: What skills and qualities (collectively referred to as competencies) do CHWs need to fulfill these roles?

Phase 1 focused explicitly on the analysis of roles and skills. Early in the Project, the team concluded CHW qualities have remained largely the same over time. For this reason, we did not emphasize the analysis of qualities. Though the Project did not propose new CHW qualities, the C3 Project team agreed that qualities are an essential element of CHW competence, and given that, we agreed that all our reporting should include reference to the central importance of qualities. Qualities, including "connection to the community served," give CHWs the networks, resources, connections, and related social capital they need to be effective in their work with the individual, families, and communities they serve. This aspect of CHWs has long been valued and stands the test of time (Rosenthal, Rush, & Allen, 2016) (see videos https://www.c3project.org/resources).

With roles and skills identified as the focus of the project's work, three major steps were undertaken in Phase 1 to answer the questions outlined above and to build CHW ownership of the contemporary roles and skills put forward by the Project.

The major steps undertaken in Phase 1 to answer those questions included:

- Data source selection
- Crosswalk analysis
- Consensus building

At each step, the project team, which included CHWs, invited other CHWs and stakeholders to participate in the process.

The goal of the data source selection process was to identify a discrete number of appropriate source documents to allow for the identification of changes over time in CHW core roles and competencies.

2.4.1.1 Looking Back at the National Community Health Advisor Study 1994–1998

The NCHAS work began in the early 1990s when a number of the current C3 Project team members designed and carried out the Annie E. Casey Foundation-funded study under the auspices of the University of Arizona. The NCHAS included four major components examining (1) CHW core roles and competencies; (2) evaluation challenges and resources; (3) strategies for developing the field overall (including youth-based programs); and (4) an examination of the changing healthcare system. All four components shared common data sources that included a majority-CHW advisory council providing oversight; a nonrandom sample national workforce survey; and a series of focus groups and discussion forums across the United States. The C3 Project built directly on that study—beginning with the core roles and competencies in the NCHAS as a starting point to compare again in looking at roles and competencies today. The NCHAS core roles and competencies have been widely used in the United States for CHW program, curriculum, and policy development and offered a great starting point for the renewal of a field-driven definition of CHW roles and competencies.

Using the NCHAS as a baseline served the C3 Project study team well. This was in part due to the widespread use of the study's recommended roles and skills as documented by Malcarney, Pittman, Quigley, Horton, and Seiler (2017), which meant that many materials reviewed were already integrating the NCHAS roles and competencies as reflected in the comment below:

> We found a high degree of consistency across competency sets, with most of the variation simply a function of a different ordering of broadly similar role categories. Indeed, all seem to reflect common roots in the seven-core CHW activity areas developed in the landmark 1998 National Community Health Advisor Study. (Malcarney et al., 2017, p. 371)

2.4.1.2   Selection of Benchmark Source Data

The next step was to identify the best comparison documents to serve as benchmarks in our analysis. The C3 Project team determined that they would use frequently cited documents at the leading edge of the field as the benchmark sources for the crosswalk comparison. The focus of the analysis was to look at what was new and distinct in these benchmark documents versus the earlier findings of the NCHAS. The team selected seven sources, including five states with emerging standards; one widely recognized curriculum; and the national Indian Health Service's Community Health Representative (CHR) Program scope of practice guidance. For each, the team identified both role and skill documents to analyze (except in the case of the CHR program as these materials were out of circulation and in development at the time of the Project). The one traditional curriculum was included in the Project was from the City College of San Francisco, as they had developed the first ever CHW textbook. Each of the other sources was important due to their ongoing use in states exploring certification and other CHW credentialing and recognition options. The states selected—Massachusetts, Minnesota, New York, Oregon, and Texas—were among the first developing statewide formal guidance on the CHW workforce, and all have leaders who have played an important role in developing the CHW workforce nationally. In some cases, the state-level guidance documents were being developed in the same timeframe as the Project, so ongoing communication was key.

2.4.1.3   The Crosswalk Analysis

The goal of the crosswalk between the NCHAS baseline documents and the newer benchmark documents was to analyze any differences between them with an emphasis on identifying innovations in the benchmark documents, indicating new roles and competencies that help CHWs to meet the challenges of contemporary health and community issues.

With both the NCHAS and the various benchmark source data in hand, the team developed a matrix table to allow for a crosswalk comparative review of all documents, using the NCHAS list of core roles and skills as the starting point. The reviewers focused on looking for new and different roles and skills. This approach was a contrast from the approach in the original NCHAS when the focus was to identify what was common among the many varied CHW roles and competencies. This focus on differences allowed for the identification and validation of innovation and responsiveness to contemporary factors. Innovations identified, even in just one site, were brought forward for review and consideration. After completing the crosswalk analysis, the full C3 Project team of staff, consultants, CHW fellows, and advisory members reviewed the crosswalk findings. From this review, they put forward an updated contemporary list of roles and skills, and they affirmed current data on CHW qualities for national review.

2.4.1.4   Consensus Building with CHW Networks and Associations

The goal of the C3 Project consensus-building process was to expand cohesion in the field and the visibility of CHWs by offering a single, national set of CHW core roles and competencies that can be referenced by those both inside and external to the field as they work to build greater support and sustainability for CHWs in all settings.

At every step, the review process sought to document and increase the consensus in the field related to the recommended roles and competencies. As discussed above, the team members doing the crosswalk analysis first compared notes and then brought their findings into alignment, and then their findings were vetted by the C3 Project staff/consultant team and by the Project's majority-CHW advisory group. Once the list was ready, the formal study plans ended, but the C3 Project team and advisors agreed that before the recommendations were distributed more widely, CHW leadership in the field needed a chance to review and refine the findings. The team then decided to undertake a bigger consensus building effort: the CHW Network/Association Review. The team invited all known U.S. CHW networks/ associations at the local, state, regional, and national levels to participate in the review, and 23 of the 45 associations identified agreed to participate. An efficient review method for this process was put forward by the C3 Project fellows that placed CHW leaders at the center of that review. As noted earlier in the discussion of participatory research, the method called for a minimum of five network/ association members to review—with four of those five members needing to be CHWs.

For the formal Network/Association Review, the C3 Project formed a second majority-CHW advisory group to lead the review; an additional CHW fellow was also brought on board to be a part of this process. A support structure to guide this voluntary review process was assembled from volunteers across the country who were eager to support the review. With many on board, technical assistance teams were formed and assigned to each network/association; each group was also assigned a buddy network/association. A series of kick-off conference calls in English with Spanish translation provided an opportunity to learn about the Project and the requested review. Support materials, including a PowerPoint in English and Spanish, were provided to all groups to support the process. Most of those who joined the C3 Project team to support the review were members of the CHW Section of the American Public Health Association. Following the national review and the subsequent integration of that feedback into the recommended roles and competencies, the C3 Project began the release of its findings in a summary and full report. The first venue for release was the CHW field's national Unity Conference; release at APHA and various other venues followed (Rosenthal et al., 2016).

2.4.2   Dissemination

With the release of the C3 Project's full report, the C3 Project CHW fellows challenged other CHWs and the field overall to carry this work forward in their opening letters of the report. They urged others to take up the charge to build a wide and full consensus around the recommended roles and competencies presented in the report.

2.4.3   Phase 2

Phase 2 (2016–2018) of the C3 Project emphasized deepening the understanding of CHW roles and skills in various work place settings and approaches to individual skill assessment—continuing efforts to build consensus about their use. Specifically, the C3 Project Phase 2 sought to answer the following questions:

1. Settings impact: What is the impact of CHWs' work setting on their roles and skill requirements? This component examined the distinction between CHWs serving in community and clinical settings.
2. Assessment strategies: What methods best assess CHW skill proficiency? This component included exploring 360° approaches to assessing CHWs for the C3 Project's 11 identified skill areas.
3. Outreach and messaging: Who needs to be a part of the review and refinement of the C3 Project recommendations on CHW roles and competencies? This component included continued national and regional consensus-building along with an exploration of what key messages are needed to secure feedback and enlist endorsement by CHWs and other stakeholders.

The major steps taken to answer those questions included:

- Gathering information about CHW roles and competencies in varied settings
- Gathering CHW assessment tools and strategies
- Outreach to stakeholders for input and consensus building

2.4.3.1   Settings Input Phase and Framework Development

The goal of the "settings" core work was to identify if place-based roles and skills were needed to strengthen CHWs' capacity to serve in both clinical and community settings among several venues. In this area, the C3 Project team also worked to identify strategies for improving understanding of and support for CHWs wherever they serve.

The team looked at the impact of workplace setting in the contexts of education and training, service and practice, and within policy and regulatory frameworks. Research began with an online survey of CHWs and stakeholders to gather input on the use and importance of Phase 1 recommended roles and skills in both clinical and community-based settings. Just over 500 individuals responded to the online survey, including over 200 CHWs. The team then hosted two open "town hall" webinar conference calls to further explore these same issues. Each call included a closing half-hour in Spanish to open access to Spanish speakers. More than 150 individuals participated in the two calls. The calls included open dialogue and an online chat feature where participants shared their questions and comments. Lastly, the settings team conducted a series of three virtual focus workshops with key informants. The first of the three workshops included stakeholders; the second included CHWs working in clinical settings; and the last was with CHWs working in community-based settings. A total of 20 key informants participated in these workshops.

2.4.3.2   Gathering Assessment Tools and Strategies

The goal of the assessment core work was to understand the ways in which CHW proficiencies in the recommended skills could be assessed to support the growth and development of individual CHWs. The assessment team worked with CHWs, trainers, and supervisors to better understand effective approaches to assessment in order to provide field-driven, evidence-based recommendations, tools, and resources for supporting a comprehensive assessment of CHWs' skills.

Research is built on the C3 Project's national survey, soliciting assessment processes and inviting volunteers to respond if they wanted to be contacted to further share their assessment tools and processes. The C3 team then conducted key informant interviews and a structured evaluation of existing assessment tools to ultimately create a field-informed toolkit to support assessment of CHWs' skill proficiencies. Specifically, two team members conducted 32 interviews with CHWs, CHW trainers, and CHW supervisors. These interviews focused on best practices in assessing CHW skills. Interviews were analyzed by three coders to identify key themes. In addition, 55 tools were collected that are used in the field to assess various CHW skills across settings; a selection of these serve as examples of assessment tools in the toolkit the team created.

2.4.3.3   Outreach to CHW Networks and Stakeholders for Continued Consensus Building

The goal of the consensus building for Phase 2 of the C3 Project was to pursue further consensus and broaden acceptance and adoption of the C3 Project recommended roles and competencies among CHW networks and various stakeholders nationwide. Varied outreach strategies were used to achieve this goal, including continued follow-up with CHW networks (including those that did not respond to earlier invitations, as well as new networks), presentations at conferences, "sign-on" announcements in national newsletters, meetings with national organizations, outreach to national health provider membership organizations, and general networking with numerous organizations. The team included a senior CHW ally policy expert and two CHWs who addressed many network and stakeholder questions. Input given by these groups on the roles and skills was noted and catalogued for future cyclical reviews. The assessment of the effectiveness of this outreach involved an online utilization survey sent to a select number of stakeholders and all known CHW networks, briefly described below.

As previously described, the Outreach Core worked to pursue further consensus and broaden acceptance and adoption of the C3 Project recommendations from Phase 1 among CHW networks and various stakeholders, including policy makers, employers, funders, and national associations as well as local, state, and federal policymakers. The work of the Outreach Core was not research but rather validation and dissemination work. The result of their efforts was feedback gathered and documented on roles and competencies and statements of support for those roles and competencies.

The Outreach Core utilized various strategies to emphasize the consensus for and adoption of the C3 recommendations among CHW networks and other key stakeholder groups. The Outreach Core strategies included:

1. Continued follow-up with CHW networks/associations who participated in Phase 1, some including those who did not have a chance participate and some who chose not to participate
2. Presentations and workshops at state and national conferences
3. Work to secure "sign-on" announcements in national newsletters and publications
4. Convening one-to-one meetings with representatives of high-priority national organizations
5. Participation in networking activities (directly and through national advisors) to reach additional high-priority national stakeholders and organizations

2.5 C3 Project Recommendations

2.5.1 Phase 1

Phase 1 of the C3 Project's findings, also referred to as recommendations, constitutes a contemporary list of CHW roles and skills as well as an affirmation of existing qualities. There are now a total of 10 roles and 11 skills. We note that roles and skills are not intended to match each other; rather, multiple skills may support several roles supporting a CHW's broad scope of practice.

This textbook has been organized around the framework provided by the C3 Project's recommended roles and skills. Through CHWs' own voices, the book highlights each CHW role, bringing to light CHWs' full scope of practice. This book also illustrates CHW's skills and expertise in relationship to those roles—all found to be foundational to CHW practice by the C3 Project. Finally, embedded in every chapter, CHWs' connection to their community served is illustrated and verified.

2.5.2 Roles

In Phase 1, the C3 Project identified ten roles applicable in many different settings; seven existing roles from the 1998 NCHAS were affirmed with slight nomenclature updates, along with one major name change for a better match to contemporary language. The newly named CHW role is "care coordination, case management, and system navigation" and was formerly known as "Assuring that People Get the Services They Need." During the 1998 study, this role had been considered, but the NCHAS Advisory Council urged us not to put forward language related to a navigation and case management role and so that request was honored by the study team at that time: thus, the 1998 role name was more broad.

Three new roles came out of the C3 Project. The first is "implementing individual and community assessments;" this was a sub-role in "building individual and community capacity" in the NCHAS. The next new role is "conducting outreach;" this role was to some degree an implied sub-role in the NCHAS's "Assuring that People Get the Services They Need" in the sub-role "case finding." Finally, the last new role is "participating in evaluation and research." Notably, during the NCHAS, this role had been considered, but the role was very newly evolving. Since that time, the role has become more commonplace for CHWs, though not yet widespread.

2.5.3   Skills

The C3 Project identified 11 core skill areas—three being new skills. As in the roles, one skill name changed to meet contemporary norms; this was formerly "organizational skills," which was newly named "professional skills and conduct." The new skills added parallel to the new roles added. New skills added include individual and community assessment skills; outreach skills; and evaluation and research skills.

The skill "knowledge base" was significantly expanded from Phase 1. Originally there were three sub-skills on knowledge including knowledge about the community, specific health issues, and the health and social service systems. Instead of those three, there are now eight sub-skills in total, including five new areas: knowledge about social determinants of health and related disparities; knowledge about healthy lifestyles and self-care; knowledge about mental/behavioral health issues and their connection to physical health; knowledge about health behavior theories; and knowledge of basic public health principles.

2.5.4   Qualities

As noted earlier in this chapter, CHW qualities were not re-evaluated in the C3 Project; instead, the project team asked for affirmation and endorsement of existing knowledge about CHW qualities, with "connection to the community served" being the most critical quality.

2.5.5   C3 Project Phase 1 Recommendations: CHW Roles and Competencies

Table 2.1 provides for an overview of the roles and competencies (skills and qualities) as published by the C3 Project team in 2016. See the C3 Project's (c3project.org) webpage's resources for a full role and competency checklist. For greater clarification of the definition of "competencies" as including skills and qualities, see Chap. 3 in this book on this topic led by Noelle Wiggins, who was the lead team member on the core role and competency work undertaken during the NCHAS and a consultant to the C3 Project in Phase 1.

Table 2.1 C3 Project Phase 1: recommended CHW roles and competencies (skills and qualities)

(1) Scope of practice
CHW roles
(a) Cultural mediation among individuals, communities, and health and social services systems
(b) Providing culturally appropriate health education and information
(c) Care coordination, case management, and system navigation
(d) Providing coaching and social support
(e) Advocating for individuals and communities
(f) Building individual and community capacity
(g) Providing direct service
(h) Implementing individual and community assessments
(i) Conducting outreach
(j) Participating in evaluation and research

(2) Competencies
CHW skills
(a) Communication skills
(b) Interpersonal and relationship-building skills
(c) Service coordination and navigation skills
(d) Capacity building skills
(e) Advocacy skills
(f) Education and facilitation skills
(g) Individual and community assessment skills
(h) Outreach skills
(i) Professional skills and conduct
(j) Evaluation and research skills
(k) Knowledge base

CHW qualities
The C3 Project recommends using existing qualities as identified in previous research, and of all qualities, a close connection to the community served is seen as the most critical quality for a CHW to possess

Source: Original publication of these findings in July, 2016 in The Report of the Community Health Worker Core Consensus (C3) Project available on C3Project.org. First in press publication in the Journal of Ambulatory Care Management 40(3):193-198, July/September 2017. E. L. Rosenthal, D. Fox. Commentary on "Community Health Workers and the Changing Workforce: No More Opportunities Lost."

2.5.6   Phase 2

The Phase 2 C3 Project findings or recommendations focus on two areas, settings and assessment; this phase also included outreach and dissemination messaging (Rosenthal, Menking, & St. John, 2018).

2.5.6.1   The Influence of Setting on CHW Roles and Scope

Based on the input received using the methods previously described, the C3 Project recommended that the core roles and competencies as defined in Phase 1 stay uniform in their application to any setting. In so doing, efforts should be made to promote the development of a full range of roles and skills for all CHWs. Related to this research, we have concluded that the physical location of where the CHW works does not define their focus. Findings reveal that CHWs work across a spectrum of locations and agencies, and at any one time, they may be more focused on the community's needs or an agency-driven (often clinical) agenda, independent of where they are based.

Setting core recommendations were further focused on various spheres or levels. All recommendations are based on themes identified in the qualitative data and advisor input. Recommendations addressed are as follows:

1. Training and education: Broad initial trainings for CHWs are recommended including preparation for all roles and skill areas, whereas continuing education and training could more appropriately be setting-specific.
2. Practice and service: Roles and skills may be tailored to selected settings, but when designing CHW programs and services, integration of a widest possible set of roles is encouraged.
3. Policy and regulations: Policies should ensure support for the full range of CHW roles and skills, including training to support CHW roles in policy advocacy—both for their own profession and in support of the individuals and families they serve.

To aid the review of the impact of settings on the work of CHWs, the settings core team and advisors developed schematic frameworks. Ultimately, three frameworks were developed and presented at various meetings in 2017; feedback on the frameworks helped in their refinement. Each was designed to target varied audiences including CHWs; allies, employers, and trainers/educators; and finally, researchers and policymakers. In gathering feedback on the three distinct frameworks, consensus determined that all audiences may benefit from exposure to each framework.

Each of the three frameworks depicts CHWs at a balance point wherein CHWs integrate opposing elements (see a hybrid of the three frameworks in Fig. 2.1; see the C3 Project Phase 2 report at c3project.org for a closer look at the three frameworks described below). The first of the frameworks, "the CHW Settings Continuum Framework," illustrates that independent of where CHWs are physically serving, they may be acting on behalf of a community, or conversely, they may emphasize health system and clinical concerns even when in a community setting. The center of the framework represents the many innovative intervention approaches in which CHW excel, such as within community-oriented primary care. This is seen as an optimal balancing point between communities and health and social systems. The second framework, the "CHWs Lens of Health Equity Framework," depicts CHWs as consistently bringing a lens of health equity and social justice to all their work. Finally, the third framework, "the Dancing CHW Framework," puts the CHW's heart as the center as she nimbly and skillfully balances determinants of health on the one hand and systems of care on the other.

As has been described earlier, the assessment core team conducted early outreach through the Project's Phase 2 online survey. From self-identified survey respondents, the team was able to reach out to these and other key informants and gather information on assessment methods along with assessment tools. From their early

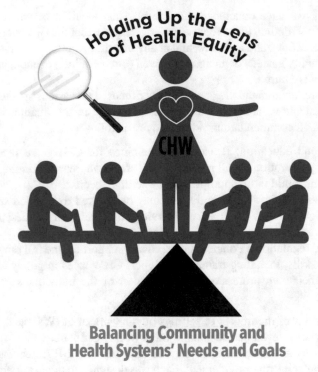

Fig. 2.1 The C3 Project integrated CHW framework. From: The C3 Project's Phase 2 report: Together leaning toward the sky. The Community Health Worker Core Consensus Project, 2018 (p. inside back cover). (Reprinted with permission from the C3 Project)

findings, the team determined that a first step to providing guidance on skill assessment was developing a solid framework around which to organize assessment approaches and resources. In response to this, they developed the multilevel framework depicted in Fig. 2.2. With this in hand, the assessment team worked to classify assessment processes and tools.

Building on their framework the team went on to develop "The Community Worker Assessment Toolkit: A Framework for the Assessment of Skill Proficiency to Promote Ongoing Professional Development." The Toolkit, released in 2018, is geared for use by program managers, supervisors, trainers, CHWs, and others in CHW supervisory roles. The Toolkit provides background about assessment and justification for the importance of assessing CHW skills. It also provides guiding principles for assessing CHW skill proficiency. The Assessment Toolkit includes recommended program elements deemed necessary to support the assessment of CHW skill proficiency. The Toolkit includes case studies of exemplary programs, featuring their approaches to improving CHW skills. More specifically, the Toolkit includes assessment tools for assessing CHW skills; a self-assessment tool for CHWs; a self-assessment tool for supervisors; a job description template for recruiting CHWs; and an interview guide to be used by hiring managers when recruiting CHWs.

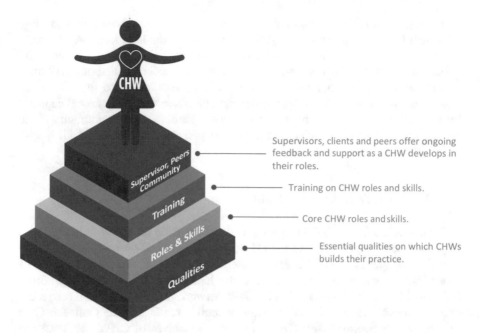

Fig. 2.2 Supporting the assessment of CHW skill proficiency: a 360° view. From the C3 Project's Community Health Worker Assessment Toolkit: a framework for assessing skills proficiency and fostering professional development, 2018, p. 7). (Reprinted with permission from the C3 Project)

The C3 Project assessment recommendations are summarized as a table in the Project's Phase 2 report. Recommendations begin by stating that "CHW self-assessment is an essential part of improving skill proficiency." To that end, the C3 Project recommends the following guiding principles be followed in assessing individual CHW skills:

- Use innovative, mixed methods, and technologies for hiring, training, and skill assessment.
- Conduct CHW assessment with cultural competency and humility.
- Use assessment throughout the lifecycle of the program.
- CHWs should play an active role in assessing themselves, their peers, and their work environment.
- Supervisors should also be assessed to continually support CHWs.
- Consider contextual factors (e.g., support from management) that may impact CHW assessment.

The C3 Project team proposes that there are numerous benefits to effectively and regularly assessing CHW skill proficiencies. Notably, this process can:

- Reduce CHW turnover
- Improve CHW capacity to deliver interventions with greater fidelity
- Enhance effectiveness in working with community members and team members (Allen, Brownstein, Cole, & Hirsch, 2018)

Ideally, the C3 Project team notes that as skill assessment contributes to more proficient CHWs, it is hypothesized that this, in turn, can help to improve patient outcomes. Assessment can also lead to better integration of CHWs into teams by expanding CHW supervisors' and other stakeholders' understanding of CHW roles and scope of practice and their skills. Ultimately in addition to these benefits, assessment of CHW proficiency in skills can contribute to organizational capacity by building recognition of "how they overcome barriers, forge community-clinic linkages, and help community members and patients reach their health goals" (Allen et al., 2018).

2.5.6.2 Outreach to the CHW Field

The work of the Outreach Core team reaching out *within* the CHW field produced important new insights on both the C3 Project content and on best approaches to ensuring the greater use of C3 Project identified roles and competencies. One of those insights was related to the need to continue to create opportunities to bring individual CHWs, CHW leaders, and CHW networks/associations from across the country together to discuss and continue to build consensus. The Outreach Core member's conversations with CHWs and representatives of CHW networks and associations highlight some of the state and regional differences in points of view. These included ways to identify and utilize the C3 Project recommendations as it relates to training standards, credentialing, and other potential "requirements." We also uncovered that there were varying levels of engagement and support of C3 Project recommendations within local and state areas and that some need time to come to a consensus before they align with the findings from a national initiative like the C3 Project. The team also learned that many states do not currently have a CHW network/association, and even in states that do, there may be independent CHWs voices that should not be discounted. The Project team determined to build consensus, engaging these leaders in addition to working with the established CHW networks and associations may be necessary.

The work of the Outreach Core team targeted *outside* the CHW field produced important new insights as well on both the C3 Project content and again on best approaches promoting C3 Project's identified roles and competencies' greater use. An early lesson learned was that national organizations outside the CHW field may be hesitant to "endorse" C3 Project recommendations due to concerns including the potential of establishing national CHW standards that could potentially encroach on their members' own scope of practice. The team also learned that the C3 Project has a lot to offer to stakeholder groups in providing a foundation for their member education on CHWs, particularly with the use of the roles and competencies that can provide basic knowledge and guidance to inform CHW integration into inter-professional teams. The team identified that new tools to provide for assessment of foundational knowledge about CHWs by those learning about CHWs may also be of value in this context.

In achieving its goals of outreach to stakeholders, there were significant accomplishments. A growing number of state policy initiatives have adopted the C3 Project recommendations as a starting point for deliberations on definitions and policies regarding CHWs—at least 20 at the time of this writing. The American Diabetes Association was one organization the Project reached out to, which resulted in the inclusion of a citation about C3 Project recommendations in their 2017 and 2018 Standards of Care. The National Association of Community Health Centers issued a support letter for the C3 Project recommendations. Federal technical assistance through the Health Resources and Service Administration to HIV/AIDS grantees working with CHWs adopted C3 Project recommendations as a standard in working with grantees. Several other key national endorsements and support letters were received, including from the American Nurses Association, National Rural Health Association, MHP *Salud*, and the National Commission for Health Education Credentialing (issuers of CHES/MCHES certification). There was also the development of a national initiative among Regional Health Equity Councils to make CHWs, as outlined by the C3 Project's role and competency recommendations, a central part of health equity strategies nationally and their National Partnership for Action plans. Finally, community prevention guide references the C3 Project and lists the C3 Project recommended CHW roles and skills in response to the findings from the Community Preventive Services Task Force that includes CHWs as evidence-based best practice in the prevention and management of several targeted health issues (Community Guide to Prevention Services. Diabetes Management: Interventions Engaging Community Health Workers n.d.).

A C3 Project utilization survey of networks/associations and stakeholders further showed that the C3 Project findings are being regularly consulted. The great majority of survey respondents were familiar with the Project and had used or planned to use its findings in their organizations. Uses and intended uses of the C3 Project's findings identified in the survey included using C3 Project CHW roles and competencies as a reference to define CHWs, to aid in securing resources and funding, to assist in educating about CHWs, to plan training or education opportunities for CHWs, and to generally strengthen existing CHW field infrastructure (Palmer, 2017).

With the release of the C3 Project's report following Phase 2, the C3 Project Advisory Chairs addressed the readers encouraging them to continue to work to move CHWs forward and to use the C3 Project work to help them with that work. In her opening letter, CHW advisory chair, Floribella Redondo-Martinez, shared that "we have been working in communities without defining our roles. We were telling our story individually, not as a profession…we are now equipped with tools that share our core roles and competencies" (with the C3 Project). She calls for the field, with these tools in hand, to carry on the efforts to build toward greater recognition of CHWs.

2.6 Holding the Door Open: C3 Project Dissemination and Ongoing Work

In wrapping up Phase 2 of the Project, the C3 Project team considered next steps for dissemination and added an additional focus to establishing a platform for ongoing dissemination. Thus, as indicated earlier, the C3 Project team positioned the findings from Phases 1 and 2 on an independent website (c3project.org) so that C3 Project resources are visible and available for future review and development. The C3 Project team worked with a communications firm to support this step. As a part of this, a representative group of C3 Project staff, consultants, advisors, and other stakeholders developed and refined a Message Map to guide our ongoing outreach and communications (St. John et al., 2018).

2.6.1 What Does This All Mean for CHWs and the Wider Development of the Field and Its Contributions to Improved Health?

Through an evidenced-based approach inclusive of CHWs, the C3 Project has worked to provide resources to serve the CHW field.

2.6.1.1 The Value of Consensus

Consensus building has traditionally been one of the strategies the CHW workforce has utilized to grow as a profession. A part of this has been related to better articulating the core roles and competencies of CHWs, as was a major focus of both the NCHAS (1998) and the C3 Project (2016). Consensus building helps to ensure agreement across a broad range of CHWs and can promote CHW self-determination, a guiding principle in CHW workforce organizing locally and nationally. While consensus can be time-consuming to build, consensus is crucial as CHWs move forward with a unified voice. Consensus building was also important in the launch of the National Association of CHWs (see Chap. 15). The C3 Project from its outset began with agreed-upon core roles and competencies put forward in 1998 in the NCHAS, which were developed with keen attention to CHW leadership and direction. With consensus building as a cornerstone, guided by CHW leaders, the C3 Project's aim to update CHW core roles and competencies was achieved.

2.6.1.2   Next Steps

Ongoing regular updates of these roles and competencies are recommended to support the future development of the CHW field. The C3 Project team is committed to this ongoing cyclical review, especially in collaboration with national CHW-led leadership. Intervals for review are under consideration.

2.6.1.3   National CHW Leadership

A notable quote about the importance of professional associations says that an association "is the cradle from which all else flows" for a profession (Hamm & Early, 1994). In the case of CHWs, a long—but recently successful—evolution of such an association (see Chap. 15) has meant that the CHW field has not had the benefit of a dedicated CHW-centered national organization to support its development. With the presence of the National Association of Community Health Workers (NACHW), that development will surely follow. Based on the examination of other health professions, there is no doubt that the process will at some point include an examination of guidelines on the scope of practice and competencies by CHWs for CHWs. Our hope is that the C3 Project and the CHW-informed and CHW-driven consensus that the C3 Project has pursued to inform this work will serve as a resource to the newly established NACHW organization and its leadership. Until that time, we will continue efforts to sustain this work and provide support in the new association's efforts to promote self-determination of the CHWs throughout the United States. Ultimately, the C3 Project team recognizes that through the increased visibility and integration of CHWs that a national association will foster, all CHWs will be better able to contribute to the health and well-being of the many individuals, family, and communities they so capably serve.

Acknowledgments

- *The C3 Project (Phases 1 and 2) engaged a diverse and competent core team of staff, consultants, and students. That team included CHWs and CHW allies. Beyond the core team, we were grateful for the guidance from numerous advisors. Acknowledgment goes to Phase 1 advisory chairs/CHW fellows Catherine Gray Haywood and Jacqueline Ortiz Miller and advisors Noelle Wiggins and Sergio Matos. Thanks also go to Phase 2 visionary advisory chairs/hermanas, Floribella Redondo-Martinez and Gail Hirsch. See C3Project.org for a complete list of all C3 Project advisors and collaborators without whom this Project could not have succeeded.*
- *The C3 Project builds on a long tradition of CHW work in the United States. Special recognition goes to all who contributed to the National Community Health Advisor Study (NCHAS, 1994–1998) that set the stage for this work, especially to Jill Guernsey de Zapien and Maia Ingram at the University of Arizona and Susan Mayfield-Johnson with the then Center for Sustainable Health Outreach. We are also grateful for continued collaborators in the C3*

Project within our core team including E. Lee Rosenthal, J. Nell Brownstein, and Durrell Fox—all three of whom played vital leadership roles in the NCHAS from 1994 to 1998. We also are grateful for continued collaboration with Noelle Wiggins, our Phase 1 advisor, who led the work on core roles and competencies in the NCHAS.

- *We acknowledge the collaborative support, leadership, and guidance from many working within the CHW Section of the American Public Health Association and at the Centers for Disease Control and Prevention (CDC). We recognize Betsy Rodriguez at the CDC for supporting Spanish language translation for various C3 Project resources.*
- *Finally, these acknowledgments recall friends now gone, with respect and fondness, we remember the University of Arizona contributors Nancy Collyer, Don Proulx, and Joel Meister. Their lasting contributions to CHW field-building projects have made a difference—improving support for CHWs and the individuals, families, and communities they serve.*

References

Addressing Chronic Disease through Community Health Workers: A Policy and Systems-Level Approach. (2015). Retrieved from https://www.cdc.gov/dhdsp/docs/chw_brief.pdf.

Albritton, E., & Hernandez-Cancio, S. (2017). *Blueprint for HEalth Care Advocacy: How Community Health Workers are driving health equity and value in New Mexico.* Retrieved from https://familiesusa.org/resources/blueprint-for-health-care-advocacy-how-community-health-workers-are-driving-health-equity-and-value-in-new-mexico/.

Allen, C. G., Brownstein, J. N., Cole, M., & Hirsch, G. (2018). *The Community Health Worker assessment toolkit: A framework for the assessment of skill proficiency to promote ongoing professional development.* Retrieved from https://www.c3project.org/.

Altman, D., & Mascarenhas, A. K. (2016). New competencies for the 21st century dental public health specialist. *Journal of Public Health Dentistry, 76*(S1), S18–S28. https://doi.org/10.1111/jphd.12190

Ashcroft, R., Kourgiantakis, T., & Brown, J. B. (2017). Social work's scope of practice in the provision of primary mental health care: Protocol for a scoping review. *BMJ Open, 7*(11), e019384. https://doi.org/10.1136/bmjopen-2017-019384

Community Guide to Prevention Services. Diabetes Management: Interventions Engaging Community Health Workers. (n.d.). Retrieved from https://www.thecommunityguide.org/findings/diabetes-management-interventions-engaging-community-health-workers.

Cosgrove, S., Moore-Monroy, M., Jenkins, C., Castillo, S. R., Williams, C., Parris, E., ... Brownstein, J. N. (2014). Community Health Workers as an integral strategy in the REACH U.S. program to eliminate health inequities. *Health Promotion Practice, 15*(6), 795–802. https://doi.org/10.1177/1524839914541442

Dean, E., Moffat, M., Skinner, M., Dornelas de Andrade, A., Myezwa, H., & Söderlund, A. (2014). Toward core inter-professional health promotion competencies to address the non-communicable diseases and their risk factors through knowledge translation: Curriculum content assessment. *BMC Public Health, 14*(1), 717. https://doi.org/10.1186/1471-2458-14-717

Hamm, M., & Early, L. (1994). Certification: Yes or no? *Association Management*, 1–6.

Islam, N., Nadkarni, S. K., Zahn, D., Skillman, M., Kwon, S. C., & Trinh-Shevrin, C. (2015). Integrating Community Health Workers within Patient Protection and Affordable Care Act implementation. *Journal of Public Health Management and Practice: JPHMP, 21*(1), 42–50. https://doi.org/10.1097/PHH.0000000000000084

Lane, D. S., Ross, V., Chen, D. W., & O'Neill, C. (1999). Core competencies for preventive medicine residents: Version 2.0. *American Journal of Preventive Medicine, 16*(4), 367–372.

Malcarney, M.-B., Pittman, P., Quigley, L., Horton, K., & Seiler, N. (2017). The changing roles of Community Health Workers. *Health Services Research, 52*(S1), 360–382. https://doi.org/10.1111/1475-6773.12657

Meeker, J., Perry, A., Dolan, C., Emary, C., Golden, K., Abla, C., … Seal, A. (2014). Development of a competency framework for the nutrition in emergencies sector. *Public Health Nutrition, 17*(3), 689–699. https://doi.org/10.1017/s1368980013002607

Minkler, M., & Wallerstein, N. (2008). *Community-based participatory research for health.* Hoboken, NJ: John Wiley & Sons.

Palmer, C. (2017). *The C3 project utilization survey.* El Paso: Paul L. Foster School of Medicine.

Rogers, E. A., Manser, S. T., Cleary, J., Joseph, A. M., Harwood, E. M., & Call, K. T. (2018). Integrating Community Health Workers into medical homes. *The Annals of Family Medicine, 16*(1), 14–20. https://doi.org/10.1370/afm.2171

Rosenthal, E. L., Wiggins, N., Brownstein, J.N., et. al (1998). *Summary of the National Community Health Advisor Study.* Retrieved from https://crh.arizona.edu/sites/default/files/pdf/publications/CAHsummaryALL.pdf.

Rosenthal, E. L., & Brownstein, J. N. (2016). The evolution of the Community Health Worker field in the United States: The shoulders we stand on. In T. Berthold (Ed.), *Foundations for Community Health Workers* (2nd ed.). Hoboken, NJ: Wiley.

Rosenthal, E. L., Menking, P., & St. John, J. (2018). *A report of the C3 project phase 1 and 2, together leaning toward the sky.* Retrieved from El Paso: https://www.c3project.org/.

Rosenthal, E. L., Rush, C. H., & Allen, C. G. (2016). *Understanding scope and competencies: A contemporary look at the United States Community Health Worker Field.* Retrieved from https://www.c3project.org/.

St. John, J., Rosenthal, E. L., Hirsch, G., Redondo, F., Rush, C., Fox, D. J., … Menking, P. (2018). *Developing communication strategies to improve the visibility of the frontline public health workforce: Lessons learned from the Community Health Worker core consensus (C3) project.* Paper presented at the American Public Health Association annual meeting, San Diego, CA.

Support for Community Health Worker Leadership in Determining Workforce Standards for Training and Credentialing, 201414 C.F.R. (2014).

Torres, S., Balcázar, H., Rosenthal, L. E., Labonté, R., Fox, D., & Chiu, Y. (2017). Community Health Workers in Canada and the US: Working from the margins to address health equity. *Critical Public Health, 27*(5), 533–540. https://doi.org/10.1080/09581596.2016.1275523

Verhagen, I., Steunenberg, B., de Wit, N. J., & Ros, W. J. (2014). Community Health Worker interventions to improve access to health care services for older adults from ethnic minorities: A systematic review. *BMC Health Services Research, 14*(1), 497. https://doi.org/10.1186/s12913-014-0497-1

Chapter 3
Roles, Skills, and Qualities of Community Health Workers

Noelle Wiggins and Keara Rodela

Like other health professionals, community health workers (CHWs) possess a set of core roles and competencies that define their contributions to communities and health and social service systems. Yet, part of what makes CHWs unique, and uniquely valuable, are the ways in which those roles and competencies are *different* from those of other health professionals. In order for CHWs to make the best possible contribution to improving health and reducing inequity, a clear understanding of how CHW roles and competencies are understood and practiced is crucial.

A fundamental way in which the CHW profession is different from other health professions is its history. The CHW profession has its roots in natural helping systems that have existed in all human communities throughout history (Jackson & Parks, 1997). These systems became formalized in areas where many people lacked health care and the conditions necessary for good health (Wiggins & Borbón, 1998). As such, from the beginning, the central role of CHWs has been to *work with communities to address and eliminate social and health inequities* (Gonzalez Arizmendi & Ortiz, 2008).

A variety of studies over the years have tried to identify the *core roles* of CHWs, including the 1998 National Community Health Advisor Study (Rosenthal, Wiggins, Brownstein, & Johnson, 1998) and the 2018 CHW Core Consensus Project (Rosenthal, Menking, & St. John, 2018). Some studies have focused on particular roles of CHWs, such as the role of advocate (Ingram et al., 2012), while others have

---

Portions of this chapter are adapted from: Wiggins, N., & Borbón, I. A. (1998). Core roles and competencies of Community Health Workers. In *Final report of the National Community Health Advisor Study* (pp. 15–49). Baltimore, MD: Annie E. Casey Foundation.

N. Wiggins (✉)
Wiggins Health Consulting LLC, Portland, OR, USA
e-mail: chwcommonindicators@gmail.com

K. Rodela
Immigrant and Refugee Community Organization, Portland, OR, USA

© Springer Nature Switzerland AG 2021
J. A. St. John et al. (eds.), *Promoting the Health of the Community*,
https://doi.org/10.1007/978-3-030-56375-2_3

tried to define roles in particular settings, such as clinics (Malcarney, Pittman, Quigley, Horton, & Seiler, 2017).

One of the hallmarks of how CHWs work, and a principal reason for their success in improving health and reducing inequities, is flexibility (Ingram et al., 2012). Based on a highly developed understanding of their communities' strengths and needs grounded in their lived experience, CHWs respond in multiple ways, from accompanying participants to medical appointments, to accessing shared cultural concepts to increase motivation, to organizing communities to shape health policy, to educating health systems about cultural norms, community strengths, and power imbalances. Thus, not surprisingly, the range of roles identified among CHWs is unusually broad when compared to other health professions.

In the current historical moment, as CHWs are increasingly integrated into health services, this broad range of roles can present challenges. Medical culture emphasizes hierarchy and specialization, both of which can be contradictory to the way in which CHWs work (Sanford, Wiggins, Reyes, & George, 2018). Even though fee-for-service reimbursement is increasingly being deemphasized, the underlying structure of alternative payment methodologies still relies on billing codes. Well-meaning attempts to find sustainable funding mechanisms for CHWs can further limit their roles. Yet multiple studies agree that the true "value added" from CHW programs is obtained when CHWs are supported to play a full range of roles (Damio, Ferraro, London, Pérez-Escamilla, & Wiggins, 2017; Islam et al., 2015; Johnson et al., 2012; Reinschmidt et al., 2006; Wiggins et al., 2013).

Some of the same studies that have explored CHW roles have also explored *core competencies*. Both research and experience suggest that the combination of qualities, skills, and knowledge CHWs need in order to be effective in their roles does not fit neatly into a conventional competency-based framework. This is not surprising when one considers how the role of the CHW has traditionally been conceptualized and practiced. One of the few defining characteristics of CHWs that has been widely agreed upon over time and throughout the world is *membership in the community in which they work* (https://chwimpact.org/download). Community membership (or cultural congruence) can be defined in various ways: shared language, race/ethnicity, lived experience, etc. (Islam et al., 2017). But none of the definitions of community membership is analogous to what have conventionally been defined as *competencies*. While it can imply a number of concrete skills, community membership is essentially a characteristic or quality. Competencies have been defined as things that people are able to do that can be objectively measured. A more flexible, less conventional definition of "competency" is required to fit a flexible, less conventional field.

A concrete example of the difficulty of using a conventional framework for describing the competencies of CHWs comes from our experience conducting the National Community Health Advisor (NCHA) Study (Rosenthal et al., 1998). Between 1995 and 1997, the first author and her colleagues conducted discussion groups and interviews with CHWs and CHW supervisors all over the country. One of our main goals was to identify the primary roles that CHWs played and the competencies they needed in order to play those roles. We defined competencies as "a combination of qualities and skills," qualities as "personal characteristics that can be enhanced but not taught," and skills as "things people can do because they have learned."

To learn about CHW roles, we first asked, "What activities do you conduct?" We usually received direct answers like, "I encourage women to get screened for breast cancer," or "We conduct support and education groups for people with diabetes," or "I bring people in my community together to talk about our most important health problems and how we can solve them."

When we started to ask about competencies, things got really interesting. We initially phrased the question, "What qualities and skills do you need to play your roles as a CHW?" Almost inevitably, CHW participants would quickly identify a long list of qualities, among them patience, being nonjudgmental, and the willingness and ability to grow, change, and learn. So we'd ask the question again, putting the emphasis on skills: "What qualities and *skills* do you need to do your work?" And the CHW participants would list more qualities: friendliness, sociability, personal strength, and compassion. So ultimately, we'd drop qualities from the question altogether, and ask, "And what *skills* do you need to conduct your work?" At this point, the CHW participants would usually start to mention some skills, perhaps communication skills or assessment skills or writing skills. But they would usually also identify additional qualities: honesty, respect, creativity, and resourcefulness. Based on the analysis of data from the interviews, we eventually identified 18 personal qualities that were essential for CHWs (along with 7 core roles and eight skills clusters).

The CHWs interviewed for the NCHA Study, speaking from their own lived experience, were articulating a fundamental principle of their work which would be reinforced through later research with community participants. Recent research by Katigbak, Van Devanter, Islam, and Trinh-Shevrin (2015); Kangovi, Grande, and Trinh-Shevrin (2015); and Islam et al. (2017) all support the idea that, while CHWs' knowledge and professionalism are important, what program participants most value are interpersonal qualities like being friendly, respectful, and nonjudgmental. An even more fundamental characteristic of the relationship between CHWs and participants is mutuality and shared power, which grow out of but are not synonymous with cultural congruence. As one CHW interviewed for the NCHA Study related, "We are not coming … from these high offices, you know, telling them what do you need, or what can I help you with … We know what they need because we've been there. Probably we are still there" (Wiggins & Borbón, 1998, p. 37). Many of the qualities identified in the recent research are the same ones identified by the CHWs and supervisors interviewed for the NCHA Study.

In the NCHA Study, and still today, we recommend that lists of essential qualities be used when recruiting and hiring CHWs. An effective recruitment and hiring process will seek to determine whether candidates possess the qualities mentioned above, often using nonconventional strategies like role playing and scenarios (Kangovi et al., 2015). List of skills can serve at least two distinct purposes. First, they can be used to determine the basic content of CHW training and capacitation courses. (Other specific topics will need to be added based on the issues facing particular communities and the program focus.) Second, these measurable skills can serve as the basis for the development of assessments to be used at the end of training series and/or to confer certificates of competence. List of roles of CHWs can and should be used to create position descriptions and class specifications for CHWs. By clearly differentiating between roles, skills, and qualities and respecting the unique importance of each, we can help to assure that CHW programs are structured for maximum impact, and that CHWs are able to make optimal contributions to communities, social justice, and health and social service systems.

References

Damio, G., Ferraro, M., London, K., Pérez-Escamilla, R., & Wiggins, N. (2017). *Addressing social determinants of health through Community Health Workers: A call to action*. Hartford, CT: Hispanic Health Council.

Gonzalez Arizmendi, L., & Ortiz, L. (2008). Neighborhood and community organizing in *colonias*: A case study in the development and use of *promotoras*. *Journal of Community Practice, 12*, 23–35.

Ingram, M., Reinschmidt, K., Schachter, M., Davidson, K., Sabo, A., Zapien, C., & Carvajal, L. (2012). Establishing a professional profile of Community Health Workers: Results from a national study of roles, activities and training. *Journal of Community Health, 37*(2), 529–537.

Islam, N., Nadkarni, S. K., Zahn, D., Skillman, M., Kwon, S. C., & Trinh-Shevrin, C. (2015). Integrating Community Health Workers within patient protection and affordable care act implementation. *Journal of Public Health Management and Practice: JPHMP, 21*(1), 42–50. https://doi.org/10.1097/PHH.0000000000000084

Islam, N., Shapiro, E., Wyatt, L., Riley, L., Zanowiak, J., Ursua, R., & Trinh-Shevrin, C. (2017). Evaluating Community Health Workers' attributes, roles, and pathways of action in immigrant communities. *Preventive Medicine, 103*, 1–7.

Jackson, E. J., & Parks, C. P. (1997). Recruitment and training issues from selected lay health advisor programs among African Americans: A 20-year perspective. *Health Education and Behavior, 24*, 418–431.

Johnson, D., Saavedra, P., Sun, E., Stageman, A., Grovet, D., Alfero, C., … Kaufman, A. (2012). Community Health Workers and Medicaid Managed Care in New Mexico. *Journal of Community Health, 37*(3), 563–571. https://doi.org/10.1007/s10900-011-9484-1

Kangovi, S., Grande, D., & Trinh-Shevrin, C. (2015). From rhetoric to reality—Community Health Workers in Post-Reform U.S. Health Care. *The New England Journal of Medicine, 372*(24), 2277–2279.

Katigbak, C., Van Devanter, N., Islam, N., & Trinh-Shevrin, C. (2015). Partners in health: A conceptual framework for the role of Community Health Workers in facilitating patients' adoption of healthy behaviors. *American Journal of Public Health, 105*(5), 872–880.

Malcarney, M., Pittman, P., Quigley, L., Horton, K., & Seiler, N. (2017). The changing roles of Community Health Workers. *Health Services Research, 52*(S1), 360–382.

Reinschmidt, K., Hunter, J., Fernandez, M., Lacy-Martinez, C., Guernsey de Zapien, J., & Meister, J. (2006). Understanding the success of promotoras in increasing chronic diseases screening. *Journal of Health Care for the Poor and Underserved, 17*(2), 256–264.

Rosenthal, E. L., Menking, P., & St. John, J. (2018). The Community Health Worker Core consensus (C3) project: A report of the C3 project phase 1 and 2. In *Together leaning toward the sky: A national project to inform CHW policy and practice*. El Paso: Texas Tech University Health Sciences Center.

Rosenthal, L., Wiggins, N., Brownstein, N., & Johnson, S. (1998). *The final report of the National Community Health Advisor Study*. Baltimore: Annie E. Casey Foundation.

Sanford, B., Wiggins, N., Reyes, M. E., & George, R. (2018). *Community Health Workers: Integral members of Oregon's Health Workforce*. Portland, OR: Oregon Community Health Workers Association.

Wiggins, N., & Borbón, I. A. (1998). Core roles and competencies of Community Health Workers. In *Final report of the National Community Health Advisor Study* (pp. 15–49). Baltimore, MD: Annie E. Casey Foundation.

Wiggins, N., Kaan, S., Rios-Campos, T., Gaonkar, R., Rees-Morgan, E., & Robinson, J. (2013). Preparing Community Health Workers for their role as agents of social change: Experience of the community capacitation center. *Journal of Community Practice, 21*(3), 186–202.

Chapter 4
Describing Results from the "Promoting the Health of the Community" National Needs Assessment

Danielle Fastring, Susan L. Mayfield-Johnson, Julie Ann St. John, and Wandy D. Hernández-Gordon

Community health workers (CHWs) make a difference. CHWs are a key part of the healthcare, public health, and social service workforce. CHWs have numerous skills, abilities, and qualities, which enable them to help others improve their health outcomes and qualities of life. This is clearly described in the previous introductory chapters. The importance of CHWs, their contributions, and roles, skills, and qualities are well studied and documented, and in fact, the framework for this textbook is the recognized roles of CHWs that arose from national studies. Further, Chap. 1 discussed the intent and purpose of this book, which is to serve as a resource for CHWs, CHW employers, CHW allies, and those interested in potentially integrating/hiring CHWs into their place of work, because, in spite of all the contributions of the CHW field, there are still employers, policy makers, professionals, and other entities who do not yet fully understand or embrace why CHWs matter and why and how CHWs contribute to improving population health status. So, the editors of this book had the task of laying out how CHWs do just that—and through what means (ten core roles). In order to set the stage for this book, the editors decided a current "snapshot" of CHWs in the United States would

D. Fastring (✉)
College of Osteopathic Medicine, William Carey University, Hattiesburg, MS, USA
e-mail: DFastring@wcu.edu

S. L. Mayfield-Johnson
Department of Public Health, The University of Southern Mississippi, Hattiesburg, MS, USA
e-mail: Susan.Johnson@usm.edu

J. A. St. John
Department of Public Health, Texas Tech University Health Sciences Center, Abilene, TX, USA
e-mail: julie.st-john@ttuhsc.edu

W. D. Hernández-Gordon
HealthConnect One, Chicago, IL, USA
e-mail: wandyhdz@healthconnectone.org

© Springer Nature Switzerland AG 2021
J. A. St. John et al. (eds.), *Promoting the Health of the Community*,
https://doi.org/10.1007/978-3-030-56375-2_4

help inform and guide its development. As such, in 2016, the editors of this book, along with collaborators, developed a survey in order to gain input for the development of a call for chapter proposal. The survey served as an opportunity to elicit contributions about roles, responsibilities, and competencies of community health workers (CHWs), CHW instructors/trainers, CHW stakeholders/allies, and CHW employers.

Survey collection occurred July 15, 2016, to February 15, 2017. During that time, the survey collected responses from 773 participants. The survey consisted of approximately 180 questions. Each participant classified themselves as either a CHW, a CHW instructor or trainer, a CHW stakeholder or ally, or a CHW employer, and they completed a subset of the overall survey that corresponded to their current role. The survey took approximately 20 min to complete. This chapter summarizes and discusses the findings of this survey, with the intent to give our readers a glimpse of CHWs across the United States and to provide context as readers proceed through each chapter with CHWs sharing their stories of how they do the work they do and the roles they conduct to serve their places of work, communities, and clients.

4.1 Demographics of All Survey Respondents

Most of the survey respondents were female ($n = 657$, 87.48%) and Caucasian ($n = 483$, 69.10%) or African American ($n = 180$, 25.75%). Approximately one-third were of Hispanic ethnicity ($n = 242$, 32.93%). Respondents most often categorized themselves as being between the ages 36–45 ($n = 184$, 24.47%) and 46–55 ($n = 185$, 24.60%). Most respondents had either a Master's Degree ($n = 206$, 27.36%) or a Bachelor's Degree ($n = 182$, 24.17%). Participants were asked to select the category that they most identified with at the time of the survey. Results from this question can be found in Table 4.1. The majority of respondents identified

Table 4.1 Self-reported category of current role related to CHWs

Category of current role related to CHWs	n	%
Community health worker Includes all terms associated with CHW	389	50.65%
CHW instructor or trainer Teach CHW curriculum or conduct trainings for CHWs	113	14.71%
CHW stakeholder or ally Supports CHWs, but may or may not directly work with CHWs	90	11.72%
CHW supervisor Directly involved in the supervision of CHWs, works with CHWs on a daily basis	81	10.55%
CHW employer Employs CHWs, but not involved in supervision or daily interaction with CHWs	27	3.52%
My current role does not fit the listed categories	68	8.85%
Total	768	100.00%

themselves as CHWs (n = 389, 50.65%), 113 (14.71%) identified as a CHW instructor or trainer, 90 (11.72%) identified as a CHW stakeholder or ally, 81 (10.55%) identified themselves as a CHW supervisor, 27 (3.52%) said they currently employed CHWs, and the remainder (n = 68, 8.85%) reported that they did not currently fit in any of the above roles, so they were excluded from the question subsets of the survey.

4.2   Community Health Workers

4.2.1   Employment Characteristics

Participants that identified as CHWs had numerous titles. Although most worked in a job where their title was community health worker (n = 188, 58.39%), other common titles included patient educator, patient navigator, outreach worker, health education specialist, or health advisor. The majority of CHW respondents reported working in paid, full-time positions (n = 265, 69.55%). Some, however, are working in an unpaid, volunteer position (n = 26, 6.82%). When asked about the level of education required for their current position, most reported a high school diploma requirement (n = 141, 49.65%) or some college coursework (n = 47, 16.55%). There were several areas in which CHWs received training before beginning employment in their current position. Areas in which more than half of respondents received training prior to employment were communication, HIPAA compliance, cultural competency, advocacy, interpersonal skills, specific health topics, and first aid/ CPR. The most common training topics addressed after employment were HIPAA compliance, disease-specific education, and motivational interviewing. Most CHWs received training provided by their employer (n = 177, 62.99%). A majority of respondents reported that they had 1–3 years of experience working as a CHW (n = 114, 35.29%). Many respondents (n = 93, 28.79%) had worked for more than 10 years in their field. Among CHWs who reported their salary information for a full-time position (n = 254), approximately half (50.79%) had a pre-tax salary between $25,000 and $34,999. About a quarter of participants (27.17%) had a pre-tax salary between $35,000 and $49,999. Approximately two-thirds of respondents (n = 207, 64.49%) felt as though they had job security in their current position. Perceived job security was most often related to the fact that CHWs reported regular and consistent work (n = 147, 75.38%) and a good work environment (n = 119, 61.03%). Among those that did not feel as though their job was secure (n = 109), most reported that potential changes in program funding or working in a grant-funded position led to a feeling of job insecurity (82.57%). When asked about employee advancement, most CHWs reported that CHWs at their place of employment did not "regularly get promotions involving a change in job role or responsibility" (n = 118, 45.74%), nor did they "regularly receive opportunities for an increase in salary" (n = 115, 44.75%).

Table 4.2 Activities CHWs currently perform as part of their job duties

Activities CHWs currently perform as part of their job duties	n	%
Advocate on behalf of clients	237	77.20%
Follow-up with clients to ensure services received	236	76.87%
Help clients identify ways to meet other needs	233	75.90%
Make referrals	224	72.96%
Schedule appointments for clients	206	67.10%
Advocate for community needs	198	64.50%
Administrative duties (answering the telephone, filing, etc.)	197	64.17%
Conduct home visits	168	54.72%
Provide health education and information in a group community setting	166	54.07%
Attend appointments with clients to provide support and/or advocacy	163	53.09%

The most frequently reported work settings for CHWs were clinics or hospitals ($n = 96$, 31.17%) and homes ($n = 71$, 23.05%). The survey asked CHWs to select activities from a representative list that they currently perform as part of their job duties. Table 4.2 depicts the ten most frequently selected activities. When asked which priority population CHWs work with most often, most responded that they either work with families ($n = 68$, 21.38%) or the elderly ($n = 62$, 20.39%), but some ($n = 46$, 15.13%) said their work was not population specific. Next, participants were asked to identify the specific disease content areas they most often worked with. Most worked with clients who had been diagnosed with diabetes ($n = 62$, 63.92%) or hypertension ($n = 43$, 44.33%).

4.2.2 Barriers to Effectiveness

One of the topic areas the survey explored was perceived CHW effectiveness while on the job. When asked about the greatest barrier to effectiveness, the most often cited answer was having a lack of funding or resources on the job ($n = 50$, 28.57%) or patient and client issues ($n = 46$, 26.29%). Participants were asked to expand their answers; their responses capture their personal experiences they feel limit their effectiveness. For example, one respondent said, "There will never be enough money for salaries and program funding." Another respondent said, "CHWs [in my organization] wear many hats. We are put on multiple projects that stretch our time so that projects cannot receive the full attention and dedication they deserve. We need more staff, but of course funding is limited, so that is not possible. We do the best we can with what we have." Many others cited limited resources as a barrier to effectively help clients, such as available affordable housing and transportation.

Some patient and client issues mentioned were "difficulty in contacting clients who have no telephone service and run out of minutes on their cellular phones early in the month" and having clients prioritize and keep appointments related to improving or stabilizing their current health conditions.

4.2.3 Supervision

Another topic area the survey explored was supervision of CHWs. We asked respondents to rate their level of agreement with several statements related to their supervisor or supervision. Most agreed that they had a "strong relationship with their supervisor" ($n = 242$, 84.32%). Additionally, the majority of respondents felt "supported and valued by their supervisor" ($n = 244$, 84.31%). Most agreed that their "supervisor had a good understanding of what CHWs do" ($n = 231$, 83.22%). Most reported that their supervisor "had experience working with CHWs" ($n = 197$, 68.64%). A majority of participants felt that their "supervisor valued their input and suggestions as a CHW" ($n = 234$, 81.82%). Most reported that the "amount of supervision they received from their supervisor was sufficient for them to do their job effectively" ($n = 233$, 81.75%). When asked to quantify the amount of supervision they received per week, the most often reported range was between 1 and 3 h per week ($n = 101$, 35.07%). Approximately one-fifth of respondents ($n = 60$, 20.83%) reported that they received less than 1 h per week. The amount of weekly supervision was highly variable, with 48 respondents reporting that they received 7 or more hours per week of supervision (16.67%).

Participants were also asked to identify areas where they disagreed with their supervisors. Thirty-three respondents said that they never disagreed with their supervisor (13.69%). Areas of disagreement between CHWs and their supervisors most often occurred in areas related to work type, strategies and methods ($n = 84$, 34.85%), salary and benefits ($n = 83$, 34.44%), and the provision of professional development opportunities that include trainings, conferences, and continuing education ($n = 68$, 28.22%).

4.2.4 Experience with Evaluation and Research

In order to examine specific activities in which CHWs engage, questions were asked with regard to experience with evaluation and research. About two-thirds of participants had experience with evaluation and research ($n = 216$, 64.29%). Among those with evaluation and research experience, 65.69% had experience in the area of "data collection and interpretation" ($n = 134$), 43.63% had experience with "sharing results and findings" ($n = 89$), and 42.65% had experience "evaluating CHW services and programs" ($n = 87$).

4.3 CHW Instructors or Trainers

4.3.1 Employment Characteristics

Of the 113 survey participants that self-identified as a CHW instructor or trainer, 100 completed surveys. When asked to characterize the organization the CHW instructors worked for, most reported that they worked at a university ($n = 38$. 38.00%) or a community-based organization with nonprofit status ($n = 29$, 29.00%). The positions were usually grant-funded ($n = 52$, 51.49%) or funded internally ($n = 33$, 32.67%). The entities that the instructors worked for primarily provided services related to outreach and education ($n = 66$, 68.04%), nutrition education ($n = 30$, 30.93%), or mental health services ($n = 28$, 28.87%). The titles most often associated with CHW instructors or trainers were program coordinator ($n = 20$, 20.41%), program manager or director ($n = 17$, 17.35%), and trainer ($n = 17$, 17.35%). Approximately half of those surveyed ($n = 52$, 51.49%) reported that they had not been formally trained to provide CHW instruction to others.

4.3.2 Training and Instruction for CHWs

Though many CHW trainers reported that the topics covered in CHW trainings were determined by their state's CHW certification program ($n = 29$, 30.21%), some instructors ($n = 37$, 38.54%) reported that they were responsible for determining training topics. Others reported that they were part of a training center responsible for determining the training topics ($n = 26$, 27.08%). The topics most often covered were communication ($n = 86$, 89.58%), cultural competency ($n = 79$, 82.29%), advocacy ($n = 77$, 80.21%), specific health/disease topics ($n = 70$, 79.17%), interpersonal skills ($n = 71$, 73.96%), and capacity building ($n = 67$, 69.79%). When asked how often the instructors/trainers involve CHWs in the development of training materials, approximately half ($n = 46$, 48.42%) reported that they "always" do, and 29 (30.53%) reported that they "sometimes" do. Forty respondents (41.67%) had previously worked as a CHW prior to becoming a CHW trainer or instructor. Almost all CHW trainers/instructors had served in roles where they assisted with evaluation and research ($n = 86$, 90.53%). More specifically, a majority of respondents had participated in "data collection and interpretation" ($n = 67$, 79.76%), "sharing results and findings" ($n = 57$, 67.86%), "evaluation and research" ($n = 56$, 65.48%), or "developing evaluation or research design and methods" ($n = 54$, 64.29%).

4.4   CHW Supervisors

There were 81 survey participants that identified as a CHW supervisor, of which 80 completed the survey. Most worked for a community-based organization with nonprofit status ($n = 29$, 36.24%) or a healthcare organization ($n = 25$, 31.25%). The majority worked in grant-funded positions ($n = 54$, 68.35%) or a position that was funded internally ($n = 29$, 36.71%). Similar to the group that identified as CHW instructors, the CHW supervisors worked primarily for entities that provided services related to outreach and education ($n = 68$, 85.00%), nutrition education ($n = 40$, 50.00%), or mental health services ($n = 31$, 38.75%). Approximately 40.00% of respondents who identified as CHW supervisors reported that they had worked in that capacity for 1–3 years ($n = 32$). Most are referred to as program managers or directors ($n = 33$, 41.25%), CHW supervisors ($n = 11$, 13.75%), or project coordinators ($n = 10$, 12.50%).

Only one-fifth of those surveyed ($n = 16$, 20.00%) reported that they had been formally trained to provide CHW supervision to others. Less than half ($n = 28$, 43.08%) had been CHWs themselves before supervising CHWs. Among those that had requested training in their position as supervisor ($n = 32$, 40.00%), 66.67% had received the training they requested. CHW supervisors were asked to describe one area of training that they would like to receive to be more effective in their jobs. Answers to this question varied, and when analyzed for trends, training needs identified were most often related to the need for administrative support, education surrounding specific disease topics, ways to work effectively with CHWs, improving interactions with patients/clients, and skill-based trainings. The most frequently listed training need was administrative and consisted of areas such as effective supervision, improving employee motivation and morale, organizational leadership, and how to more efficiently recruit and retain CHWs. Training needs related to providing chronic disease management and trauma-informed care were also common. Many supervisors mentioned that they work with an incredibly diverse population, and they would benefit from diversity or cultural competency training. Skill-based trainings noted were primarily in the area of program evaluation and data management.

The amount of time that CHW supervisors interact with the CHWs they supervise varies greatly. Most ($n = 32$, 49.23%) interact with the CHWs they supervise on a daily basis. Approximately one-third interact with CHWs that they supervise from 2 to 3 times per week ($n = 20$, 30.77%). When asked how they interact, almost all CHW supervisors reported that they used a cellular phone ($n = 64$, 98.46%), met face to face ($n = 63$, 96.92%), or interacted via email ($n = 60$, 92.31%). Texting was also a popular way to interact ($n = 54$, 83.08%). When asked to identify the primary means of communication, face-to-face contact was the most common way for supervisors to interact with the CHWs they supervised ($n = 36$, 55.38%). This was also the method of communication preferred by most CHW supervisors ($n = 52$, 80.00%). CHW supervisors were asked to identify sources of conflict with the CHWs that they supervise. The most often reported conflict was over differing roles, tasks, and responsibilities ($n = 28$, 49.12%), differing personalities ($n = 27$, 47.37%), and, to a lesser extent, work quality and work quantity ($n = 16$, 28.07%).

Next, CHW supervisors were asked how often the CHWs in their organization conducted specific activities. Activities most frequently reported as being conducted "Always" or "Often" were individual or community outreach and education ($n = 60$, 88.24%), promoting healthy lifestyles (e.g., nutrition, exercise, etc.) ($n = 57$, 83.82%), and care coordination (e.g., referrals) ($n = 55$, 80.89%). CHWs most often linked individuals to chronic disease management community resources in the areas of diabetes self-management ($n = 50$, 75.76%), diabetes prevention ($n = 44$, 66.67%), or blood pressure self-management ($n = 38$, 57.58%). CHW supervisors were asked to identify special populations that the CHWs in their organization most often worked with. They reported that their organizations most often work with uninsured individuals ($n = 52$, 76.47%), individuals who lacked a primary care provider ($n = 48$, 70.59%), families ($n = 47$, 69.12%), and women ($n = 45$, 66.18%).

Most CHW supervisors that responded to the survey had served in roles where they assisted with evaluation and/or research ($n = 57$, 89.06%). For example, most had been involved with data collection and interpretation ($n = 53$, 83.33%), the majority had been involved with evaluating CHW services and programs ($n = 41$, 68.33%), or sharing results and findings ($n = 36$, 60.00%). Most were involved in a local or state CHW network or association ($n = 48$, 73.85%).

4.5   CHW Stakeholders, Supporters, or Allies

There were 90 survey participants that identified as a CHW stakeholder, supporter, or ally, of which 87 completed surveys. Most worked for a state government agency ($n = 23$, 28.40%), university or college ($n = 18$, 22.22%), or a community-based nonprofit organization ($n = 18$, 20.99%). Many of the survey respondents in this category had been in their role for 1–3 years ($n = 31$, 37.80%), and approximately one-fifth of survey respondents ($n = 16$, 19.51%) had been in that role for 10 years or more. People serving in this role may have the job title of program manager or director ($n = 23$, 28.05%), project coordinator ($n = 16$, 19.51%), or executive director ($n = 9$, 10.98%). Survey participants serving in this role provide support in several different capacities. Among 81 people who responded to the question, most provide advocacy support on behalf of CHWs ($n = 63$, 77.78%), educate or inform the workforce about CHWs ($n = 61$, 75.31%), or provide technical support and assistance to CHWs ($n = 48$, 59.26%). Most work directly with CHWs ($n = 66$, 78.57%) and depending on the stage of the project, may interact with CHWs quarterly ($n = 10$, 17.86%), monthly ($n = 11$, 19.64%), or more frequently ($n = 21$, 37.50%). Approximately one-third of respondents had previously worked as a CHW ($n = 26$, 34.67%). The majority had served in roles where they assisted in evaluation and/or research ($n = 58$, 76.32%). For the most part, the roles involved sharing results and findings ($n = 47$, 66.20%), collecting and interpreting data ($n = 46$, 64.70%), and, to a lesser degree, identifying priority issues and evaluation/research questions ($n = 37$, 52.11%). More than half were involved with a local or state CHW network or association ($n = 44$, 58.67%).

This group of respondents was asked to identify the biggest challenge that CHWs face. Most often, those challenges were identified as having a general lack of recognition and respect in the workplace, having such varying roles and responsibilities, identifying their place within a healthcare system, lack of standardization of training with regard to curriculum requirements for certification, and salary-related issues such as few paid employment opportunities, paid opportunities with substandard wages, and a high number of grant-funded positions that lack sustainability. In fact, salary-related issues were the most frequently cited reason that stakeholders, supporters, and allies gave for the high turnover rate of CHWs ($n = 38$, 52.78%).

4.6 Employers of CHWs

Twenty-seven respondents identified as employers of CHWs, of which 25 completed surveys. Most worked at community-based nonprofit organizations ($n = 13$, 52.00%) or at a healthcare clinic such as a hospital or clinic ($n = 6$, 24.00%). Most respondents who identified with this category held the title of executive director ($n = 9$, 36.00%) or program manager/director ($n = 6$, 24.00%). Twenty employers provided information regarding the number of CHWs employed by their organization. Employers categorized the CHW employees as working full-time, working part-time, or as uncompensated volunteers. The number of full-time CHWs ranged from 1 to 66 (median = 7) CHWs per organization. The number of part-time CHWs ranged from 0 to 24 (median = 4) CHWs per organization. Lastly, the number of uncompensated volunteers ranged from 0 to 40 (median 7) CHWs per organization. Approximately half of the respondents indicated that their organization utilized electronic health records (EHRs) ($n = 12$, 48.00%). Among those organizations utilizing EHRs, all but one organization allowed CHWs to access patients' EHRs. Specifically, they were able to utilize the EHR to read the patient registry list, to post notes in the EHR, and to look up information in the patients' records to identify needed/completed tests, appointment information, and the like. All employers provided supervision for CHWs, most often provided by the program manager/director ($n = 11$, 52.38%), or a senior level CHW ($n = 5$, 23.81%). Care teams involving CHWs most often include other CHWs ($n = 15$, 75.00%), a case manager ($n = 11$; 55.00%), the program manager/director ($n = 10$, 50.00%), and a registered nurse ($n = 9$, 45.00%). Within those care teams, CHWs most often receive and make patient referrals or assignments (e.g., for education sessions, home visits, etc.) ($n = 18$, 94.74%), assist in developing and implementing care plans ($n = 12$, 63.16%), and attend regularly scheduled meetings ($n = 12$, 63.16%).

Employers of CHWs ($n = 20$) agreed that their organization values the work CHWs do ($n = 19$, 95.00%). Most also agree that CHW work is understood by CHW supervisors ($n = 18$, 90.00%) and by teams they work with ($n = 17$, 85.00%).

Additionally, employers felt as though CHWs at their organization had opportunities for promotion ($n = 17$, 85.00%). Most employers require that prospective CHWs have a high school diploma or GED equivalent ($n = 16$, 80.00%). Employers were asked to categorize the salaries of CHWs working at their organization. The most frequently cited salary was $30,000–$40,000 ($n = 8$, 40.00%), followed by $20,000–$30,000 ($n = 5$, 25.00%). Half of the employers surveyed reported that salaries had been increasing over time ($n = 10$, 50.00%). Benefits provided to CHWs varied widely. Three-fourths of employers surveyed provided paid leave for training/education ($n = 15$, 75.0%); 70.00% of employers provided paid time off in the form of vacation time, sick time, or personal time; 65.00% provided mileage or parking reimbursement ($n = 13$); and 60.00% provided health or dental insurance ($n = 12$). Other benefits provided were not the norm. Childcare was provided by 10.00% of employers, tuition assistance was provided by 35.00% of employers, and 50.00% of employers provided a pension or retirement plan ($n = 10$). When filling CHW positions, most employers were looking to hire someone who was bilingual or multilingual ($n = 14$, 70.00%), who had knowledge of community services or resources ($n = 14$, 70.00%), and who had a similar background as the population being served ($n = 14$, 70.00%). Additionally more than half of respondents indicated that CHWs should have skills and roles related to advocating on behalf of clients, conducting home visits, following up with clients to ensure services were received, identifying ways to meet client needs, providing health education and information either individually in a home setting or for a group in a community setting, advocating for community needs, providing peer education, making referrals, assisting client enrollment in health plans, and identifying ways that clients can pay for their health care.

4.7 Conclusion

The findings from this survey, in terms of the roles of CHWs and the expectations of what CHWs do from CHW employers, support and align with the findings and recommended roles of the National C3 project, which serves as the framework for the rest of this book. The next ten chapters each include an introduction to and explanation of each role (including their sub-roles), followed by two examples by diverse CHW teams (meaning diversity in geographical setting, population served by the CHW teams, topic/focus of the CHW work, etc.) across the United States that tell the stories of how their team performs in the respective role, their strategies, challenges, successes, lessons learned, and advice.

Part II
CHWs Describe Their Roles Through Their Stories

Chapter 5
Cultural Mediation Among Individuals, Communities, and Health and Social Service Systems

Caitlin G. Allen*, **Diane Garzon Arbelaez, Cinthia Arechiga, Anastasia Belliard, Juan Carlos Belliard*, Megan Daly, Yaminette Diaz-Linhart*, Emily Feinberg, Ivys Fernandez-Pastrana, Gail R. Hirsch, Alejandra Morales, Niem Nay-Kret, Silvia Ortega, Floribella Redondo-Martinez, and Carl H. Rush**

5.1 Introduction

Caitlin G. Allen, Carl H. Rush, Gail Hirsch and Floribella Redondo-Martinez

Our experience of illness and injury and the care we receive is shaped by our cultural background. The same symptoms can be a very different experience for two people with differing cultural beliefs. Major life experiences, like childbirth and end of life, are profoundly influenced by cultural expectations and values. As individuals, we also often receive medical services from providers whose cultural background is different from our own. This can lead to miscommunication about expectations and preferences. Community Health Workers (CHWs) often serve as cultural "brokers" or intermediaries who understand or are at least sensitive to both sides in cross-cultural encounters.

Authorship is organized alphabetically in ascending order by surname.

C. G. Allen (✉)
CGA Consulting, Charleston, SC, USA
e-mail: caitlin.gloeckner.allen@emory.edu

D. G. Arbelaez
Boston Medical Center, Boston, MA, USA

C. Arechiga
San Bernardino County, San Bernardino, CA, USA

A. Belliard · J. C. Belliard (✉) · M. Daly · A. Morales
Loma Linda University Health, Loma Linda, CA, USA
e-mail: jbelliard@llu.edu

© Springer Nature Switzerland AG 2021
J. A. St. John et al. (eds.), *Promoting the Health of the Community*,
https://doi.org/10.1007/978-3-030-56375-2_5

The first core role, cultural mediation[1] among individuals, communities, and health and social service systems, addresses how CHWs play a role in informing individuals' experiences and interactions with health and social service systems. This role incorporates three sub-roles: educating individuals and communities about how to use health and social service systems; educating systems about community perspectives and cultural norms; and building health literacy and cross-cultural communication.

Since its original conceptualization during the National Community Health Advisor Study in 1998, this role has largely remained unchanged, demonstrating its prominence in the CHW field.[2] This role is further supported by recent national funding efforts designed to promote linkages between community and clinical settings, which require cultural mediation. National efforts, including the Centers for Disease Control and Prevention's funding announcements,[3] specifically included strategies that engage CHWs as an opportunity to improve community-clinical linkages and assist with cultural mediation between communities and the health and social service systems. Ongoing support for CHWs in this role will be vital as public

---

[1] Defined as the process of building bridges between cultural and social realms, and building new relationships across political, cultural, and public spheres. Citation: https://www.culturepourtous.ca/en/cultural-professionals/cultural-mediation/

[2] https://crh.arizona.edu/sites/default/files/pdf/publications/CAHsummaryALL.pdf

[3] State Public Health Actions to Prevent and Control Diabetes, Heart Disease, Obesity, and Associated Risk Factors and Promote School Health (DP13-1305)

Y. Diaz-Linhart (✉)
Brandeis University, Waltham, MA, USA
e-mail: ydiazlinhart@brandeis.edu

E. Feinberg
Boston University, Boston, MA, USA

I. Fernandez-Pastrana
Boston Medical Center, Lowell, MA, USA

G. R. Hirsch
Massachusetts Department of Public Health, Boston, MA, USA
e-mail: gail.hirsch@state.ma.us

N. Nay-Kret
Lowell Community Health Center, Lowell, MA, USA

S. Ortega
Jurupa Unified School District, Jurupa Valley, CA, USA

F. Redondo-Martinez
Arizona Community Health Workers Association, Douglas, AZ, USA
e-mail: floribella@azchow.org

C. H. Rush
Community Resources, LLC, San Antonio, TX, USA
e-mail: carl@chrllc.net

health and health care continue to promote creative ways to collaborate with communities to improve health and health care.

In the following two sections, authors describe how CHWs engage as members of the healthcare team to promote cultural mediation, providing examples of how CHWs thrive in this role and evidence for the continued support of CHWs in cultural mediation.

5.2 A Dose of Cultural Humility: Cultural Mediation and CHW/Promotores' Contribution to Health Care[4]

Juan Carlos Belliard, Anastasia Belliard, Cinthia Arechiga, Alejandra Morales, Silvia Ortega and Megan Daly

In its broadest sense, mediation is the act of being an intermediary, liaison, or mediator between differing parties in order to help bring about alignment and mutual understanding. Cultural mediation refers to the facilitation of mutual understanding between people from different cultures. Culture refers to a set of practices and beliefs shared by members of a particular group that distinguishes that group from others (Spector, 2017). Culture does not only refer to ethnicity or language but also occupation, social groups, or religious groups, which shape our values, worldview, and identity. We each relate to multiple identities based on gender, religion, ethnicity, and/or place of residence. Community Health Workers (CHWs) serve as cultural mediators in health care and bridge the worldview gap between patients and providers.

CHWs or *Promotores de Salud* are not a new concept, especially for those who have worked or lived in the *Global South or in low and lower-middle-income countries.* The declaration of Alma-Ata in 1978 at the International Primary Care Conference recognized the need for community members to assist health systems in order to achieve their goals of improved health, quality of health care, and increased access to health care. The developing world has successfully engaged CHW/Ps as a fundamental part of health and social services for decades. However, in the United States, the popularity of CHW/Ps has grown significantly in the past few decades and most significantly since the Affordable Care Act and health care's increased focus on population health. The promotor's role has expanded from community-based organizations to their integration into healthcare and social services teams. This relatively new awareness of who CHW/Ps are and what their role is in the United States has placed decision-makers and healthcare providers in the beginner seat in terms of the utilization and integration of CHW/Ps into our

---

[4]This section focuses on the CHW/P's role of cultural mediation and specifically how the CHW/P's strength of cultural humility fits into that role and its importance in health care. We use the terms Community Health Worker, CHW, and promotor(a) together as CHW/P. Promotores' names in this section have been changed to protect anonymity.

healthcare system. The simple fact that the "developed" world is now learning from the "developing" world frames the topic of this section perfectly. To even entertain the idea of co-learning or providers learning from lay health workers requires humility. The concept of cultural humility has been defined as an "ability to maintain an interpersonal stance that is other-oriented (or open to the other) in relation to aspects of cultural identity that are most important to the [person]" (Hook, Davis, Owen, Worthington Jr, & Utsey, 2013). Cultural humility is foundational to the work of CHWs/*promotores*, especially in their role as cultural mediators, and, in our opinion, is one of the most important contributions that this emerging healthcare workforce has to offer.

The US healthcare system, with its diverse populations and growing cultural and socioeconomic differences between healthcare providers and patients, requires a more intentional focus on bridging these cultural gaps and health inequities. The need for cultural mediation places the CHW/P in a position where he or she can make a significant difference in the quality of and access to health care. While cultural mediation is one of the CHW/Ps' most important roles, cultural humility is one of their most important strengths. Effective cultural mediation requires an attitude and understanding of cultural humility.

The role of cultural mediation becomes especially useful when integrating CHW/Ps into the clinical setting, which is what we are doing at Loma Linda University Health, where we cross-train *promotores* about the clinical world and clinical staff about *promotores* and then integrate CHW/Ps as colleagues. Healthcare systems throughout our region hire graduates from our program. The experiences shared by CHW/Ps in this section represent experiences from various healthcare systems which will remain anonymous.

With the help of community partners like the El Sol Neighborhood Educational Center, and some courageous and passionate *promotores*, we created the Promotores Academy that trains CHW/Ps to work within healthcare systems, from primary to tertiary care settings. This was done in part because we, like many others, recognized CHW/Ps are an effective strategy in addressing the triple aim of improving population health, lowering healthcare costs, and improving patient experience (Institute for Healthcare Improvement, 2017).

However, we found that among others doing this work, several seemed to focus on what the CHW/Ps had to offer the system and how they could make health care easier to deliver, more efficient, or cost-effective. In our work, the central question is: How do CHW/Ps benefit? Historically, CHW/Ps have done their work in a community-based setting, often as volunteers, and rarely with benefits or guaranteed hours. Because of this reality, we decided that our primary focus for training CHW/Ps would be workforce development, which is one of the most significant social determinants of health. Despite the challenges, benefits of seeing CHW/Ps becoming financially stable, able to support their families, and potentially helping improve a broken healthcare system make this initiative worthwhile.

Yami gives an example of the challenge of integrating traditional grassroots CHW/Ps with a heart for their work into a very structured healthcare system with many rules and regulations:

I just can't let people suffer when I know I can help them. Like this one lady I was working with who was very sick and not able to get out much. Every time she would come to the clinic, she would be very pale and not much energy, and if the team would offer her a granola bar, she would eat it right away. You could see that she was very hungry, and I knew from visiting her at home that she wasn't eating much or eating healthy. So, I started bringing her fresh food when I would do my home visits. My supervisor got mad and told me I couldn't do that. But I just can't let people be hungry when I know of places that give the good food for free. She can't go out and get it herself or even lift a box of food. She needs the help to get healthy.

Yami's story illustrates how the CHW/P pushes traditional boundaries of patient care and focuses on the patient's immediate need, regardless of their eligibility to receive help or if certain criteria are met.

Yami adds:

You know there are lots of people who can't get those services because they don't have SSI or insurance. And that means they don't even qualify to have me work with them, so I feel bad. They don't eat well and they need medical care. But they (clinical supervisors) told me they don't qualify so I can't work with them. So, on my own I was able to help a couple of patients like that to connect with some resources and get them signed up for some things, and I brought it to my boss and showed them so they could help, and now we have got them both with some coverage and able to get some of the help they need.

For CHW/Ps to be effective cultural mediators in a clinical environment, they need to understand not only the patient population but also the healthcare system and the professionals providing the care. This training process required careful thought and planning to ensure that the CHW/P was trained enough to navigate the complex healthcare system while maintaining their community essence. The ability to effectively navigate this tension between professional and community spaces is what makes the CHW/P, in a sense, bicultural and an effective cultural mediator. However, to be an effective cultural mediator also requires an attitude of cultural humility.

Most workplaces now require some form of cultural competence from their staff, but we argue that CHW/Ps working effectively as cultural mediators in the clinic go beyond cultural competency and instead bring both patients and providers better outcomes because of their approach and ability to understand both sides. While cultural competence focuses on a set of skills needed to work effectively cross-culturally, we expand this concept to support the idea that an attitude of cultural humility precedes and supersedes the skill of cultural competence and is an important ingredient in effective cultural mediation. Cultural humility does not seek a higher level of expertise or knowledge about a culture but represents an open approach of continuous learning from others and acknowledging other ways of knowing (Hook et al., 2013). On its own, cultural competence could be inadvertently mistaken for a discrete checklist of beliefs, values, or skills to be mastered and applied to its respective group of people. Checklists oversimplify the complexities of human behavior and culture.

Cultural competence focuses on what we should and should not do, what behaviors to expect, and what values guide those behaviors. We run the risk of operating based on stereotypes, which may be well meaning but, at best, might be ineffective and, at worst, damaging and biased. Cultural humility creates a different relationship—shifting from a relationship of the expert and the studied or the healer and the diseased to one of collaborators and co-learners.

Cultural humility is a characteristic CHW/Ps bring to the hierarchal world of health care. CHW/Ps naturally display cultural humility to healthcare staff when interacting with them as well as with patients. This is one reason CHW/Ps are so effective in their role as cultural mediators and why providers benefit from CHW/Ps' help in the clinical setting. A CHW/P's relationship with a patient is most effective when the relationship embraces collaboration and openness where the CHW/P learns from the patient. Although CHW/Ps may not necessarily be able to define or even recognize the term cultural humility, they expertly model this characteristic. CHW/Ps, like all of us, have biases, but they approach patients as peers, not from a place of power or expertise. They show respect for the patient as a person and can empathize with their situation and their challenges.

Luisa illustrates this well when she tells of working with a patient as a CHW/P whose doctor had told her she needed to urgently lose weight and change her diet.

Yeah, I had this lady that I worked with who needed to lose weight, and she was so discouraged, telling me she had tried everything and nothing worked. So, I said, you know what? I need to lose some weight too. Let's do it together, then we can keep each other on track and help each other stick to it. So, I decided to make some major changes not only for myself but to help her see that we could do it together. I started making my own lunches every day, eating more healthy. And then I told her, you know, we need to get your A1C levels down, let's stop eating sugar. So, I took all sugar out of my diet. But you know, eventually she stopped doing it and gave up, but I kept on going to show her it could be done and because everyone was watching me now to see if I could do it. Later when she saw how much weight I had lost, she was so surprised and said, "hey, that could have been me if I had stuck to it with you", so she started back up again and has lost 6 pounds so far.

The patient clearly understood the doctor's instructions and goals for her health. She even understood why she needed to lose weight and change her diet. She did not need more expertise in diagnosis, imaging, or treatment. She did not need a translator. What she needed was help following through on what she already knew she should be doing. Luisa understood that knowledge does not necessarily lead to behavior change, therefore her role as a cultural mediator was simply to come alongside her patient and help her carry out those doctor's instructions and journey with her through the experience. This required humility on her part, acknowledging her shortcomings with the patient. She did not judge or lecture. She literally put herself in her patient's shoes and humbly became a fellow learner in true solidarity. She accompanied her through the tough work of making difficult decisions day in and day out, helping her figure out how to make progress toward a healthy lifestyle, even amidst an environment full of barriers to health in which she lived. She also earned her patient's respect by *accompanying* or going with the patient to her appointments or to seek resources. Eventually Luisa was able to demonstrate to her patient that it was possible and that she could continue trying even after having given up. This gave her patient the hope she needed to persevere.

CHW/Ps understand patients are a key part of the solution, and they listen to their patients' perspectives with the hopes of discovering important pieces of the puzzle. *CHW/Ps* tend to have empathy—not judgment of the patient's situation and behavior, because they themselves, or those close to them, have similar struggles. *CHW/Ps* do not feel the need to establish credibility based on performance, knowledge, or expertise but rather their ability to listen and have compassion. Their role is not to have all the answers and recommendations for the patient but instead to help the patient navigate and achieve the answers that providers have set before them or that they as patients have set for themselves. *CHW/Ps* have often had similar challenges, socioeconomically and clinically, and identify with being in the patient's shoes. They relate to why following doctor's orders is not always easy and have experienced being "invisible" when clinicians talk about you and around you but not to you. A shared lived experience gives them both empathy and respect for the patient, and their communication with them reflects both.

A healthcare provider's focus and expertise are typically on the clinical diagnosis and remedy, which leads to their gathering only the cliff notes regarding the social issues confounding medical goals. Even social workers often see a narrow picture of the patient's social issues due to time and productivity restraints. Further, a majority of providers do not share the lived experience of their patients and truly have no idea what a day in the life of their more at-risk patients is like and just how difficult something as simple as "losing weight," "arriving on time to an appointment," or "eating more healthy" can be when faced with multiple social determinant barriers. Because of this, falling into an attitude of paternalism or cynicism toward patients is easy. Providers often discuss their cases in rounds among themselves and often subconsciously reinforce the "us and them" mentality. Due to a lack of success or solutions, providers often lower their expectations for the patient and write off their lack of adherence as a character trait or a lack of effort or desire to improve by the patient.

Yami, a CHW/P newly introduced to a clinical care setting, tells the story of her work with a single, elderly patient with congestive heart failure and poorly controlled diabetes, who had recently had his leg amputated. This is unfortunately a common occurrence in health care, where if the clinicians had had better training in a CHW/P's role or on what cultural humility is and if she had been allowed to play a more significant role as a cultural mediator, things may have gone differently. Identifying Yami's empathetic attitude toward her patient is easy. Also enlightening is seeing how Yami views the healthcare providers through her eyes and, by proxy, those of her patient's.

> *I started working with a [clinical] team... I would hear them talk about the patient a lot but finally I got to meet the patient myself. He had CHF [congestive heart failure], DM2 [diabetes type II] his sugar levels out of control, and he had lost one of his legs already.*
>
> *First visit with patient, nurse and social worker trying to see what's going on with patient and trying to see how they can help him out, so they talk to him; they explain the program, and they told him you need to take your medication. Towards the end, patient finally talked and asked if someone can help him apply for IHSS. SW [social workers] said ok, we can help you. Then we had to leave.*

Second visit: As soon as we got to the home, we can totally tell patient was very angry, and he kept saying, 'I went to the doctor, but he didn't listen to me or what I had to say', and he kept trying to say more but one of the professionals stated 'ok but now I need you to check your sugar'. Patient apologized and did it; his sugar levels were over 500. Patient tried to talk again about what was happening. They let him talk for a little bit (professionals looking at each other making faces rolling eyes), then they continue to explain to him about his sugar being so high and why they refer him to a diabetes class. Patient stated 'I will go'.

During the week I hear the team talk about the patient saying he is not being adherent with medication. 'He is not listening'. 'He didn't go to the diabetes class.' And someone else stated, 'two more visits, if not we drop him".'

Over the weekend, patient went to the emergency room, and he was released to skilled nursing facility. The social worker and I went to visit him, and finally I was able to talk to him alone, not even five minutes, but I was able to talk to the patient. I was able to explain really quick what I do, and he opened up. He started telling why he was so mad and upset and how he lost his leg. He had no support system what so ever. He was alone. Then my co-worker was making faces to me like 'hurry up, cut it and let's go.'

That's when I realized working in the clinical setting, it was not going to be easy. On my way out, I was telling my co-worker he needs support. He said, 'yeah, I know'. But I didn't say much more because his response was not too nice.

Then later in the day, he asked me, 'why do you think he needs support?'. I told him what the patient shared with me, and he said, 'next time we visit him, you can take resources for him.'

The next day the nurse care manager was upset because patient didn't make it to his appointment, and later during the day, patient called, and he didn't want to see no one anymore. The team agreed to drop him from the program. All I heard was that, 'in less than three months he will be in a better place'. That was very sad to hear. All he wanted and needed was someone to listen. And I told the social worker, but she said, 'he is out of the program.'

This patient was struggling after the loss of his leg. He never had counseling for that. He was mad and angry, and he was alone he had no one to talk to. During those visits, I can see him crying for help but he didn't get it. All he heard was people telling him what to do instead of asking 'how do you feel?' 'How do you cope with not having a leg?' or even asking how you lost your leg? Patient had so much to share, but no one listened. I was very limited in what I could do. It was a learning experience; not what I was expecting, but I learned that my job is very important and that my community needs us CHWs.

"All he heard was people telling him what to do instead of asking, 'how do you feel?'." The wisdom in these words are critical and should be a lesson learned in the delivery of health care. CHW/Ps get to the root of the issue, empathy and the ability to listen. The culture of health care has become productivity-based and professionalized. Healthcare providers are often more comfortable talking about or to their patients rather than listening to or trying to understand them. CHW/Ps can be that unorthodox colleague that models a different way of engaging patients, because of their shared struggles with those they serve.

A neonatal intensive care unit (NICU) setting that served a largely under-resourced, urban, and immigrant population hired a *promotora* named Irma. Nurses there had seen everything—drugs, gangs, domestic violence, homelessness, and undocumented immigrants. One nurse had even been physically intimidated by a patient's parent. Most NICU nurses sign up to work with premature babies, and not necessarily to deal with difficult or stressed adults. Years of working in this setting had understandably led to an attitude of cynicism and discouragement on the part of some staff on the unit. This combined with cultural, educational, and socioeconomic differences led to some less than cordial interactions between frustrated staff and frustrated parents of patients. Irma came into this setting with a very different worldview and lived experience than the staff, one that was more similar to the patients' experiences. She was not intimidated by or quick to judge the parents in the NICU, because she had family and friends who looked and talked a lot like them. She knew where they came from and what they were going through. Because of Irma's training, she also saw things from the clinician's point of view. She was prepared for this dichotomy of worldviews, and instead of choosing one, she was able to appreciate both and treat all involved with respect and dignity as she mediated between the two cultures of health care and at-risk patients. Time after time, she did this not by lecturing or providing cultural competency trainings to the staff or the parents but by modeling empathy, respect, and active listening with the parents at the bedside. Cultural humility is contagious when genuine and from the heart. Criticizing or behaving rudely to a patient is much more difficult after observing a colleague treats that same patient with compassion and respect.

Studies clearly document that over time, clinicians frequently face burnout and may experience compassion fatigue (Shanafelt, 2009). The demands for quality, safety, and patient care outcomes placed on providers lead to a stressful work environment that demands time they do not have. However, we have seen some of the most fatigued clinicians, who demonstrate cynicism and sometimes callousness, soften when CHW/Ps model cultural humility. The CHW/Ps help remind clinicians of why they went into health care in the first place.

Modeling cultural humility is often an indirect but effective means of culturally mediating between provider and patient. Yami, a CHW/P who works in an acute setting, expresses this in her own words:

> You know, the therapist I work with really gets it too. She sees the stuff these patients are going through, and I think she really cares and has a heart to help them. Sometimes some of the other staff doesn't really seem to care. You hear them talking all about these patients and their problems and the bad decisions they are making. And sometimes it makes me angry, but you know what I have started doing? I just say something nice or positive about the patient and then they [staff] don't feel comfortable talking bad about the patient after that. And you know, I think it's making a difference, they are really starting to change and really showing a heart for the patients also.

In order to learn cultural humility (or other attributes) from CHW/Ps, healthcare providers need a dose of cultural humility. Learning from someone lower down the hierarchy of health care means effectively admitting to not having all the answers, despite having more education and formal training. When clinical staff are able to get past this and see the strengths that CHW/Ps bring to the clinic, everyone wins.

Yami gives a good example of a physician who has learned from and appreciates her CHW/P with the following story:

> You know, I just love my doctor, well I call her my doctor, but you know, the doctor on our team. We really work great together, and she gets it. Now that we have been working together all this time, she really understands what we do as community health workers, and she is always wanting me to see so many of her patients. But then, unfortunately, the team

tells me I can't see them unless they are qualified with their insurance and stuff. But, anyway this doctor is so great, and she really has the heart to help her patients. I told her, 'you know, you are practically a community health worker yourself,' because she is always going the extra mile to help her patients. Sometimes she even brings in gift cards for food and things like that because she really cares about her patients and now she sees that they have all these other needs besides what they come to her for.

What CHW/Ps have to teach providers about the concept of cultural humility is that an attitude of openness and learning addresses difficult and less talked about issues of power, privilege, and equity. Tervalon and Murray-Garcia (1998) define three key elements of cultural humility that guide this section's discussion: (1) critical reflection and lifelong learning; (2) addressing power imbalance (equity); and (3) institutional accountability.

5.2.1 Cultural Humility: Promotes Critical Reflection and Lifelong Learning

Cultural humility is an essential component of effective cultural mediation. Continuous learning is essential in cross-cultural settings, because culture is dynamic, always changing, and there is always room for individuality within cultural generalizations. Understanding how culture shapes the way we operate and view the world is an important element in developing an attitude of cultural humility where we are always learning from others.

A good example of cultural differences is communication style. Some cultures depend less on verbal cues to communicate. In these cultures, most of what is communicated is contextual and nonverbal; these are known as high-context or low-verbal cultures. In contrast, low-context cultures rely significantly on verbal expression. When members from different cultural groups meet, there is potential for much misunderstanding. A person from a high-context culture may feel that someone from a low-context culture is disrespectful in his or her communication style, perhaps too loud or verbose. A simple positioning of the body or look can communicate negative or positive messages. Because of their cultural affinity with the patient, CHW/Ps can be helpful in interpreting messages and communicating in a positive way with the patient. Their ability to read nuanced verbal and nonverbal cues is an asset that enriches the healthcare team. Cultures also differ in that some cultures are more goal oriented, like many modern western cultures, and others are relationship oriented. The clash between relationship and goal priorities is also very common.

Luisa, a CHW/P working with diabetes patients, demonstrates this in her interaction with a frustrated and "difficult" patient when she states, "Le deje ver mi postura" ("I let her see my body language"), or when she refers to nurses' "dirty looks" toward a patient's mother who came to visit her dressed in sweat pants. CHW/Ps often, perhaps because of their shared experience with their patients, demonstrate a deep sense of empathy and are less likely to judge.

Cultural humility prevents judgment and helps providers learn from and about their patients. Understanding cultural worldviews becomes essential to effective health care. Culture shapes not only how we communicate and understand each other but also how we view health and illness, our explanation of what causes us to get sick, and guides what steps we think should be taken to restore health. This health worldview can cause tension between patients and providers, and we must seek to understand and reconcile these differences to seek optimal health outcomes.

Medical anthropologists differentiate between *disease* and *illness*. Healthcare providers diagnose disease through tests and patient symptoms, often seen as objective and evidence-based. Illness describes the patient's experience and how he or she explains the loss of health (Winkelman, 2009). Disease and illness often represent contrasting and distinct health worldviews. The more similar the disease is to the illness, the better outcomes from the patient/provider encounter. Modern medicine's effectiveness depends on the patient's belief in the power of the prescribed and the prescriber. CHW/Ps are more likely to share illness perspectives and narratives with the patient. With proper training, CHW/Ps in healthcare settings can reconcile the differences between disease and illness. They can also listen to and understand the patient's story, which can help them find the road back to health (Winkelman, 2009).

Yami illustrates this with her story of a patient suffering from depression:

Another woman I was working with who was going through a lot of hard stuff, and she was suffering from depression, so the doctors put her on some medication, but she was wanting to stop taking them, so they asked me to see if I could help. When I went to see her for the first time, I introduced myself and told her I was a community health worker and that I was here for the community and here for her. When I said that she almost started to cry, and she took my hand and said, 'you know, just by you telling me that I already feel much better.' I reassured her that I really was here for her, and we started to talk about her problems and eventually about her medicine. She told me everything she was going through, and then she said there was no way she was going to take those medications anymore because they made her feel like a zombie, so she stopped. I convinced her to see the therapist for some counseling at least, but she didn't really open up to her or take it too seriously. She said she preferred to just talk with me, because she felt more comfortable with me, but I told her that I was not a counselor, and I didn't have the tools that a counselor had to help her. She ended up stopping therapy as well as medicines. The next time she went to the doctor she started crying, and the doctor ended up referring her to a psychiatrist. She called me saying, "I'm not crazy. They want me to go see someone 'pero no soy loca!' (but I'm not crazy!) You know how Hispanics are like that about these things. I tried to calm her down and explained just like if you had a problem with your toe like fungus or something, they would send you to a podiatrist because that is what they specialize in. There are doctors who specialize in all parts of the body, even the brain. It doesn't mean you are crazy. But she couldn't get past it. Hispanics don't really like any of this mental health stuff. So then I tried to bargain with her that if she wouldn't go to the psychiatrist, then at least she should go to a therapist to talk about things. Sometimes I tell my patients a little bit about my experiences just so they don't feel like they are the only ones going through hard stuff. So I told her how I had gone through a lot of depression in the past and counseling had helped me. I told her the therapist would have lots of tools for her to use when she feels down and could help her learn to manage her emotions, and that if she didn't want to take medications or see a psychiatrist, then she should at least consider trying the therapist again. So in the end that is what she decided to do.

Yami was able to be a very effective cultural mediator in this case because she identified the difference between worldviews and between disease and illness and because she identified with the patient's worldview.

It is important to allow the patient to own his or her experience by eliciting their own *illness narrative* and not solely have a disease ascribed to him or her. (Kleinman, 1988). Patients benefit when they connect with a community of individuals experiencing the same disease and can reconstruct that experience in a tale of heroics and struggle, regardless of the outcomes. Because of their shared experience with the patient, CHW/Ps are more likely to allow the patient to create and share those illness experiences, therefore complementing the assigned evidence-based diagnosis that, while effective, may feel cold and insensitive to a suffering and fearful patient. CHW/Ps bring the gifts of time and patience that allow hope to grow and not just a hope for healing but a hope for dignity and respect. This is very different from the evidence-based world that we have created in health care, where truth is found through the scientific process and all things outside of that process are questioned (Kleinman, 1980).

Another element cultural humility teaches us is the importance of the art of listening in the provider-patient exchange. The CHW/Ps' ability to listen and the added time they spend with patients contribute significantly to improved health and healthcare outcomes. Their listening skills allow them to build trust and engage in ways that allow them to help the person take a next step toward health behavior change or identify a resource that may help them overcome a challenge. Luisa shares her experience as a CHW/P that illustrates this point:

> Luisa: *We had a case where a Dexcom* blood sugar monitor was connected to a patient's body to measure her insulin. The patient was upset because she didn't understand how that worked or how to use it. No one had explained anything about it to her.*
>
> Patient: *'Que me expliquen para que es y como funciona!' ('They should explain what this is for and how it works'). 'You speak Spanish? Por fin! (finally!), 'I want this out, what if it ends up in my stomach?''*
>
> Luisa: *She expressed her frustration and said that she was ready to go to the emergency to have that thing removed. I listened, 'tiene toda la razon (you are completely right).*
>
> Patient: *Mi hija es enfermera. Tengo 30 a[Equation]picandome el dedo. (my daughter is a nurse. I have been pricking my finger for 30 years).*
>
> Luisa: *I tried explaining but she wasn't ready. So I continue to listen.*
>
> Patient (after calming down, apologetically): *At that moment I was mad, hungry and didn't understand what they were doing.*
>
> Luisa: *I told her that I understood that sometimes it is difficult to deal with all the new technology, but we would help her, if she was willing to come to the clinic to have it removed. If in the beginning someone would take the time to explain to her what it was for, how to use it, maybe she would be convinced or at least more flexible to try to keep it in place.*
>
> *[The Dexcom is a glucose monitor that is inserted into the skin to monitor glucose levels on diabetic patients. This form of monitoring avoids having to stick fingers and draw blood as is done in the conventional way of glucose monitoring.]

Active listening, empathy, and the approach of not pressuring the patient to comply worked well for Luisa in this example. "She wasn't ready, so I continue to listen." The power of listening has become an underutilized therapeutic tool in health care. The results of this approach are significant, because later, the patient was not only willing to have the monitor placed again, once she felt she understood the process and the purpose, but also Luisa saved the hospital an unnecessary emergency department visit from a frustrated and confused patient. This started with Luisa's willingness to listen to the patient's story. While this added time may be unrealistic for most clinicians, the CHW/P's role of cultural mediation is to do exactly that.

Irma summarizes the need to listen, stating that providers "often hear, but they don't listen." The Cambridge Dictionary describes hearing as an event, something that happens to us naturally. Hearing is passive. Listening is described as action. In other words, you can hear sounds, but you must actively listen to try to understand a message being delivered to you. There is a big difference between passive hearing and active listening. CHW/Ps master this skill quickly and artfully apply listening to their patients. Time is the medicine.

Yami exhibits these skills when interacting with her patient:

Yami can't contain her smile as she tells about one of her patients who was also the mom of an 8-year-old boy with epilepsy. Previously, the son had 3 seizures per day on average, and doctors were not able to control the seizures with medication, so they approached the mom about doing a surgical procedure, which she agreed to. But unfortunately, the procedure made his condition worse and now he has an average of 8–10 seizures per day. He is often hospitalized for his conditions when things get bad, and this is very stressful for the mom, who is Yami's patient. Yami started working with this mom because she has diabetes and is not taking her medications. After getting to know the mom and establishing rapport with her, Yami approaches the topic of medications. Instead of reprimanding her for not taking them or preaching to her about how important they are, she actively listens as the mom opens up about how she feels overwhelmed by her son's needs and feels that her own needs are not as important. She feels it would be selfish to take medicine for herself when her son is suffering so much. Yami uses her motivational interviewing techniques to reflect back to the mom what she hears her saying and affirms her feelings. She provides emotional support and a listening ear first and foremost, all the time gathering more information about the needs and barriers this mom has to her own self-care, demonstrating genuine concern, not only for her, but also for her son. By working with her, listening to her and helping to meet her expressed needs, Yami was able to develop a relationship, gain her trust and earn the right to offer advice and influence her health behaviors in a positive way. Yami reminded the mom how she herself had said that no one else could help her son except her, she was the boy's main caretaker. She then went on to suggest that if something happened to her health, her son would be worse off. And that by taking care of her own health, she was not at all being selfish but doing what was best for herself and for her son. Little by little, she was able to help her patient see this truth. Soon, the patient was willing to start taking her medications regularly, and Yami is keeping her accountable and inspired to do that as well as continue with other health behavior changes. The reason that Yami feels like she was able to get through to the mom, and not the other healthcare providers, is because she had the time to really listen and develop a relationship with her. Yami also genuinely cared about this patient, not only in the context of her diabetes getting better, but in the context of her whole life and all the other problems she had to deal with, some of which were more important to her than her own health. Yami demonstrated this care by regularly visiting the son whenever he was in the hospital and supporting the mom emotionally when he is having medical issues in ways that may not always fit neatly into an hour session between 8 and 5, Monday through Friday.

5.2.2   Cultural Humility: Addresses Power Imbalance and Equity

The ability cultural humility has to expose power imbalances or equity issues is another important reason why CHW/Ps are good ambassadors of cultural humility in health care. CHW/Ps are not typically clinically trained, usually have less of a formal education than most clinical staff, may not have English fluency, and may struggle with technology. These characteristics can create workplace inequities. These inequities heighten the sense of "otherness" about this new healthcare team member and colleague. However, their "otherness" is what makes CHW/Ps so effective at patient engagement. Irma shares her introduction to this issue of education and pedigree:

> One of the first questions I was asked was 'what was my background, what I had studied for?' Well, my background is in business, but I fell in love with health, and the [Promotores] Academy gave me that opportunity. Anyone can take the classes. Yes, I was able to get the diploma but for me it is just a paper. As Alex Fajardo says, 'The community gives you the certificate.' It is true. That is why I won a place on the School District board, because I gave so much to my community and they needed someone to represent them, and they chose me.

Integrating this new healthcare team member, with unconventional credentials and cultural differences, can challenge the conventional clinician because the presence of the CHW/P helps expose a culture of hierarchy within healthcare staff, as well as implicit bias toward patients who are often of different cultural, linguistic, and socioeconomic backgrounds from the clinician. In this hierarchy, power and respect are gained from length of formal education, professional status, and technical skills. Biomedical culture places medical specialists at the top, and patients are often found at the bottom. This disconnect between providers and patients becomes magnified when CHW/Ps are added to the team. Bias or prejudice is more harmful when manifested by someone in a position of power, for example, from provider to patient.

In addition to workplace inequities, societal inequities directly affect the quality of patient care and are central to the work of the CHW/P who often interacts with the most marginalized patients, seeking to address the root causes of disease and health inequities. The social determinants of health expose our society's inequities in education, housing, workforce, access to health care, etc. and are what CHW/Ps are known for addressing effectively (Page-Reeves et al., 2016). John, a faculty member at a university health system, observes the following:

> I teach medical students about the social determinants of health and explain how their future patients often continue to return or can't adhere to their instructions because they have basic needs that are not being met (housing, food, transportation, etc.). A frequent response I get, mainly from the fourth-year students, is 'but what can we do address these complex issues? These aren't medical problems.' The social determinants of health are outside of the healthcare provider's scope of work, not to mention the time that it would require to address these complex needs. What is initially not understood by these medical students is that physicians don't have to do it alone. They should rely on others who may have less training but more time and experience in this area. CHWs can assist the healthcare provider, adding a personal touch to the patient experience. The fact that medical students

can't see a solution outside of their own ability to respond is telling. The health professions have a culture of fixing, and helping others, and not necessarily collaborating with those affected to address the issues of concern. The idea of relying on the community to address community needs is often foreign to those of us who have been trained to single handedly solve problems and assess needs. In contrast, the promotor comes in, often struggling with English, without a healthcare title or much formal education and collaborates with the patient, engaging them in ways that we haven't been able to accomplish before.

Acknowledging limitations in knowledge and skills requires cultural humility on the part of the providers. Cultural humility also requires a willingness to "share" some of the power with the CHW/Ps and allow them access to "their" patient to address the social determinants of health.

5.2.3   Cultural Humility: Institutional Accountability

Fisher-Borne, Cain, and Martin (2015) suggest cultural humility moves us from a position of *mastery* to one of *accountability*. Besides demonstrating how CHW/Ps naturally model cultural humility in their interaction with patients and healthcare colleagues and how providers can learn cultural humility from CHW/Ps, we find the role of the institution in promoting cultural humility equally important. As we have learned through our work at the *Promotores* Academy, training and readiness have to occur on both sides: the CHW/P and the employing staff/institution. There is a need for staff and organizational readiness to learn and incorporate new models of health care to address ongoing challenges that health care has faced with diverse patient populations and increasing chronic diseases linked to social determinants of health (Rogers et al., 2018). The definition of cultural humility helps us understand key factors in this transformation of a system that is expertise-driven, hierarchical, and familiar with teaching into one engaged in reciprocal learning. We find cultural humility to be a well-fitting framework for the integration of CHW/Ps into large, complex, and hierarchical healthcare systems where value and power are associated with titles, education levels, and professional pedigrees. Luisa shares her experience working as a clinic-based CHW/P when asked about her experience as an immigrant (she had some college education outside of the United States):

For me, it was very difficult. I came with an accent and with a degree that was from another country. I have a degree in psychology from Mexico, but here it is not recognized. The questions are, 'where did you get your degree? For how many years? What did they teach you there?' The quality of that kind of study, psychology, is not valued. At some point they have the right to know where you have worked on that field, what were your experiences, etc. But for the work we do as CHWs, as Irma mentioned, the community is the one that can tell how efficient and professional we are. The result of the work will be our resume.

Our western or American worldview often places an individual's value on what they do, and in our society, what one does depends on his or her level and area of education. Luisa realizes that her studies in Mexico mean little in her new setting and that her value comes from the community rather than the system. Her comment,

"The result of the work will be our resume," shows her confidence in her belief that her impact as a *promotora* will serve as her credentials. How we ensure that the workforce values CHW/Ps is also important. There needs to be institutional policies and an institutional culture that facilitates fair treatment of CHW/Ps that allows them to function optimally. By doing this, everyone benefits, including the patient.

5.2.4 Cultural Humility and Healthcare Professionals

In training *promotores*, clearly, as an institution, we have much to learn from CHW/Ps and from the process of integrating them into the healthcare setting. Learning to see health care from the eyes of the patient is a gift that CHW/Ps bring. Sometimes we are unaware of how our clinical processes can negatively impact the patient. Luisa shares how she sees some of these patient-provider interactions:

> The physician has few minutes to review the chart; then he/she has many people getting involved as the assistants, nurses, etc... For me, it is not necessary to have the patient go through all this process since the patient probably has many other issues going on besides the chronic disease. The patient gets overwhelmed with all the health professionals that get in the room... they will tell him: you need to do this and that, if not, some bad consequences can happen with you, for example as having an arm or leg amputated, or your life can be cut shorter. This can give much anxiety to the patient. The patient will reject all the instruction or help that have been proposed.

CHW/Ps and healthcare professionals both share the goal of helping the patient restore health and improve their quality of life, but they may approach the process very differently. Both can learn from and complement each other. However, in order for healthcare professionals to learn from CHW/Ps, not only must they themselves demonstrate cultural humility, but the administration of the clinic in general must be open to new methods of patient interaction.

Luisa shares how she and a nurse from her team decided to do joint home visits since they were both accustomed to doing home visits on their own and wanted to learn from each other. They quickly identified the difference in their respective approaches. According to Luisa, the nurse focused only on the clinical needs of the patient, while Luisa describes her home visitation as being "patient-led," "focused on his priorities," using simple words, and building trust. Subsequently, this patient was more concerned with losing his house than in his follow-up medical appointments or taking his medications appropriately. This is a good example of how CHW/Ps can play a critical role in patient activation, where they build the capacity of the patients, meeting them where they are, so patients can take an active role in their health care. By assisting him with his housing needs, his healthcare needs were eventually addressed. Cultural mediation presents itself in various forms but is always closing a gap, which, in this case, included closing the gap between clinical priorities and the patient's social determinants of health.

Even clinicians' admission that they need a cultural mediator to work with their patient requires a certain amount of openness to learning. To allow the mediator to be a non-licensed, non-professional, and sometimes English as a second language person who, for all purposes, appears to be in the same situation economically and educationally as their patient takes a significant dose of cultural humility. Taking this dose requires humility and being secure in one's role. Moreover, this may also require changes in policy, protocol, and productivity models, which need to begin from the top, with institutional leadership that supports this approach (Rogers et al., 2018).

Ideally, CHW/Ps represent, look, dress, talk, and act like patients. We as healthcare providers do not always identify with our patients, and we certainly do not learn from them as much as we could. The fact that CHW/Ps often look and think more like our patients than providers creates an interesting dynamic. What appears to the healthcare professional as a disadvantage may actually be the secret to CHW/Ps' success as cultural mediators. Their non-professional vernacular and shared lived experiences make them more relevant and accessible to many patients. They develop rapport and a trusting relationship with the patient when given the time and freedom to do so. If embraced by the institution, cultural humility can help transform healthcare professionals, and CHW/Ps can effectively serve as cultural mediators and close the growing cultural gap between healthcare providers and patients. We have seen healthcare professionals and systems who realize this and become open to new ways of providing care. We have also seen healthcare systems who do not embrace cultural humility and refuse to listen to or learn from the CHW/Ps and resist change, despite having a CHW/P on the team.

This is a common pattern when integrating CHW/Ps into the clinic. When put into a system that often lacks cultural humility and is unwilling to learn from the CHW/P or open to new ways of doing things or to share power with the CHW/P, CHW/Ps often are challenged in doing their work. This ultimately limits the capabilities of the CHW/P and the outcomes of the patient. In order for CHW/Ps to shine, they need freedom, respect, and time with patients, all necessary to establish trust and truly address the root causes of the situation.

Yami shares an example of when she was given this freedom and time to address the patient's most pressing priorities, which were in the peri-clinical world of social (not medical) determinants of health. Because staff in her healthcare system valued what she said and did as a CHW/P, she was able to establish a trusting relationship with the patient and eventually earn the ability to influence the patient's medical priorities:

> I had another patient who was going through a divorce with his wife. He was the first patient I have ever had that really got on my nerves, because he was so negative. And I don't know what happened between him and his wife, and I don't ask or try to take sides with him or with her, but I just know that this divorce was really stressing him out, and he was so sad and down, and he was really nervous and anxious about going to court. He was also the type who had never done a thing by himself before, and he didn't know what to do. I tried to help him with a lot of things and show him how to do it himself. So, he asked me if I could represent him and I said, no, I'm not an attorney. Then he said, well can you come and be my translator, and I said no, they have special people who do that for a living, but we can ask for one of them to help you. What I can do is go with you and be there in the building to support you. So I did, and he was so thankful and grateful and appreciated it so much. I

could see that it gave him the confidence he needed to face such a hard thing. I continued to support him through this and reminded him of the positive things he was doing that were great. Little by little he started to gain confidence and believe what I told him and believe in himself. But then later, his daughter testified against him and that just sent him over the edge. He went into so much depression and was having a really hard time. The realtor who was working with him on selling the house saw him one day when he was so down that he was saying he didn't even want to go on, so she asked him who he had who could help him and he gave her my card. So I get this call from her, and she tells me what is going on, so I went to meet with him to try to talk him into going to the therapist or doctor, but you know we Hispanics don't really believe in those things too much, so he didn't want to, but eventually I was able to convince him to get help because I already had a relationship with him from before so he trusted me and listened to what I told him.

Yami was able to be an excellent cultural mediator in this case because she listened to the patient's needs instead of presenting her own goals for the patient. Her colleagues showed cultural humility by giving her freedom and access to the patient outside of the clinic setting, as well as trusting her to do what CHW/Ps do, instead of limiting her to the clinical space.

This often requires systemic change, a new way of looking at productivity and thinking outside the box. CHW/Ps are very resourceful and can bring helpful ideas to make things work when listened to and given the opportunity. This requires institutional support, accountability, and a change in the institutional culture.

Irma tells the story of working with parents of a baby who had been hospitalized since birth and whose doctors were trying to convince them of the need for a medical procedure before being discharged [story paraphrased]:

The doctors were frustrated with the parents' refusal to consent. The case managers were frustrated with the delay in discharge. And the administrators were frustrated with the cost of keeping the infant in the hospital unnecessarily. Irma, who works for the hospital as a CHW, understood the staffs' frustrations and goals. With an attitude of cultural humility, she acknowledged the institution's needs to her supervisor and was given the freedom and time she respectfully requested with the baby's parents. As such, she was able to intervene as a cultural mediator and learn from parents the root cause of their indecision, which was fear and lack of trust, as well as not completely understanding the baby's situation. With a good grasp on priorities of all involved, she was able to work with the parents to do some popular education style teaching using a doll and language they understood to reinforce what the nurses had already explained in more technical terms. She was also able to introduce these parents to other parents in the hospital who had recently gone through a similar procedure with their child, so that they could hear firsthand if what the doctors were telling them was true or not. In the end, the procedure was done, everyone was happy, and the baby benefited from the best outcome. If her unit had not listened to her as she explained things from the parents' point of view or given her the freedom to address their needs in a new and unconventional way, the story may have ended quite differently.

When healthcare professionals and administrators demonstrate cultural humility and are willing to be learners, they allow CHW/Ps access to their patients, and they respect and listen to what CHW/Ps have to say about the patients. By doing this they enable CHW/Ps to do the important work of cultural mediation. We have seen healthcare administrators adopt this vision and provide support and funding to begin to find the best way to utilize this exciting and emerging workforce in their unit or institution. When this happens, everyone wins, especially the patient. This not only makes sense in terms of mission but also makes business sense. Margin and mission do not have to compete.

5.2.5   Next Steps/Conclusion

In closing, some of the lessons CHW/Ps have taught us on this endeavor to integrate them into the clinical setting include the following:

1. Cultural mediation between healthcare providers and patients is necessary for optimal outcomes.
2. CHW/Ps are uniquely qualified to provide cultural mediation due to their shared lived experience. This is and should be one of their main roles.
3. Cultural humility is what makes CHW/Ps innately effective cultural mediators. This is one of their most important strengths.
4. Cultural humility differs from and goes beyond cultural competency.
5. Cultural humility is an attitude, not an intervention.
6. Cultural humility can and should be modeled to clinicians and administrators.

Our recommendations based on these lessons learned include:

1. Strategically train clinicians and other healthcare staff about CHW/Ps' role as cultural mediators and their strengths in cultural humility prior to introducing CHW/Ps in the clinic.
2. Integrate CHW/P training in health professions curricula so that every provider is well versed in CHW/P work and utilizes them effectively.
3. Strategically train CHW/Ps to see potential areas of conflict or misunderstanding in the clinic from the clinician's viewpoint as well, since this will not be inherent knowledge for them.
4. Approach the integration process with an attitude of cultural humility as well, leaving room to learn from CHW/Ps and patients, and be flexible to make changes to the system based on their input.

Cultural humility provides an attitudinal framework that provides a foundation for effective cultural mediation and increases the quality of health care to the increasing numbers of patients from diverse backgrounds. We affirm that clinic-based CHW/Ps are excellent *promotors* of cultural humility through their role of cultural mediation because of their standing as lay workers imbedded in clinical teams. They model lifelong learning, expose power and equity issues within the healthcare workforce and at the patient and community level, and require institutional support and accountability. These are exciting times for health care with opportunities and innovative strategies like acknowledging that some of the key solutions to chronic disease management and social determinants of health reside with the community. While there is a lot of discussion and deliberation about CHW/P training and if they should be credentialed or certified, perhaps a more important question is how we should train our existing healthcare professionals to be able to effectively welcome the CHW/P into the healthcare field and provide true patient-centered care.

How we do this work of integrating these new members into the healthcare team is critical because CHWs will either help change how we deliver health care or they will be assimilated into a system that has not been shown to be effective with chronic care or addressing root causes of disease and illness.

References

Fisher-Borne, M., Cain, J. M., & Martin, S. L. (2015). From mastery to accountability: Cultural humility as an alternative to cultural competence. *Social Work Education, 34*(2), 165–181.

Hook, J. N., Davis, D. E., Owen, J., Worthington, E. L., Jr., & Utsey, S. O. (2013). Cultural humility: Measuring openness to culturally diverse clients. *Journal of Counseling Psychology, 60*(3), 353.

Institute for Healthcare Improvement. (2017). *The IHI triple aim.* Retrieved from http://www.ihi.org/Engage/Initiatives/TripleAim/Pages/default.aspx.

Kleinman, A. (1980). *Patients and healers in the context of culture: An exploration of the borderland between anthropology, medicine, and psychiatry* (Vol. 3). Berkeley, CA: University of California Press.

Kleinman, A. (1988). *The illness narratives: Suffering, healing, and the human condition.* New York: Basic Books.

Page-Reeves, J., Kaufman, W., Bleecker, M., Norris, J., McCalmont, K., Ianakieva, V., … Kaufman, A. (2016). Addressing social determinants of health in a clinic setting: The WellRx pilot in Albuquerque, New Mexico. *The Journal of the American Board of Family Medicine, 29*(3), 414–418.

Rogers, E. A., Manser, S. T., Cleary, J., Joseph, A. M., Harwood, E. M., & Call, K. T. (2018). Integrating Community Health Workers into medical homes. *The Annals of Family Medicine, 16*(1), 14–20.

Shanafelt, T. D. (2009). Enhancing meaning in work: A prescription for preventing physician burnout and promoting patient-centered care. *JAMA, 302*(12), 1338–1340.

Spector, R. (2017). *Cultural diversity in health and illness* (9th ed.). New York: Pearson.

Tervalon, M., & Murray-Garcia, J. (1998). Cultural humility versus cultural competence: A critical distinction in defining physician training outcomes in multicultural education. *Journal of Health Care for the Poor and Underserved, 9*(2), 117–125.

Winkelman, M. (2009). *Culture and health. Applying medical anthropology* (pp. 2–3). San Francisco: Jossey-Bass.

5.3   Community Health Workers and Behavioral Health Prevention

Yaminette Diaz-Linhart, Ivys Fernandez-Pastrana, Diane Garzon Arbelaez, Niem Nay-Kret, and Emily Feinberg

> *When I first met a young mother who was expecting her second child, she was not going to routine prenatal appointments, was traveling back and forth between two living arrangement, trying to figure out a housing transfer and had just disclosed depression and anxiety symptoms during a clinic appointment. We met to talk about "problem-solving education," a program designed to strengthen problem-solving skills and reduce stress by decreasing symptoms of depression. After a few more sessions, she told me she met with the social worker and went to her scheduled prenatal appointment; she said "it wasn't as bad as I had anticipated. The sessions felt very similar to our problem-solving sessions, and I think I will go back to see her." Each week, she seemed more willing to do what she needed to do—to make changes in her life and the lives of her children. She realized that most problems do not disappear overnight but "doing more" about her problems instead of avoiding them was helping her move in the right direction. As a community health worker, I find it rewarding to problem solve with families and guide them through the resources they need to chip away at the challenges they are facing.*
> *—Diane, Community Health Worker*

5.3.1   Introduction

Community Health Workers (CHWs) play a vital role in behavioral health prevention, including working directly with individuals and families to engage, identify, and advocate for their behavioral health needs. The current behavioral health workforce is not adequate to meet the demand for services. As a result, there are emerging opportunities to develop new models of delivering behavioral health services targeted to both prevention and treatment (National Academies of Sciences, Engineering, and Medicine, 2017). Using CHWs to promote behavioral health requires redesigning models of care. CHWs play an important role in mediating how communities understand behavioral health and are able to access and engage in behavioral health services. A 2018 systematic review of CHWs and mental health interventions found evidence for both feasibility and effectiveness of mental health interventions delivered by CHWs, especially for underserved communities (Weaver & Lapidos, 2018). Additionally, CHWs have been integrated into clinical care teams to promote integrated behavioral health.

Malcarney, Pittman, Quigley, Horton, and Seiler (2017) described four types of integration of CHWs, with the most common type of integration as "direct hire," whereby CHWs are hired directly and integrated into health systems to "bridge the gap between the healthcare system and the community" (p. 369).

Even with emerging evidence for the feasibility, effectiveness, and advantages of CHW-led behavioral health interventions, CHWs are generally underutilized for behavioral health services. Their potential to contribute to the prevention of behavioral disorders has been largely unexplored, despite the need for increased prevention-focused interventions. In 2009, the National Research Council and Institute of Medicine reported on the importance of utilizing a public health prevention and promotion framework to promote well-being and prevent the onset of behavioral health disorders. Behavioral health prevention interventions differ from treatment because the intervention may not be specifically tied to a diagnosed behavioral health disorder. Behavioral health prevention focuses on interventions that promote mental health through population-level work (promotion and universal prevention), as well as interventions that target subgroups of populations to reduce the risk of development of behavioral health disorders (selective and indicated prevention) (National Research Council and Institute of Medicine. Division of Behavioral and Social Sciences and Education, 2009). In 2013, the Substance Abuse and Mental Health Services Administration (SAMHSA) reported on behavioral health workforce issues and partnered with the Health Resources & Services Administration (HRSA) to fund grants for both paraprofessional and professional training programs to develop and expand the behavioral health workforce. Of note, a 2014 SAMHSA-HRSA report noted the promising role of CHWs as culturally responsive team members in the behavioral health workforce core competencies (Hoge, Morris, Laraia, Pomerantz, & Farley, 2014). Since there is strong support for the efficacy of CHW interventions in primary care, chronic disease management, cost savings, and reduced inappropriate healthcare use, extending CHW interventions for behavioral health promotion and prevention builds on existing efficacy research (Centers for Disease Control and Prevention, 2014; Jack, Arabadjis, Sun, Sullivan, & Phillips, 2017; Kangovi et al., 2018; Kim, Choi, et al., 2016; Kim, Kim, et al., 2016; Viswanathan et al., 2009; Whitley, Everhart, & Wright, 2006). Bridging CHW prevention and promotion work into behavioral health is an important step for the CHW field.

This section highlights several different Boston-area CHW behavioral health prevention and promotion projects (healthcare and community-based) using a dual-generation approach in pediatric settings to highlight the importance of CHWs as cultural mediators. Dual-generation approaches emphasize strategies that target economic, social, developmental, and health needs of both parents and children to improve outcomes for the entire family system (Chase-Lansdale & Brooks-Gunn, 2014). Projects include three different research studies (one in an Early Intervention setting and two in Head Start settings) and two clinic-based projects (one in a Developmental and Behavioral Pediatric clinic of a safety-net hospital and a large initiative in pediatric primary care of three community health centers).

5.3.2 Roles of Community Health Workers in Behavioral Health Prevention

Working in the Clinical Pediatric Primary Care setting as a CHW, I was called to assist a behavioral health clinician (BHC) and pediatrician who were seeing a patient with special needs and the family spoke Khmer. Due to the language barrier during the appointment, the BHC and pediatrician thought that I could help interpret during the visit. As I in interpreted, the BHC and pediatrician had referred the patient to go to the Center for Children with Special Need (CCSN) [for an assessment of the child's development]. The mother stated that she looked up the word "autism" on the internet and the definition that she learned was the word "crazy." During this visit, I had the opportunity to speak with the patient's family about the meaning of the word "autism" and the different words used for behavioral health issues, including what a "development delay" means and that "autism" is one word that used to describe the growth and development of a child. The word "autism" does not really exist in the Khmer language and if the disabled child can access services at all or if any services in Cambodia, it would be at a "mental health" facility. During the visit, we shared what "autism" means as part of how the child needs support growing and developing. After this, the family was open to learning about the referral, and I continued to work with the family on how to best support their child's growth.
—Niem, Community Health Worker

In our work, CHWs serve as cultural and linguistic mediators for families struggling with identifying, engaging, and advocating for their behavioral health needs across clinical and community-based settings. CHWs provide health education, individual support and coaching, advocacy and help navigate complex medical and community-based systems. CHWs used evidence-based interventions that integrated behavioral health principles and strategies into the work with families. The interventions were developed for each project and documented in detail. This process, referred to as manualization, helps ensure uniformity and consistency of intervention application. CHW interventions spanned from the prevention to treatment continuum within community-based and healthcare settings (Fig. 5.1). Tasks varied by population needs. Interventions incorporated improvement methods, such as Plan-Do-Study-Act cycles, to develop and improve the interventions directly with the intervention team.

Interventions were pilot-tested in both community-based and healthcare settings to tailor CHW interventions for population, setting, and CHW core competencies. One key component included capacity building within sites to develop systems of support for behavioral health. For example, in Early Intervention and Head Start settings, direct-service employees were trained on depression screening, symptoms, and referrals. In healthcare settings, building capacity included building awareness and structural processes for multi-system coordination. For instance, during the screening process, structures were developed to establish standardized links from community-based sites to specialty clinics. Additionally, CHWs developed standardized checklists to help families access recommended services after diagnostic assessments.

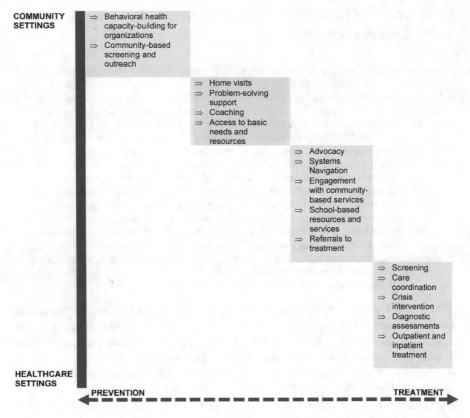

Fig. 5.1 CHW behavioral health intervention continuum. (Published with kind permission of © Yaminette Diaz-Linhart 2021. All Rights Reserved)

5.3.3 CHW Behavioral Health Prevention Interventions

Problem-Solving Education (PSE): PSE is an intervention to prevent depression, build problem-solving skills, and target current stressors. PSE was adapted from Problem-Solving Therapy (Feinberg et al., 2012; Feinberg et al., 2014; Silverstein, Cabral, et al., 2018; Silverstein, Diaz-Linhart, et al., 2018), an evidence-based treatment for depression. Mothers were screened for depression risk in community-based settings. CHWs delivered 4–6 in-person sessions via home visits designed to reinforce a problem-solving strategy. CHWs engaged in weekly group supervision to review cases and fidelity to the intervention.

Engagement Interview and Navigation: Depression Navigation is an intervention to help mothers access and engage with formal behavioral health services and informal emotional support adapted. Depression Navigation was adapted from the Engagement Interview (Diaz-Linhart et al., 2016; Grote et al., 2015; Grote et al., 2017). Mothers were screened in community-based childcare settings with validated clinical measures to identify depression. CHWs met on average twice across a

6-month period to help mothers identify the impact of depression and to create action plans to increase support and decrease depression symptoms for mothers.

Family Navigation (FN): FN is an intervention to coordinate individual- and systems-level developmental, health, and social needs of children and their families. FN intervention integrated behavioral health needs of children and families across multi-systems coordination (Blenner, Fernández, Giron, Grossman, & Augustyn, 2014; Broder-Fingert et al., 2018; Broder-Fingert et al., 2018; Broder-Fingert et al., 2018; Feinberg et al., 2016). Family navigators supported screening, met with families for coaching and support, worked directly with service providers to coordinate appointments, and helped families engage in services after diagnostic resolution.

Pediatric Primary Care Integrated Behavioral Health: Through a multi-community health center initiative, we developed and implemented a core behavioral health curriculum spanning eight different behavioral health disorders. Workbooks were designed for CHWs working within primary care pediatric team-based care (Teamupforchildren.org). CHWs were trained as part of a 2-year multidisciplinary learning community. CHWs worked directly with behavioral health clinicians, pediatricians, nurses, and medical assistants to target needs within five different areas tailored to each health center's needs: basic needs and community resources; support for screening and referrals; care coordination; population health management; outreach and education.

5.3.4 Impact on Using Community Health Workers for Behavioral Health Prevention

"Jomar[5]" is a 3-year-old boy with cognitive delays and autism. His family faced multiple barriers to access care, government and community resources. I began working with his mother, a non-English speaking single mother with 4 children aged 3 to 18. They were facing homelessness and food insecurity. Jomar's older sister had cognitive delays and aggressive behaviors, which led to police involvement and a restraining order. These multiple issues created a severely fragmented family. Due to his medical and behavioral health conditions, Jomar had very limited or non-existent progress in all developmental areas: language skills, social skills, adaptive skills, behavioral self-regulation skills. He made very little progress at school due to inconsistent attendance, disrupted sleeping patterns at home, medication side effects due to inconsistent administration of medications by his mother. Due to his medical and social complexities, Jomar had a multidisciplinary medical and social team which included 14 different providers across several healthcare and community-based settings.

My role as a Family Navigator focused on coordinating different services and providers by bridging the goals identified by Jomar's mother and by the service providers. Initially, I focused on problem-solving social determinants, such as homelessness, food insecurity, and legal advocacy. After being called to the emergency room several times when his mother and the school teachers would bring Jomar because they could not help him calm down, we

---

[5] Name has been changed to protect privacy and confidentiality.

focused on special education advocacy. I led and coordinated directly with CHWs from Jomar's primary care team and with his medical providers to advocate for an out of district school placement where more intensive and consistent services could be provided. Although this was a difficult decision for his mother, she felt it was the best possible option for her son. After 3 years of coordinating services and special education advocacy, Jomar was placed in a residential program. When I went to visit Jomar with his mother a week into his placement, Jomar said "mama" for the first time and had also started to use the potty. Since the successful placement, Jomar's mother has been consistently able to care for her other children, and she started English classes. I will never forget when I ran into her in the community, and I didn't even recognize her—she was finally optimistic about her life. This has been one of the most powerful experiences as a Family Navigator.
    —Ivys, Family Navigator and Supervisor

Results of research studies and clinic-based projects demonstrated significant impacts on individual families and organizations (Table 5.1). CHWs in behavioral health prevention have reduced parenting stress, reduced depression symptoms, prevented depressive episodes in mothers, increased appropriate screening and diagnoses for children at risk for developmental and behavioral health disorders, and increased family and patient access to services and resources. In our integrated pediatric behavioral health initiative, our CHW curriculum has successfully incorporated CHWs within team-based integrated pediatric behavioral health care.

Personal stories by CHWs demonstrate the impact of CHWs in behavioral health prevention and promotion. Diane worked directly with mothers to problem-solve and chip away at current challenges mothers are facing, which she understands firsthand as a mother of four children. Niem served as a cultural mediator with Cambodian families for behavioral health conditions within and outside of the health center. Ivys served as a connector and mediator across healthcare and community-based service providers, including the school system, to promote the development and behavioral health of children and families. In our work, CHWs— also known as "experience-based experts"—served as cultural mediators in behavioral health prevention through their personal and professional lived experiences (Gilkey, Garcia, & Rush, 2011). Leveraging CHW expertise in cultural mediation is a unique feature of promoting emotional well-being for families across community and health system settings.

By elevating the role of CHWs in behavioral health prevention, our work has included capacity building for the CHW role by incorporating practice transformation initiatives in hiring, training, fidelity, and supervision. Our research studies report on high levels of fidelity to the interventions by CHWs. In some of our work, CHWs co-lead supervision with licensed social workers and other behavioral health providers. While our work was conducted within the context of research studies and implementation projects, we believe integrating CHWs in behavioral health by leveraging their expertise as cultural mediators extends to broader practice settings. Our focus on enrolling a diverse population representative of real-world settings and on integrating CHW interventions in health system workflows supports integrating CHWs in behavioral health prevention and promotion. Our work demonstrates feasibility and acceptability of expanding the CHW role in behavioral health prevention. Balcazar et al. (2011) emphasized cultural mediation and

Table 5.1 CHW roles and impact in behavioral health prevention

Project and population	Intervention	CHW role	Results
Mothers of children recently diagnosed with autism in early intervention settings[a] Funded by: NINR K23 NR010588	Problem-Solving Education (PSE) Home visits	Cultural and linguistic mediation Health education Individual support and coaching Building individual and community capacity	Significant reductions in parenting stress and mean depression symptoms for mothers (Feinberg et al., 2014)
Depressed mothers in Head Start[a] Funded by: NIMH R21 MH097925	Engagement Interview and Navigation Home visits	Cultural and linguistic mediation Health education Care management and system navigation Building individual capacity Outreach Evaluation	Significant increase in engagement with mental health care (Diaz-Linhart et al., 2016)
Head Start Randomized Control Trial[a] Funded by: NIMH R01 MH091871	Problem-Solving Education (PSE) Home visits	Cultural and linguistic mediation Health education Individual support and coaching Building individual and community capacity	Significant reductions in depression symptoms (Silverstein et al., 2017) Significant reductions in perceived stress (Silverstein, Cabral, et al., 2018; Silverstein, Diaz-Linhart, et al., 2018) Significant engagement with specialty mental health services (Silverstein, Cabral, et al., 2018; Silverstein, Diaz-Linhart, et al., 2018)

(continued)

Table 5.1 (continued)

Project and population	Intervention	CHW role	Results
Developmental Behavioral Pediatric Clinic in Safety-net Hospital Funded by: NIMH R01 MH104355	Family Navigation Home visits Healthcare visits School and Special Education visits Federal and State entitlement program visits	Cultural and linguistic mediation Health education Care management and system navigation Coaching and support Advocacy Building individual and community capacity Outreach	Significant increases in screening and diagnosing children at risk for autism (Feinberg et al., 2016) Significant increases in family access and engagement with developmental services and entitlement programs (Broder-Fingert, Carter, et al., 2018; Broder-Fingert, Qin, et al., 2018; Broder-Fingert, Walls, et al., 2018)
TeamUp for Children Integrated Behavioral Health Initiative in three Federally Qualified Community Health Centers Funded by: Richard and Susan Smith Family Foundation	CHW Integrated Behavioral Health CHWs assigned to address prevention, access, and engagement of behavioral health needs	Cultural and linguistic mediation Health education Care management and system navigation Coaching and support Advocacy Direct service Outreach	Successful training in core CHW behavioral health curriculum Successful integration of CHW role in behavioral health in clinical teams Successful practice transformation of three health centers

[a]Completed

experience-based expertise of CHWs as what separates CHWs from other social and healthcare professionals. This differentiation is especially important in behavioral health since traditional medical training dismisses experience-based expertise.

5.3.5 Challenges

Acceptance of CHW role and ability as cultural mediators in behavioral health: Organizations and other professional roles remain skeptical of the appropriateness of expanding the CHW role to behavioral health prevention and promotion. While CHWs learn about the specifics of behavioral health disorders, they do not engage in "treatment" of those conditions. CHWs partner directly with behavioral health clinicians and other medical provider when families require clinical assessments and interventions. The work itself may be experienced as therapeutic for families due to the ongoing relationship families develop with CHWs. Several of our interventions successfully laid the foundation for families to engage with behavioral health treatment, serving almost as a way to help families know what to expect from behavioral health services because of CHWs' ability to serve as cultural mediators.

Supervision and support: Due to the nature of behavioral health work, CHWs may face crises with families. As a result, CHWs were trained to identify suicidal ideation, psychosis, and other common crisis needs based on the population and intervention. Behavioral health providers were on call and available for urgent needs, especially when CHWs conducted home visits. Group supervision was an integral part of the work and included weekly case reviews and review of fidelity for the intervention. CHWs were also encouraged to debrief with their supervisors at any point, not just during supervision times. As part of the supervision process, CHWs were encouraged to take turns leading supervision directly with the behavioral health clinician. In doing so, CHWs were able to develop their collective supervision skills to create broader and more sustainable support within organizations.

Defining populations for CHW behavioral health prevention: Expanding the CHW role into behavioral health prevention required identifying populations that would be best served by culturally appropriate CHW interventions. Using the Mental Health Intervention Spectrum, our work focused on developing roles for CHWs within the "promotion" and "prevention" areas of the spectrum (O'Connell, Boat, & Warner, 2009). For example, CHWs working in integrated pediatric primary care have tasks within promotion and universal prevention (i.e., social determinants resources, screening). CHWs in our problem-solving research within Head Start only worked with mothers who screened for depression symptoms (indicated prevention). By conceptualizing and identifying tasks within the promotion and prevention spectrum, interventions have focused on a specified population with a specific set of systematic tasks that are culturally appropriate. As a result, our work has incorporated multiple methods, including pilot testing, efficacy testing, and effectiveness research of our interventions to assess and determine CHW behavioral health prevention by leveraging CHWs as cultural mediators.

5.3.6 Lessons Learned

Behavioral health prevention and promotion interventions through CHWs' expertise as cultural mediators are a novel approach to support underserved children and families in both community-based and healthcare settings. Our work highlights the unique contributions by CHWs through cultural mediation, both through CHWs' own lived experiences as cultural insiders and through their unique understanding of the behavioral health needs of different populations served. As our research and clinic-based work continue, CHWs are central in how we continue to develop and implement behavioral health prevention for improved child and family health.

References

Balcazar, H., Rosenthal, E. L., Brownstein, J. N., Rush, C. H., Matos, S., & Hernandez, L. (2011). Community Health Workers can be a public health force for change in the United States: Three actions for a new paradigm. *American Journal of Public Health, 101*(12), 2199–2203. https://doi.org/10.2105/AJPH.2011.300386.

Blenner, S., Fernández, I., Giron, A., Grossman, X., & Augustyn, M. (2014). Where do we start? Using family navigation to help underserved families. *ZERO TO THREE, 34*(6), 4–8.

Broder-Fingert, S., Carter, A., Pierce, K., Stone, W. L., Wetherby, A., Scheldrick, C., … Feinberg, E. (2018). Implementing systems-based innovations to improve access to early screening, diagnosis, and treatment services for children with autism spectrum disorder: An autism Spectrum disorder pediatric, early detection, engagement, and services network study. *Autism*, 1362361318766238. https://doi.org/10.1177/1362361318766238.

Broder-Fingert, S., Qin, S., Goupil, J., Rosenberg, J., Augustyn, M., Blum, N., … Feinberg, E. (2018). A mixed-methods process evaluation of family navigation implementation for autism spectrum disorder. *Autism*. https://doi.org/10.1177/1362361318808460.

Broder-Fingert, S., Walls, M., Augustyn, M., Beidas, R., Mandell, D., Wiltsey-Stirman, S., … Feinberg, E. (2018). A hybrid type I randomized effectiveness-implementation trial of patient navigation to improve access to services for children with autism spectrum disorder. *BMC Psychiatry, 18*(1), 79. https://doi.org/10.1186/s12888-018-1661-7.

Centers for Disease Control and Prevention, D. of H. and H. (2014). *Policy evidence assessment report: Community Health Worker policy components* (p. 13). Retrieved from Department of Health and Human Services website: https://www.cdc.gov/dhdsp/pubs/policy_resources.htm.

Chase-Lansdale, P. L., & Brooks-Gunn, J. (2014). Two-generation programs in the twenty-first century. *The Future of Children, 24*(1), 13–39.

Diaz-Linhart, Y., Silverstein, M., Grote, N., Cadena, L., Feinberg, E., Ruth, B. J., & Cabral, H. (2016). Patient navigation for mothers with depression who have children in head start: A pilot study. *Social Work in Public Health, 31*(6), 504–510. https://doi.org/10.1080/1937191 8.2016.1160341.

Feinberg, E., Abufhele, M., Sandler, J., Augustyn, M., Cabral, H., Chen, N., … Silverstein, M. (2016). Reducing disparities in timely autism diagnosis through family navigation: Results from a randomized pilot trial. *Psychiatric Services, 67*(8), 912–915. https://doi.org/10.1176/appi.ps.201500162.

Feinberg, E., Augustyn, M., Fitzgerald, E., Sandler, J., Ferreira-Cesar Suarez, Z., Chen, N., … Silverstein, M. (2014). Improving maternal mental health after a child's diagnosis of autism spectrum disorder: Results from a randomized clinical trial. *JAMA Pediatrics, 168*(1), 40–46. https://doi.org/10.1001/jamapediatrics.2013.3445.

Feinberg, E., Stein, R., Diaz-Linhart, Y., Egbert, L., Beardslee, W., Hegel, M. T., & Silverstein, M. (2012). Adaptation of problem-solving treatment for prevention of depression among low-income, culturally diverse mothers. *Family & Community Health, 35*(1), 57–67. https://doi.org/10.1097/FCH.0b013e3182385d48.

Gilkey, M., Garcia, C. C., & Rush, C. (2011). Professionalization and the experience-based expert: Strengthening partnerships between health educators and community health workers. *Health Promotion Practice, 12*(2), 178–182. https://doi.org/10.1177/1524839910394175.

Grote, N. K., Katon, W. J., Russo, J. E., Lohr, M. J., Curran, M., Galvin, E., & Carson, K. (2015). Collaborative care for perinatal depression in randomized trial. *Depression and Anxiety, 32*(11), 821–834. https://doi.org/10.1002/da.22405.

Grote, N. K., Simon, G. E., Russo, J., Lohr, M. J., Carson, K., & Katon, W. (2017). Incremental benefit-cost of MOMCare: Collaborative care for perinatal depression among economically disadvantaged women. *Psychiatric Services, 68*(11), 1164–1171. https://doi.org/10.1176/appi.ps.201600411.

Hoge, M. A., Morris, J. A., Laraia, M., Pomerantz, A., & Farley, T. (2014). *Core competencies for integrated behavioral health and primary care* (p. 24). Retrieved from SAMHSA-HRSA Center for Integrated Solutions website: https://www.integration.samhsa.gov/workforce.

Jack, H. E., Arabadjis, S. D., Sun, L., Sullivan, E. E., & Phillips, R. S. (2017). Impact of community health workers on use of healthcare services in the United States: A systematic review. *Journal of General Internal Medicine, 32*(3), 325–344. https://doi.org/10.1007/s11606-016-3922-9.

Kangovi, S., Mitra, N., Norton, L., Harte, R., Zhao, X., Carter, T., ... Long, J. A. (2018). Effect of community health worker support on clinical outcomes of low-income patients across primary care facilities: A randomized clinical trial. *JAMA Internal Medicine, 178*(12), 1635–1643. https://doi.org/10.1001/jamainternmed.2018.4630.

Kim, K., Choi, J. S., Choi, E., Nieman, C. L., Joo, J. H., Lin, F. R., ... Han, H.-R. (2016). Effects of community-based health worker interventions to improve chronic disease management and care among vulnerable populations: A systematic review. *American Journal of Public Health, 106*(4), e3–e28. https://doi.org/10.2105/AJPH.2015.302987.

Kim, K. B., Kim, M. T., Lee, H. B., Nguyen, T., Bone, L. R., & Levine, D. (2016). Community Health Workers versus nurses as counselors or case managers in a self-help diabetes management program. *American Journal of Public Health, 106*(6), 1052–1058. https://doi.org/10.2105/AJPH.2016.303054.

Malcarney, M.-B., Pittman, P., Quigley, L., Horton, K., & Seiler, N. (2017). The changing roles of Community Health Workers. *Health Services Research, 52*(S1), 360–382. https://doi.org/10.1111/1475-6773.12657.

National Academies of Sciences, Engineering, and Medicine (2017). Training the future child health care workforce to improve the behavioral health of children, youth, and families. In: *Proceedings of a workshop.* https://doi.org/10.17226/24877.

National Research Council and Institute of Medicine. Division of Behavioral and Social Sciences and Education. (2009). *Depression in parents, parenting, and children: Opportunities to improve identification, treatment, and prevention. Committee on Depression, Parenting Practices, and the Healthy Development of Children. Board on Children, Youth, and Families.* Washington, DC: The National Academies Press.

O'Connell, M. E., Boat, T., & Warner, K. (2009). *National Research Council and Institute of Medicine. (2009). Preventing mental, emotional, and behavioral disorders among young people: Progress and possibilities. Committee on the Prevention of Mental Disorders and Substance Abuse among children, youth, and young adults: Research advances and promising interventions.* Washington, DC: The National Academies Press. Retrieved from https://www.ncbi.nlm.nih.gov/books/NBK32789/.

Silverstein, M., Cabral, H., Hegel, M., Diaz-Linhart, Y., Beardslee, W., Kistin, C. J., & Feinberg, E. (2018). Problem-solving education to prevent depression among low-income mothers: A path mediation analysis in a randomized clinical trial problem-solving education to prevent depression among low-income mothers problem-solving education to prevent depression among low-income mothers. *JAMA Network Open, 1*(2), e180334–e180334. https://doi.org/10.1001/jamanetworkopen.2018.0334.

Silverstein, M., Diaz-Linhart, Y., Cabral, H., Beardslee, W., Broder-Fingert, S., Kistin, C. J., ... Feinberg, E. (2018). Engaging mothers with depressive symptoms in care: Results of a randomized controlled trial in head start. *Psychiatric Services, 69*(11), 1175–1180. https://doi.org/10.1176/appi.ps.201800173.

Silverstein, M., Diaz-Linhart, Y., Cabral, H., Beardslee, W., Hegel, M., Haile, W., ... Feinberg, E. (2017). Efficacy of a maternal depression prevention strategy in head start: A randomized clinical trial. *JAMA Psychiatry, 74*(8), 781–789. https://doi.org/10.1001/jamapsychiatry.2017.1001.

Viswanathan, M., Kraschnewski, J., Nishikawa, B., Morgan, L. C., Thieda, P., Honeycutt, A., ... Jonas, D. (2009). Outcomes of community health worker interventions. *Evidence Report/Technology Assessment, 181.* 1-passim.

Weaver, A., & Lapidos, A. (2018). Mental health interventions with Community Health Workers in the United States: A systematic review. *Journal of Health Care for the Poor and Underserved, 29*(1), 159–180. https://doi.org/10.1353/hpu.2018.0011.

Whitley, E. M., Everhart, R. M., & Wright, R. A. (2006). Measuring return on investment of outreach by Community Health Workers. *Journal of Health Care for the Poor and Underserved, 17*(1 Suppl), 6–15. https://doi.org/10.1353/hpu.2006.0015.

Chapter 6
Providing Culturally Appropriate Health Education and Information

Caitlin G. Allen*, Arika Makena Bridgeman-Bunyoli, Teresa Campos Dominguez, Francis Kham, Ella Miller, Katie Miller, Sue Miller, Linda J. Nisley, Alix Sanchez, Lizdaly Cancel Tirado, Doretta Thomas, Melissa K. Thomas*, Kelly Volkmann, and Noelle Wiggins*

6.1   Introduction

Noelle Wiggins and Caitlin G. Allen

Sharing culturally centered health education and information is among the oldest and most fundamental roles of community health workers (CHWs). A primary function of the "aunties," sobadores, wise women, curanderos(as), and other

---

Authorship is organized alphabetically in ascending order by surname.

C. G. Allen ✉
CGA Consulting, Charleston, SC, USA
e-mail: caitlin.gloeckner.allen@emory.edu

A. M. Bridgeman-Bunyoli
Portland Children's Levy, Portland, OR, USA

T. C. Dominguez
Multnomah County Health Department, Portland, OR, USA

F. Kham
Immigrant and Refugee Community Organization, Portland, OR, USA

E. Miller · K. Miller · S. Miller · L. J. Nisley · D. Thomas
Center for Appalachia Research in Cancer Education, Whipple, OH, USA

A. Sanchez
Multnomah County Department of Human Services, Portland, OR, USA

L. C. Tirado · K. Volkmann
Benton County Health Services, Corvallis, OR, USA

M. K. Thomas (✉)
Ohio University Heritage College of Osteopathic Medicine, Athens, OH, USA
e-mail: thomasm5@ohio.edu

N. Wiggins (✉)
Wiggins Health Consulting LLC, Portland, OR, USA
e-mail: chwcommonindicators@gmail.com

© Springer Nature Switzerland AG 2021   87
J. A. St. John et al. (eds.), *Promoting the Health of the Community*,
https://doi.org/10.1007/978-3-030-56375-2_6

traditional healers who were the ancestors of CHWs was to provide information about health to community members in ways that were accessible and understandable (Wiggins & Borbón, 1998). Often, these trusted community members were filling a gap left by the formal health system, because of either lack of resources, linguistic and cultural differences, or specific intent to deny education and information.

6.1.1   History of CHWs as Health Educators

Some of the earliest articles about CHWs in the US public health literature focus on their role as health educators (Cauffman, Wingert, Friedman, Warburton, & Hanes, 1970; Chase, Larson, Massoth, Martin, & Niernberg, 1973; Conn, 1968; Young & Hamlin, 1969). In fact, a common title for CHWs during the late 1960s and early 1970s was some variation of "Health Education Aide." Studies occurred in both urban (Cauffman et al., 1970) and rural areas (Chase et al., 1973). Some studies from this period compared CHWs' ability to share health education to the ability of formally credentialed health professionals such as doctors and nurses; at least one study included rudimentary cost-benefit analysis (Cauffman et al., 1970). The results of multiple studies suggested that CHWs "performed as well as physicians and nurses" and could successfully "fill important roles in health education" (Cauffman et al., 1970, pp. 1908 and 1904). Rationales provided for involving CHWs as health educators included a lack of formally trained health professionals, cultural congruence between communities of focus and CHWs, and CHWs' ability to educate systems about community perspectives and needs.

Notable reviews of the CHW literature over the last 20 years have continued to emphasize the importance and effectiveness of CHWs as health educators. Witmer, Seifer, Finocchio, Leslie, and O'Neil (1995), in a still-influential 1995 review, cited CHWs' ability to "teach concepts of primary or secondary prevention and improve access to prenatal care" (p. 1056). Swider (2002), in a rigorous 2002 review, found some evidence of improvements in knowledge, health behavior, and health outcomes associated with CHW health education interventions. In a 2009 evidence review on outcomes of CHW interventions, almost all the outcomes studied—health knowledge, health behavior, health outcomes, and healthcare utilization—were strongly related to CHWs' role as health educators (Viswanathan et al., 2009). A 2013 review by the Institute for Clinical and Economic Review (ICER) (2013) found that six of eight studies that compared experimental groups receiving CHW health education interventions to control groups with usual care and access to educational materials showed significant positive outcomes for the experimental groups, including improvements in HbA1c and improved self-reports of dietary changes. These reviews reflect the plethora of studies that have focused on CHWs' role as health educators since the 1960s.

6.1.2 Definition of the Role[1]

Based on interviews, focus groups, and a survey with CHWs and their supervisors around the United States, "Providing culturally appropriate health education and information" was identified as a core role of CHWs in the 1998 National Community Health Advisor Study (Rosenthal, Wiggins, Brownstein, & Johnson, 1998). It was reaffirmed in the 2018 report of the C3 Project (Rosenthal, Menking, & St. John, 2018).

CHWs' ability to provide culturally centered health education derives from their understanding of community norms, idioms, and worldviews, combined with their knowledge of health issues. CHWs make health education culturally centered by providing education in an appropriate language, or from a trusted source, or both. Cultural centeredness also depends on employing appropriate methodology. Many CHWs around the country use methods derived from popular or people's education (PE). (More information about PE will be discussed in one of the subsequent chapters.) Cultural centeredness can also mean going to where the people are, by tabling at community events, going door-to-door, facilitating health education classes in community centers, organizing health fairs, and conducting home visits.

The C3 study explains CHWs' role in health education in terms of two functions:

Conducting health promotion and disease prevention education in a manner that matches linguistic and cultural needs of participants or community

As culturally adept and aware public health professionals, CHWs help to keep people healthy and intervene so that existing problems do not get worse. For example, CHWs promote health by teaching people about the value of exercise and a healthy diet. They prevent disease by encouraging people to reduce risk factors such as smoking and alcohol consumption. In both cases, they raise awareness about the underlying social conditions that can make it hard to eat well, get exercise, and stop smoking and how people can work together to address these conditions.

Specific topics of CHW health education run the gamut from dental health to domestic violence. Among the most common topics are perinatal health, sexually transmitted infections including HIV/AIDS, and cancer screening and treatment. Education provided by CHWs reflects a broad definition of health and can include life skills training, budgeting, and many other topics.

Providing necessary information to understand and prevent diseases and to help people manage health conditions (including chronic disease)

Another focus for health education by CHWs is management of chronic diseases such as diabetes and hypertension. For example, an Oregon program offered "Cooking Class Support Groups" where Latina women with diabetes or at risk of

---

[1] This section is adapted from Wiggins, N., and Borbón, I. A. (1998). Core roles and competencies of community health advisors. In Final report of the National Community Health Advisor Study (pp. 15–49). Baltimore, MD: Annie E. Casey Foundation.

developing it could participate in an interactive class, do exercises geared to their ability, and prepare a familiar and nutritious meal. All these activities were directed at achieving good diabetic control. CHWs also work one-on-one to help individuals manage their chronic illnesses.

The following two sections describe CHWs' role in health education, including ways CHWs have helped address breast cancer using culturally appropriate health education in Amish Country and examples of CHWs using PE in Oregon.

References

Cauffman, J. G., Wingert, W. A., Friedman, D. B., Warburton, E. A., & Hanes, B. (1970). Community health aides: How effective are they? *American Journal of Public Health, 60*(10), 1904–1909.

Chase, H., Larson, L., Massoth, D., Martin, D., & Niernberg, M. (1973). Effectiveness of nutrition aides in a migrant population. *The American Journal of Clinical Nutrition, 26*(8), 849–857.

Conn, R. H. (1968). Using health education aides in counselling pregnant women. *Public Health Reports, 83*, 979–982.

Rosenthal, E. L., Menking, P., & St. John, J. (2018). The Community Health Worker core consensus (C3) project: A report of the C3 project phase 1 and 2. In *Together leaning toward the sky: A national project to inform CHW policy and practice*. El Paso: Texas Tech University Health Sciences Center.

Rosenthal, L., Wiggins, N., Brownstein, N., & Johnson, S. (1998). *The Final Report of the National Community Health Advisor Study*. Baltimore: Annie E. Casey Foundation.

Swider, S. (2002). Outcome effectiveness of community health workers: An integrative literature review. *Public Health Nursing, 19*(1), 11–20.

The Institute for Clinical and Economic Review. (2013). *Community Health Workers: A review of program evolution, evidence on effectiveness and value, and status of workforce development in New England*. Retrieved February 15, 2020, from http://icer-review.org/wp-content/uploads/2011/04/CHW-Draft-Report-05-24-13-MASTER1.pdf.

Viswanathan, M., Kraschnewski, J., Nishikawa, B., Morgan, L. C., Thieda, P., Honeycutt, A., … Jonas, D. (2009). *Outcomes of community Health Worker interventions. Evidence report/technology assessment no. 181. AHRQ publication no. 09-E014*. Rockville, MD: Agency for Healthcare Research and Quality.

Wiggins, N., & Borbón, I. A. (1998). Core roles and competencies of community health workers. In *Final report of the National Community Health Advisor Study* (pp. 15–49). Baltimore, MD: Annie E. Casey Foundation.

Witmer, A., Seifer, S. D., Finocchio, L., Leslie, J., & O'Neil, E. H. (1995). Community health workers: Integral members of the health care work force. *American Journal of Public Health, 85*(8 Pt 1), 1055–1058.

Young, M. M., & Hamlin, G. P. (1969). People workers-a local health department's experience with health education aides. *American Journal of Public Health, 59*(10), 1845–1850.

6.2 Providing Culturally Appropriate Health Education in Amish Country

Melissa K. Thomas, Ella Miller, Linda J. Nisley, Doretta Thomas, Katie Miller, and Sue Miller

We all are like pieces in a puzzle, and when we come together, we make a beautiful picture. Each piece is important...one is not bigger than the other.
—Doretta Thomas, C-CHW, Ohio

6.2.1 Introduction

The Center for Appalachia Research in Cancer Education ("CARE") officially became a nonprofit organization in 2011 and serves as the organizational support for programs and services addressing health disparities in rural and Appalachia Ohio (and surrounding states).

The mission of CARE is to reduce the burden of cancer in Appalachia and rural communities by providing culturally competent health care and health education; educating healthcare professionals about the distinct cultural and healthcare needs of communities; and researching, planning, implementing, and evaluating effective health interventions to achieve health equity in cancer education, screening, diagnosis, treatment, and survivorship (The Center for Appalachia Research in Cancer Education, 2018).

The cornerstone of CARE's work in rural and Appalachia Ohio is the Amish and Mennonite-led breast health program named Project Hoffnung[(sm)] (Hope in German): The Amish and Mennonite Breast Health Project. Established in 1997, Project Hoffnung emerged in an effort to address the lack of culturally competent breast cancer education and access to life-saving breast cancer screening services for Amish and Plain communities. Research efforts by Project Hoffnung and the Project Lead and Community Health Worker (CHW) Dr. Melissa Thomas uncovered disproportionately higher breast cancer mortality rates in two of the world's Amish settlements, located in Ohio (Thomas, Hiermer, Indian, & Sickle-Santanello, 2005). Project Hoffnung serves the entire state of Ohio and parts of Indiana, Kentucky, and Pennsylvania in delivering culturally competent breast health information, free women's health screenings, and the support needed to navigate the healthcare system. Additionally, CARE is responsible for the development and implementation of a national biennial conference on "Addressing the Health Care Needs of Amish and Plain Communities." A dedicated committee of Amish, Mennonite, and Appalachian community members and leaders plans this 3-day peer-reviewed conference, which provides a unique learning experience where community members have a chance to share their own experiences and recommendations with healthcare providers about how to improve healthcare delivery.

6.2.2   Background

On any given day in over half of the states in North America, a quiet backcountry road may reveal a glimpse into what seems a moment stuck in time. Horse and buggies roam the gravel roads, large farmhouses paint the hillsides, and children work beside their parents in fields and kitchens. In fact, Amish communities reside in 31 states in the United States with a total population of over 336,000 and 2489 church districts. Ohio alone is home of 2 of the world's largest Amish settlements, 593 separate church districts, and over 76,000 Amish members (2019 population rates) (Amish Population, 2019). Additionally, the Amish population is growing at a rate faster than any other subculture in North America, with a doubling time of 20.5 years. Such estimates would lead us to expect a total Amish population of over a half-million by mid-2030 and a million by 2050 (Donnermeyer, 2015).

From their early beginnings in sixteenth-century Europe, the Amish have continued to thrive in a world of persecution and oppression for their strong religious beliefs and passive lifestyle against war (Kraybill, Johnson-Weiner, & Nolt, 2013). The Amish are a Christian sect and can trace their roots back to sixteenth-century Europe during the Protest Reformation, where the Anabaptist movement brought forth the new belief in adult baptism and separation of church and state. Their beliefs in nonconformity, maintaining a separation from mainstream society, are based on their biblical views, and decisions regarding the acceptance of modern conveniences such as telephones, cars, and electricity differ from church district to church district (Kraybill et al., 2013). Throughout the years, differences regarding religious beliefs and acceptance of technological advances have created many divisions in the Amish community, and dozens of Amish and more conservative Mennonite communities exist throughout North America (Nolt, 2003).

Access barriers found in most underserved populations, coupled often with a lack of trust or acceptance of the "English" (or non-Amish) way of life, have created the following barriers in addressing cancer issues in these rural communities:

Language: Many Amish are trilingual, speaking Pennsylvania Deutsch (pronounced "Dutch" in the United States) in their communities, German in religious ceremonies, and English in the non-Amish world. While most Amish are proficient in English, there are language barriers in written and spoken educational programs administered in the communities especially when it comes to medical and/or technical terms. Additionally, their native language, a dialect of German, is mostly an oral language, creating additional barriers when seeking to communicate in a written format (Kraybill et al., 2013). Not surprisingly, Amish community members in Appalachia Ohio had lower literacy levels when compared to non-Amish residents (Katz, Ferketich, Paskett, & Bloomfield, 2013).

Education: Typically, the Amish limit education to an eighth grade level, which the US Supreme Court recognized as a legitimate school system (Kraybill et al., 2013). Lower literacy levels and a known rejection of technology (e.g., computers, smartphones, etc.) may lead to an even greater lack of cancer information than that which already exists in most rural, underserved regions.

Financial burdens: The Amish rarely possess traditional forms of health insurance. While most do pay all levied taxes except Social Security, they often will not accept Medicare or Medicaid benefits (Kraybill et al., 2013). In many Amish settlements, women will not participate in the Breast and Cervical Cancer Early Detection Program (BCCP) or the Affordable Care Act's insurance program due to the government-funded services the program provides. Many also rely on paid drivers for transportation needs, often a cost of 50 dollars or more per round trip visit to a hospital or clinic.

Disproportionately high breast cancer rates: A systematic review of breast cancer and rural regions showed that women in rural areas had higher overall rates of late-stage breast malignancies than their urban counterparts (Williams, Jeanetta, & James, 2016). Although limited data exist on the risk of cancer in Amish communities, research funding awarded to Founding Director and Certified CHW Dr. Melissa Thomas and colleagues by the National Susan G. Komen for the Cure revealed higher mortality rates in both Geauga and Holmes County settlements (Thomas et al., 2005). In Holmes County, which contains the largest Amish settlement in Ohio, the researchers noted a 53 percent increase in female breast cancer mortality between 1991 and 1997 versus a ten percent decrease in all Ohio women during the same time period (Thomas, Indian, & Chan, 1998). Additionally, the study team estimated that breast cancer was the leading cause of death among Amish women under the age of 60.

Underutilization of breast cancer screening: In another Komen-funded study of a random sample of 334 Amish women in the Holmes County settlement, participants greatly underutilized mammography screening, even though 74% of respondents reported knowing someone who had breast cancer. Almost 60% of the sample reported having had a mammogram sometime in the past, but less than one-third (28%) reported having had a mammogram in the past year (Thomas, Menon, & Kuebler, 2002). When replicating the study 10 years later, while more women had reported hearing of a mammogram (72.4% vs 59.1%), fewer women were compliant with recommended breast cancer screening guidelines in 2013 when compared to 2002 results (44.3% vs 60.1%, respectively) (Thomas, Thomas, & Miller, 2017). Katz et al. (2011) noted similar results in a study conducted in 2011 that Amish women had lower rates of breast cancer screening compared to non-Amish females (24.8% vs 53.7%, respectively).

Lack of knowledge of breast cancer: Numerous surveys conducted at Amish women's health screenings in Ohio revealed that the majority of women underestimated breast cancer risk and believed many myths associated with the causes of breast cancer (Thomas, Thomas, Miller, Cech, & Dustman, 2017; Thomas, Thomas, Miller, & Fraser, 2016). One of the most pervasive myths was that mammograms cause breast cancer due to radiation and the pressure placed on the breast. Some women also believed that bumping or bruising the breast causes breast cancer. Many of these beliefs do have some level of truth, making breast health messaging a unique challenge. For example, we know that high levels of radiation can cause cancer, and finding a way of communicating levels of radiation in a mammogram can be difficult without providing a complex scientific explanation. Also, some women stated that they knew somebody who fell or bruised their breast, only to discover a breast cancer diagnosis after following up with a healthcare provider. While explaining that more than likely such an act just provided a focus to that particular part of the body, word of mouth and anecdotal evidence can be quite compelling when compared to evidence-based research.

Concern about cancer: In the 2013 cluster random sample of Amish church districts in the Holmes County settlement, almost one-third (29.1%) of the respondents cited cancer as their number one health concern, the most common response listed on the open-ended survey question (Thomas, Thomas, & Miller, 2017).

6.2.3 Program Description

Project Hoffnung is a community-led initiative where community members serve as the guides and provide direction of the programs and services provided (Fig. 6.1). There are six key components of the program: (1) development, delivery, and evaluation of a culturally competent breast health education program; (2) access to a no-cost women's health screening day, including mammograms, clinical breast exams, pelvic exams, Pap tests, and other health screening services when available from local hospitals and health departments; (3) patient navigation support for any woman in need of follow-up services for abnormal screening findings; (4) survivorship support including home visits, breast prosthesis fittings, and financial aid assistance; (5) cultural competency training for hospitals and agency settings who serve Amish and Mennonite communities; and (6) research that identifies health disparities, addresses health concerns and issues, evaluates programs and services provided, and disseminates results for replication and enhanced support to other agencies serving Amish and Mennonite communities.

For the past 22 years, CARE provides a bridge between the cultures of rural communities and health care with the creation of Project Hoffnung. After first discovering knowledge, attitudes, beliefs, and behaviors surrounding breast cancer and estimating breast cancer incidence and mortality rates among Amish women in two of the world's largest Amish settlements, the Project Hoffnung team began testing the effectiveness of culturally competent breast health education programs based on the Champion Health Belief Model (Champion, 1984). Multiple national presentations made at scientific peer-reviewed conferences provided opportunities to disseminate evidence-based strategies for successful health education and screening interventions (Thomas, Riegel, Thomas, Cech, & Miller, 2015; Thomas, Thomas, & Miller, 2017). In 2011, researchers presented at the International Cancer

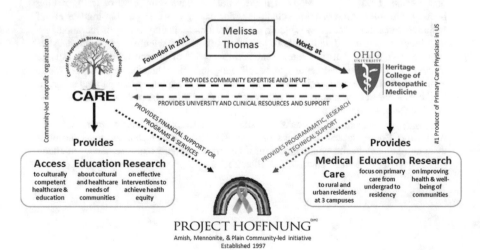

Fig. 6.1 Project Hoffnung

Education Conference about one such intervention. All women received a 15-minute education program prior to participating in the screening and included a knowledge scale adapted from Champion's Health Belief Model Scale (CHBMS) (1984). Findings included the following: the program significantly increased breast cancer knowledge among Amish and Mennonite women who attended a women's health day screening ($Z = -4.828$, $p < 0.001$) (Thomas, Thomas, & Hiermer, 2011). In addition to showing that knowledge increased after the delivery of the education program, women who participated in the Project Hoffnung program were more compliant with recommended breast cancer screening guidelines even after a 10-year period ($p = 0.001$) (Thomas, Thomas, & Miller, 2017).

The framework of the services portion of the program has been adapted from the Pathways model, which was developed in 2001 by Drs. Mark and Sarah Redding in Ohio and recently adapted by the Oregon Affiliate of Susan G. Komen for the Cure for breast health (Applegate et al., 2016). The "Project Hoffnung Pathways" model measures success based on successful completion of key steps: (1) the screening completion step of comprehending breast screening results and/or (2) the patient navigation completion step of attending all appointments and addressing support needs. While much effort is initially placed on the outreach and partnership development to both communities and agencies to establish a screening day, the bulk of activity centers on the screening days themselves that are held in some of the most remote and/or resource-starved sections of the states served. Referred to as the "Three Cs of Screening Days," community members prefer to attend Project Hoffnung programs for the cultural sensitivity (all staff/volunteers are female and most are community members), the convenience (this is the only location where mammograms and a visit with a healthcare provider can be scheduled at the same time at locations that are chosen by the community to provide easy access by horse and buggy), and the cost (grant funding and donations cover most costs, and prices are negotiated at a substantially lower rate for other services at local healthcare systems).

Project Hoffnung has office space in the heart of Amish Country, Holmes County, Ohio, and CHWs staff the office in person 2–3 days per week. A toll-free call forwarding system ensures that staff members are accessible regardless of the location of program activities. Many women still prefer to write to schedule appointments and/or share updates or needs with team members, due in part to access to telephone service and the preference of sharing in the form of written letters. The nurse practitioner on the program is available 24 h a day to accommodate the various schedules and accessibility issues with the communities we serve.

In 2017, a new partnership formed with the Heritage College of Osteopathic Medicine at Ohio University, located in Appalachia Ohio, which provided additional opportunities to provide clinical and research support to Project Hoffnung. While serving in a research faculty position, CHW Melissa Thomas also saw a truly synergistic relationship between a community-led program and a medical school that gives medical students and faculty first-hand knowledge of how community-engaged research can be applied and enhanced through the leadership and experience of community health workers.

Project Hoffnung team members developed a cultural sensitivity training that has been delivered to community agencies, volunteers, hospitals, and other healthcare organizations over the years that provides best practices and historical/cultural background information from one of the Amish or Mennonite CHWs. After noting the increase of "docu-drama" television series regarding Amish communities from large networks more commonly known for their science and fact-based shows (e.g., The Discovery Channel, National Geographic, etc.), community members shared concern over the false representation and incorrect lifestyles shared by tourists when visiting popular Amish locations based on these shows. The CHWs grew increasingly concerned that such activity increased the stigma and stereotypes surrounding Amish communities, possibly negatively impacting their treatment in business and healthcare settings. While many books have been written about the Amish, some by individuals who were previously members, there were no books written specifically by the Amish that gave them a voice in what they wanted to communicate regarding their beliefs and values. In 2014, Project Hoffnung CHWs and volunteers launched a 4-year project that utilized a unique spin on the qualitative research method photo-voice (Sutton-Brown, 2014). The result of their community-led work was a photo book published in 2018 titled *Life Through Their Lens: A Photo Collection of Amish and Mennonite Communities* (Life Through Their Lens, 2018; Thomas, 2018). Medical students are currently reviewing the book in a research study exploring its impact on increasing cultural sensitivity and intercultural communication. Additionally, all proceeds of the book fund the women's health screening programs and follow-up care for Amish and Mennonite women.

6.2.4   Roles of the CHW

Project Hoffnung is led and coordinated by a team of seven CHWs: three members of the Amish community, two from the Mennonite community, and two who are Appalachian. Additionally, a support team of four year-round volunteers and dozens of site-specific Amish, Mennonite, and rural champions provide financial guidance, mentorship, and even administrative assistance for key mailings and projects. Several leaders of the community, including Bishops and elders, serve as a sounding board and guide for all activities. Figure 6.2 depicts the CHW team, role, length of service, and relationship between all members of the project. It is important to note that the organizational structure is not hierarchical in that there are no leadership positions among the core CHW staff. Rather, the team works as a collective group where decision-making is shared with input from all CHW members. While not obvious on paper, the one distinction between CHW roles is that of Ella Miller, who is known unofficially as the "Mother" of the project for all of her wisdom, advice, and experience as a 31-year breast cancer survivor and lifetime member of the Amish community. When asked about her "Mother" title, Ella laughed and said "I don't see myself like that. I don't feel I would deserve that. It doesn't bother me, but yes, it's sometimes embarrassing that I'm that old, but that's okay. I don't mind."

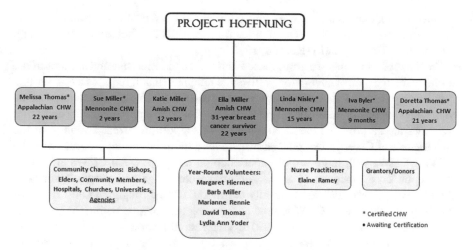

Fig. 6.2 Project Hoffnung organizational chart

In 2001, the Project Hoffnung staff and volunteers developed a 21-item outreach model that identified the key components of a successful program serving Amish and Mennonite communities. Using the traditional horse and buggy road safety sign as the visual presentation of the model, the program itself is identified as the buggy. The CHWs sit inside the buggy, but the Amish and Mennonite CHWs are the drivers; the Appalachian CHWs are the passengers.

Making this distinction is important because while no person is given higher leadership authority on the project, deference is still made to the CHWs from within the community. One of the biggest mistakes noted by the team members was that often organizations place funding as the "horse," or driving force, of the program. However, to be successful, the culture and the religion of a community must be understood and respected to lead the program. Sustainability is the cornerstone of Project Hoffnung's vision, so much so that funding was identified as the "cushion" inside the buggy; it makes the ride more comfortable, but it is not necessary to get where one needs to go (Thomas, Thomas, Ferguson, Sharpe, & Hiermer, 2002). The Project Hoffnung outreach model has cross-cultural applicability and provides best practices learned that still apply after 19 years of development.

According to the output of the Community Health Worker Core Consensus (C3) Project, all ten roles and multiple sub-roles are fulfilled by the CHWs of Project Hoffnung (Rosenthal, Rush, & Allen, 2016). While providing culturally competent education and access to health services (Roles 1–4, 7), CHWs play a direct role in outreach activities to identify Amish and Mennonite communities and go door-to-door to talk with women about their cancer concerns (Role 9). CHWs also serve as the voice of the project and present at local, state, and national conferences about the issues facing their communities and recommendations on how to improve healthcare practices (Roles 5, 6). Finally, five of the seven CHWs have been directly engaged in community assessments and research activities that include serving as co-investigators on studies that require completion human subjects training of the Collaborative Institutional Training Initiative (CITI) (Research Ethics and Compliance Training, n.d.) (Roles 8, 10).

While most activities are group-based and utilize the expertise and support of the entire team, the patient navigation pathway is unique in that it requires a one-on-one relationship between the community member and CHW. Phone calls, letters, home visits, and attendance at hospital appointments, healthcare appointments, and other activities are all provided based on the level of support preferred. Training for the specific role of CHW patient navigator involves a train-the-trainer program with the existing CHWs with more senior experience on the project. All CHWs are cross-trained on core functions to allow for unexpected staff and program changes. Additionally, four CHWs are currently certified CHWs through the Ohio Board of Nursing, and the newest CHW will be completing certification within the year. The two Amish CHWs are not eligible for CHW certification per Ohio guidelines because a high school diploma or General Education Development/High School Equivalency (GED) certificate is required.

Six of the seven members of the CHW team were interviewed regarding their experiences and lessons learned through the years. Their input is provided below.

6.2.5 Part of the Community

Linda: *"I think it's very important [being a member of the community] because for any culture and any place when you speak with the same language there's a trust there that is built right away whereas if you're not from the community it's going to be a longer process to build that trust. When you're not from the community or even if you're from the community you may not understand all the aspects of it, but you're going to have a better idea of how the community and how their wants are and how they like to do things."*

Ella: *"One thing is because you speak their language, there are people still out there that can't understand all the English words you do. I don't either, but I use the dictionary when I don't."*

Katie: *"It's important…very. I think that is where I get respect from the people that I try to help out and work with. They can trust me, not that I'm trying to be bragging, but if they trust me with whatever it could be that's where it stays. So be trustful and make sure that they know that you're there for them."*

Sue: *"Well just today, I had multiple calls and every time I asked do you speak Pennsylvania Dutch and they'd say yes, then I would switch to the Pennsylvania Dutch language and I could instantly feel how they relaxed and it just became easier for them to say what they want to say. They trust me and understanding where they're coming from helps, too."*

"Sometimes I can tell that they just want to make an appointment and go but then last week I had a lady and we made her appointment and we got to chatting and then she told me she lost like 120-some pounds I think since last fall and how she's changed. I mean she talked for almost 20 minutes just sharing what's happening in her life and in her community. I can't wait to meet her."

Doretta: *"There's no hardship in that whatsoever [not being Amish or Mennonite]. A lot of my life was spent growing up as a child in what they do to this day: the farming; we butchered hogs, we butchered beef, we had around chickens, we had our own eggs, we had* ducks. *At one time my dad was an avid game hunter. My mother and I canned everything we could get our hands on. My parents had a huge garden, and we were all involved with all of the gathering of the crops, the canning, and what we couldn't can we froze. We had an outhouse. We had to carry the water from the kitchen sink into the bathtub. So you know I share so much of what was a part of me growing up is still practiced to this day so I have always felt very connected to the community...So it's just never been anything that I think any differently. It just was such an easy transition for me, and that's why I think there's that strong bond and connection there between us."*

Melissa: *"I have often said that you do not have to belong to a community to help, but you do have to know your place. While I have been blessed to work with dozens of Amish and Mennonite communities throughout a multi-state region over two decades, I am still not a member of these communities, and it is important to recognize the experience and culture of community members who serve Project Hoffnung. When asked to present about our program and/or develop courses and conferences, I make every effort to include Amish and Mennonite members as part of the planning committee and as co-presenters. I continue to learn and am humbled with every encounter I have with members in these communities. I am happy to share best practices and lessons learned, but I do not feel I have a right to tell others who they are. To me, one of the most dangerous roles to play as an outsider is that of a self-described 'expert' of a culture that is not your own."*

6.2.6 Rewards

Linda: *"The most rewarding...there's so many things. Definitely the education alone has been very rewarding and very helpful in my own personal life. Just the relationships you get to build with the ladies in the community. One of the most rewarding things is if you've had a lady that you've been able to be there for her and support her though all of her diagnosis and it does end up being good and you have that relationship, that reward, and seeing what she's been able to do and what she can do now."*

Ella: *"Seeing people survive after diagnosis and out there living a normal life. It's very rewarding to go out and help people."*

Doretta: *"I would have to say the friendships that I've acquired along the way with the Amish and Mennonite people and the fact that I know that we have saved lives that might have been lost to breast cancer had we not been there for them. That's a very gratifying experience to know that in some small tiny way I helped save a human life."*

Linda [teamwork]: *"The great value of being a team member is just the support that you get as an individual and having that support of being able to guide the community member into having more answers. As a CHW you don't have all the answers and you don't give medical advice but being able to have that connection to someone where you can ask questions and having that support from other team members in just approaches and how to process. When there's a difficult day to be able to go back to your team members and share your day and get advice from them and get help from them. That has been huge."*

Melissa: *"There's no denying that one of the most rewarding aspects of this project and being a CHW is knowing that we have made an impact in reducing the burden of cancer in Amish and Mennonite communities. There are so many diseases and health conditions that we can't control or prevent, but there is nothing more devastating to me than to realize that someone has died of a disease that could have been prevented had s/he had access to lifesaving culturally sensitive education and access to quality health care. That's what we do....we use research and implement community-led outreach and programs that don't just provide these services....we empower communities with the tools they need to take charge of their health. The greatest reward in the end is that our program is no longer needed anymore, that we have provided that bridge between the culture of health care and the culture of these communities so that trust and support have been established and built from within."*

Doretta [educating]: *"It's the best part of it all because I'm one of the first people that they see and get to talk to. They don't really get to communicate that much when they're filling out all that paperwork, so when they come to me and it's been a year since I've seen them and most of them I've been seeing for twenty years so they know me quite well and I know them quite well. They cannot wait to talk to me and catch up over things that's been going on with them over the past year. They'll tell me how their year has been...you know, they broke a leg, someone in the family's had a baby. It's just a very personal time for us that we can catch up and they're very interested in my life as well...you know, how's my health and how have I been but mainly they want to talk to me about their life in the past year. I can't even tell you what that means to me that they think that much of me to share that with me and so excited to tell me about that. We have even exchanged recipes in the mail. It's just a special, special bond that we share that is just amazing."*

6.2.7   Challenges

Linda: *"The most difficult part probably is when there is someone that has a diagnosis that you know there is medical treatment out there for them and they choose not to take that medical treatment immediately. They choose to wait and do alternative medicine or just wait because they can't make a decision right away. That probably has been the most difficult."*

Melissa: *"I think one of the biggest challenges is working with healthcare systems, providers and grant-funding agencies who think they know what's best for communities without ever including them in the conversation. I continue to be amazed at the lack of cultural humility that some organizations have that result in policies and practices that are not sensitive to those who may need help the most. It seems that the most prejudiced individuals we've encountered are those who live just around the perimeter of Amish communities, where they know just a little about the culture and make assumptions about the rest. Thankfully, these experiences have been the exception rather than the rule, and they have helped shape our educational programs to partners. While we've made great strides in educating providers and agencies with the creation of Project Hoffnung, I know that our work is still ongoing to increase quality of care in our rural regions."*

Doretta: *"It thankfully doesn't happen very often, but it's very hard when a lady refuses to seek further medical help and she chooses the route of herbs and then as the disease progresses the herbs and her treatments and salves don't work. Then she wants to come back and get help and it's too late. That's very sad. That is still to this day a big challenge for us and we're very limited in how we approach this situation. So it's a very delicate matter because we like for them to be able to do their own choosing. We cannot control their choices. We can just offer what we have and then we have to back away, but it's very hard when we know that there's treatment there that could probably save their life."*

Ella: *"Convincing people they need to do a mammogram...that's a big challenge because there's that myth out there that a mammogram causes cancer. If I don't have cancer, I'll have it after that."*

"This last winter, there was a lady that called me and she said she had seen her doctor three different times and he wanted her and gave her papers to get a mammogram. She said there was a lady in church who said that's what causes cancer. And she said 'I went home,

put the paper in the drawer. I was afraid of it. Afraid of not doing it but I felt guilty to do it...because of what she said.' And there she was. She was diagnosed with cancer. She had depression problems besides that. It's a sad story. But what can you do, if people are out there telling others? That's a big challenge."

6.2.8 Importance of Education/Certification

Sue: *"It has been very helpful in understanding the role that I play as a CHW. Totally broadened my horizons. It's really just having more knowledge about how to go about doing my job."*

Linda: *"I was excited because it was truly a time for me that I was going back to college and I was going to get an education and a degree to a certain extent that was going to be very helpful to me and my community work that I was doing. It was scary that I was going to a university but also exciting, a great experience. People in class and instructors were very helpful. I felt like I gained a lot of insight in specifically what my role as a CHW is and guidelines. I feel very honored and privileged."*

Melissa: *"I had already had my PhD when I went back to get my CHW certification, and I felt it was important to 'walk the talk' and show how much I valued the process [of certification]. I had no idea how much I would learn and how connected I felt to all of the students in my program. We came from all walks of life with so many diverse experiences, but I felt in that room that I had found my tribe, that no matter what, we all were there for one another and had so many life experiences to share. I walked away with so many tools and collective knowledge that have made me a better CHW, a better listener, a better person."*

Doretta: *"This experience [becoming a certified CHW] turned out to be one of the most amazing things for me. I was VERY reluctant to do this because of my age. 73 is not when most people go back to school. I didn't want to be with a bunch of very young and smart college kids. I only have a high school diploma so you can see my reluctance. First day of class my fears were quickly erased...only two young people and all the rest were middle-aged and looking to advance their careers. The instructors were so kind and patient. So I not only got a certification but I also got to experience college life to some degree and made wonderful new friends. I gained so much knowledge to take back to my communities to help make them stronger and more knowledgeable about their health. I learned a valuable lesson which I wasn't prepared to learn: don't be afraid to try new learning experiences. Grasp all the knowledge you can and go for all the wonderful things that come your way NO MATTER HOW OLD YOU ARE!"*

6.2.9 As a Survivor

Ella: *"I think it makes people aware that the years since diagnosis that it is necessary to do the mammogram. A lot of them say they didn't realize I was a survivor."*

6.2.10   Lessons Learned

Linda:
"*One of the lessons learned is to never assume that the lady knows or does not know. I know for me that's been a big lesson to not assume that she doesn't know what she wants to do or that she wants my help but to wait and let her know that I'm here to help her and then to wait until she tells me she wants my help.*"

"*Another lesson learned is to ask questions, too. Once they tell you they want your help, to ask questions to find out what do they know and what do they want your help to do-not just assume that they want you to help them with every process but to continue to ask 'Would you like me to help? What do you need me to do?'. Try to empower the lady, not do everything for her but to empower her to give her the tools she needs to make the decision that's right for her even if it's not the decision I wish she would make.*"

"*I think the media has had a huge role in what people think about the Amish and Mennonite community, and I think people tend to watch the documentaries and the shows and then they put everybody in that same category instead of realizing that is only a very small population of the people or very small group that is doing those documentaries and that a lot of those are people already out of the community and not part of the community. People tend to believe what they see on TV. It's easy to just think that's how the community is when in reality that's not how the community is. And I think that goes for any culture.*"

"*I learned a lot. I was from the community and thought I would know how the community is and learned that as I went out to the different Amish communities that in fact they are not all the same and in fact Amish communities are a very diverse group and have different ways of doing things and different beliefs. So try to learn about the community and be sensitive how their community is, how they do things, what they believe and how they want healthcare to be for them as that community.*"

Ella: "*I guess being relaxed with people and not being overly protective. People know when they call you that you can give your opinion…that you're not there to judge them, either. It's their choice, not mine, although a lot of people want me to make their choices, to tell them what to do but I'm very careful with that. I don't want them to think that I'm telling them what they can do and can't do.*"

Melissa: "*I learned not to assume the values or priorities of a community. When we first developed our breast health education program, the gold standard was 'train the trainer' programs where we trained community members who in turn would train others. After training two Amish women and providing instructions on setting up community programs to teach others about breast health, they simply would not go out and educate. Frustrated, I finally asked why, and the community members told me that they loved learning about breast cancer but did not feel comfortable teaching others…that it made them feel 'higher' than the rest of the community. They actually preferred if we 'English' would be the teachers. We could have saved so much energy had we just asked in the first place instead of following 'best practices' at the time.*"

6.2.11   Advice in Working with Amish and Mennonite Communities

Linda: "*To remember that we are just like any other people. We have feelings, we have emotions, just like anybody else. Treat us the way that you want to be treated. Don't make any assumptions about us because here again you don't like when people make assumptions about you so don't do that to others.*"

Sue: *"Respect their culture. Cultural humility. Even if you don't understand it, respect it."*

Katie: *"I think you have to be willing to accept what you might meet, which might not always be pleasant. You have to be open with what people have to say. You can't just go in there and say this is what I want, this is where I'm coming from. It's what I call a two-way street. I am here to help you. What do you want? I feel that's what I have to do if I want to go out there. That would be the way for me to start things to be open-minded and see what really do these people need. What really would they expect from me?"*

Ella: *"Don't say everything you know, because you are going to get yourself into trouble. People will repeat what you said and you know that might get you in trouble. Like with giving people advice on what to do. Do this or do that and now look what happened. Be very careful with that."*

Katie: *"Well we're humans just like everybody else. There used to be mostly farmers in the area. Anymore there's carpenters, there's masons, many different mix. A lot of people have their own shops at home. I would say a lot of people, even though not everybody, but a lot of people like to be self-sufficient on their farms on their homes, gardens."*

Ella: *"What I really think is important is going out and seeing the ladies and tell them down the road it's not as bad as it looks."*

Sue: *"We're just people like everyone else. We may dress different and that's just the way of life that we've chosen born out of our convictions. It's not our salvation."*

Melissa:

"Always keep in mind ownership/ethical issues that surround any program, especially when working with diverse population groups. For example, this project does NOT belong to us. One of my biggest pet peeves is to hear people say 'My' patients, 'my' staff, 'my' people'. The sense of ownership that hides behind that one adjective takes away the rights and voice of a community."

"After receiving a big national research grant, my employer, a large nonprofit hospital system, was eager to promote the great news in the large urban newspaper. Before accepting to be interviewed, I decided to ask one of the Amish bishops who lived about an hour from the city what he thought publishing this story. His response has guided me throughout my entire career. He informed that he and his community members also had access to the large city newspaper, and if he saw a big article that the hospital received this big grant, he would wonder…'Are you doing this for us, or are you doing this for you?' Action without permission equals exploitation."

"Choose your partners wisely. In the first few years of our program, we were desperate for help and support, so we naively agreed to partner with any person or agency who wanted to work with us. We soon realized that not all partners shared our same value set in the respect and community-led approach we had to developing and implementing our breast health initiatives. We now use MOUs (Memorandum of Understanding) with new partners and develop guiding principles for individuals as part of volunteer training. There are times that non-Amish volunteers and partners want to lead or direct our work, and we have to remember that the community guides this program, not the other way around."

Doretta: *"Just be yourself. Be sincere and don't try to pretend to be something you're not. Just be you and they will accept you for who you are and respect you. Don't go in there with the attitude that you know what's best for them because you don't know what's best for them. They're not going to accept you like that. You've got to go in there and earn their trust and then you will accomplish your goals."*

6.2.12   Conclusion

Throughout these past two decades, rural and Appalachian CHWs have been at the forefront of a movement to reduce the burden of breast cancer among Amish and Mennonite women. What started out as simply a question as to why these communities were not participating in mobile mammography screenings has evolved into a nationally recognized program that credits its success on putting CHWs at the heart of all planning, implementation, and dissemination activities. Community-led initiatives are complex and constantly changing, and training CHWs to lead such programs takes a unique commitment to ensure success by increasing self-efficacy in serving as team members and advisors. Six components comprise Project Hoffnung's efforts to serve as a bridge between the cultures of community and health care, and sustainability has been accomplished through a statewide partner and volunteer base committed to achieving health equity in cancer care.

All too often researchers and healthcare professionals focus on the "what" in a community and move directly to the "how." In the case of breast cancer, once Project Hoffnung staff discovered disproportionately higher breast cancer mortality rates among Amish women, numerous evidence-based strategies pointed to how to effectively deliver education and programs. However, no research existed on the "why"—why were Amish women dying at higher rates when compared to their non-Amish neighbors? Strategies implemented over 22 years have helped answer that question, focusing on education, access, cultural sensitivity, and health factors contributing to a predisposition to cancer. The key to answering the "why" is the community, and empowering CHWs has led to a tremendous understanding of what the community wants and needs to address their health concerns. The "why" phase provides the framework to "how"—how we address the community's concerns.

The lessons learned from Project Hoffnung are not unique to serving Amish and Mennonite women. Anybody serving communities can benefit from the advice and lessons shared by the CHWs in this section. When allowing the cultural values of a community to guide the work, even if at times those values may differ wildly from outside team members, the community can easily integrate the support and information offered. While respecting one of the core values of Amish life— humility—a transformation occurred over the years that led to more effective programs, increased acceptance, and enhanced personal lives that blurred the lines between "us" and "them." A new community formed out of this common bond, one that shared so many similar values in wanting to be respected and being heard. By incorporating the values of the community, by placing CHWs not just at the table but also giving them a voice to guide and share, lives have not only been saved but also supported, changed on all sides of the cultural landscape that makes Project Hoffnung a voice of hope to all.

References

Amish Population. (2019). *Young center for Anabaptist and Pietist studies*. Elizabethtown College. Retrieved May 8, 2020, from http://groups.etown.edu/amishstudies/statistics/population-2019/.

Applegate, M., Brennan, L., Kuenkele, V., Redding, S., & Redding, M. (2016). Pathways community HUB manual: A guide to identify and address risk factors, reduce costs, and improve outcomes. Agency for Healthcare Research and Quality. (AHRQ Publication No. 15(16)-0070-EF). Available from: https://innovations.ahrq.gov/sites/default/files/Guides/CommunityHubManual.pdf

Champion, V. L. (1984). Instrument development for health belief model constructs. *Advances in Nursing Science, 6*, 73–85.

Donnermeyer, J. (2015). Doubling time and population increase of the Amish. *Journal of Amish and Plain Anabaptist Studies, 3*(1), 94–109.

Katz, M., Ferketich, A., Paskett, E., & Bloomfield, C. (2013). Health literacy among the Amish: Measuring a complex concept among a unique population. *Journal of Community Health, 38*(4), 753–758. https://doi.org/10.1007/s10900-013-9675-z

Katz, M. L., Ferketich, A. K., Paskett, E. D., Harley, A., Reiter, P. L., Lemeshow, S., … Bloomfield, C. D. (2011). Cancer screening practices among Amish and non-Amish adults living in Ohio Appalachia. *The Journal of Rural Health, 27*(3), 302–309. https://doi.org/10.1111/j.1748-0361.2010.00345.x

Kraybill, D., Johnson-Weiner, K. M., & Nolt, S. M. (2013). *The Amish*. Baltimore: Johns Hopkins University Press.

Nolt, S. (2003). *A history of the Amish*. Intercourse, PA: Good Books.

Research Ethics and Compliance Training. (n.d.). *Pathways Community HUB Manual: A guide to identify and address risk factors, reduce costs, and improve outcomes*. Rockville, MD: Agency for Healthcare Research and Quality (AHRQ); January 2016. AHRQ Publication No. 15(16)-0070-EF. Replaces AHRQ Publication No. 09(10)-0088. Retrieved from https://about.citiprogram.org/en/homepage/.

Rosenthal, E.L., Rush, C., & Allen, C.G. (2016, April). *Understanding scope and competencies: A contemporary look at the United States Community Health Worker Field Progress Report of the Community Health Worker (CHW) Core Consensus (C3) Project: Building national consensus on CHW core roles, skills and qualities*. Retrieved from https://www.c3project.org/resources.

Sutton-Brown, C. A. (2014). Photovoice: A methodological guide. *Photography and Culture, 7*(2), 169–185. https://doi.org/10.2752/175145214X13999922103165

The Center for Appalachia Research in Cancer Education. (2018). Retrieved from www.appal-care.org.

Thomas, M. K. (2018). *Life through their lens: A photo collection by Amish and Mennonite communities* (Vol. I). Whipple, OH: Center for Appalachia Research in Cancer Education.

Thomas, M.K., Hiermer, W., Indian, R., & Sickle-Santanello, B. (2005, December). *Estimating breast cancer incidence and mortality rates among the Amish*. Poster presented at the American Public Health Association annual meeting, Philadelphia, PA.

Thomas, M. K., Indian, R., & Chan, W. (1998). *Female breast cancer incidence and mortality among Amish women in Northeast Ohio*. Unpublished raw data.

Thomas, M. K., Menon, U., & Kuebler, P. (2002, June). *Delivering effective health promotion programs to the Amish: Key findings of the Amish breast health project*. Poster presented at the Susan G. Komen Breast Cancer Foundation annual mission conference, Washington, DC.

Thomas, M. K., Riegel, H., Thomas, D., Cech, A., & Miller, B. (2015, November). Does four minutes make a difference? Delivering culturally competent breast cancer education to *Amish & Mennonite women*. Paper presented at the American Public Health Association, Chicago, IL.

Thomas, M. K., Thomas, D., & Miller, B. (2017, September). *The use of tailored interventions in delivering breast cancer messages to Amish and Mennonite women*. Paper presented at the international cancer education conference, Cleveland OH.

Thomas, M. K. Thomas, D., Miller, B., Cech, A., & Dustman, S. (2017, November). *Impact of social influence on breast cancer education among Amish and Mennonite women.* Paper presented at the American Public Health Association annual meeting, Atlanta, GA.

Thomas, M. K., Thomas, D., Miller, B, & Fraser, H. (2016, November). *Knowledge and beliefs surrounding breast cancer among Amish and Mennonite women in rural Ohio.* Poster presented at the American Public Health Association annual meeting, Denver, CO.

Thomas, M. K., Thomas, D. K., Ferguson, S., Sharpe, J., & Hiermer, M. (2002, May). Project Hoffnung outreach model: Strategies for effective health promotion programs in Amish communities. Paper presented at the 3rd biennial cancer, culture and literacy symposium of the Moffitt Cancer Cancer, Clearwater Beach, FL.

Thomas, M.K., Thomas, D.K., & Hiermer, W. (2011, September). *Project Hoffnung (HOPE): Lessons learned from delivering culturally competent breast cancer education to Amish and Mennonite communities in rural Ohio.* Poster presented at the 2011 international cancer education conference, Buffalo, NY.

Williams, F., Jeanetta, S., & James, A. S. (2016). Geographical location and stage of breast cancer diagnosis: A systematic review of the literature. *Journal of Health Care for the Poor and Underserved, 27*(3), 1357–1383. https://doi.org/10.1353/hpu.2016.0102

6.3   Community Health Workers: Trauma-Informed, Culturally Centered, Decolonizing Popular Educators

Arika Makena Bridgeman-Bunyoli, Teresa Campos Dominguez,
Lizdaly Cancel Tirado, Francis Kham, Alix Sanchez, Kelly Volkmann, and
Noelle Wiggins

6.3.1   Introduction

In this section, we first survey the range of health education approaches and then provide a thorough introduction to popular/people's education (PE) as an approach to health education that is both effective and consistent with the history and intent of the CHW model. We explain how PE, when practiced genuinely and mindfully, is also trauma-informed, culturally centered, and decolonizing. The heart of our section is three case studies written by CHWs (and one ally) who use PE to share health education and information in a variety of communities and settings and across several levels of the socio-ecological model, from individual to group to community. Our intent throughout the section is to demonstrate how CHWs, when properly chosen, trained, and supported, can be uniquely skilled and qualified health educators.

6.3.2   The Spectrum of Health Education Approaches

Approaches to sharing health education and information lie along a continuum. On the one end lie extremely formal, top-down approaches based in the belief that knowledge exists and must be conveyed from teacher to student. Freire (2003), a well-known advocate of the popular (people's) education approaches we will discuss, called this type of education, where knowledge is deposited into the head of the student by the teacher, "banking education." Further along the spectrum lie participatory approaches based in the idea that knowledge is constantly developing and is created in the interaction between teachers and students. This type of education is associated with adult learning theory and the "andragogy" of Knowles (1988). At the far end of the spectrum reside the popular and critical approaches to education. These approaches are based on the idea that, rather than preserving the status quo, education should serve to liberate and create a more just and equitable society.

Based on their location within systems and their own inclinations, community health workers (CHWs) can be found using all these approaches to education as well as others. However, our experience in Oregon and around the world suggests that the approaches to education most consistent with the CHW model are those on the liberatory end of the spectrum. One reason for this is history; the CHW model formalized in response to many of the same conditions of oppression that produced popular and emancipatory education. The liberatory approaches to education also share many key principles with the CHW model. For example, both models propose that people, and especially people most affected by inequities, are the experts about their own experience. They also emphasize that the knowledge we gain from life experience can be just as important as, and, in some cases, more important than, the knowledge we gain through formal study. Using the CHW model and popular education together often seems to have a multiplicative effect, since the models reinforce and strengthen one another. For these reasons, we strongly support use of popular (people's) education in CHW programs. The next section introduces popular (people's) education and shows how, when practiced correctly, PE supports the principles of trauma-informed, culturally centered, and decolonizing education.

6.3.3   Introduction to Popular (People's) Education[2]

Popular education, a philosophy and methodology that creates settings in which people most affected by inequities can identify problems and underlying causes and develop solutions, has been a cornerstone of CHW programs around the world for decades. The word "popular" in "popular education" derives from the Romance languages and refers to something belonging to or arising from the vast majority of common people who lack political and economic power (Wiggins, Hughes, Rios-Campos, Rodriguez, & Potter, 2014). A viable English translation is "people's education."

While strongly influenced by Brazilian educator Paulo Freire (1973, 2003), popular education (PE) predates Freire and has continued to develop since his death in 1997. Popular education has been widely used for health promotion and has been associated with increased empowerment and improved health (Wallerstein, 2006; Wiggins, 2012). A few recent studies have systematically compared PE to conventional education as methods for increasing knowledge and empowerment, with hopeful results (Wang, Chao, & Liao, 2011; Wiggins et al., 2014).

---

[2]This section is adapted from Wiggins, N., and Pérez, A. (2016). Using popular education with health promotion students in the USA. *Health Promotion International.* doi: https://doi.org/10.1093/heapro/dav121.

6.3.4   History and Definition of Popular (People's) Education

Indigenous communities around the world identify similarities between PE and indigenous ways of knowing and being (Sosa, personal communication, 1999; Cochran et al., 2008). Latin Americans trace PE's formal roots to nineteenth-century efforts to extend primary education to all, to workers' universities organized by students influenced by socialism in the late nineteenth and early twentieth centuries, and to adult education efforts that accompanied revolutionary movements throughout the twentieth century (Gómez & Puiggrós, 1986). Workers' universities are also a feature of PE history through a European lens, as are correspondence societies in eighteenth-century France, the nineteenth-century Chartist movement, and Scandinavian folk schools (Chatterton, 2008; Crowther, 1999).

Examples of attempts to make education at all levels "popular" (i.e., accessible to those to whom it had been denied) in the African American community in the United States include clandestine schools in the nineteenth and twentieth centuries, Freedom Schools in the 1960s, and the convention movement and Black newspapers from the seventeenth century to the present (Chilcoat & Ligon, 1994). Other traditions of PE indigenous to the United States include the practice developed at the Highlander School in Tennessee (Horton, 2003) and applications and extensions of that practice by leaders of the Civil Rights Movement (Tippett, 2013) and the Labor Movement (Delp, Outman-Kramer, Schurman, & Wong, 2002). hooks has been an especially influential proponent of PE in the United States and a link between PE and feminist post-structural pedagogy (hooks, 2003). South Africa, the Philippines, and many other places around the world have their own histories of PE (Walters & Manicom, 1996).

Taking these influences together, PE can be described as a philosophy and methodology that arises in response to conditions of systematic oppression and attempts to change those conditions by creating situations in which people most affected by inequity can (re)discover their individual and collective capacity and use it to solve problems, shift power, and create more equitable communities (Wiggins et al., 2014).

6.3.5   Methodology in Popular (People's) Education

Methodology in PE is crucial because it supports and embodies the core principles of this approach to teaching and learning. Common methods in PE include:

- *Dinámicas* used to build trust and create community
- A variety of *brainstorming techniques* used to draw out what participants already know
- A range of drama-based techniques (*radio plays*, *sociodramas*, and *role plays*, among others) used to share new information, spark discussion about controversial topics, and provide practice in using new skills

- *Problem-posing*, a classic Freirian technique, used to identify and analyze problems and develop solutions
- *Cooperative learning methods* that help participants develop the skills they need to work collectively (Wiggins et al., 2014)

Similarities in methodology across diverse PE settings suggest that educators seeking to undo social inequity and build critical thinking skills come organically to similar strategies.

6.3.6 Popular (People's) Education: Trauma-Informed, Culturally Centered, and Decolonizing

As an educational philosophy and methodology developed in response to systematic oppression and the trauma that oppression can cause, popular education embodies many of the principles and practices of trauma-informed care: safety; trustworthiness and transparency; peer support and mutual self-help; collaboration and mutuality; empowerment, voice, and choice; and cultural, historical, and gender issues. (More information about these principles can be found at https://store.samhsa.gov/system/files/sma14-4884.pdf.)

As a starting point for any educational intervention, popular educators seek to create an environment of *safety and trust* so that participants will feel comfortable sharing their ideas and experiences. Starting with people's and communities' experience is inherently *strengths based* and validates and values participants' *cultural knowledge and historical experience*. Techniques like problem-posing are used to involve those who have the greatest stake in any decision in making that decision, ensuring *transparency*. Popular educators use techniques such as cooperative learning to further *develop participants' ability to work as a collective*, and they emphasize people working together and *helping one another*. Techniques such as dinámicas and setting group agreements are used to *balance power and assure that everyone's voice can be heard*. The ultimate aim of popular/people's education is *empowerment*, from the individual to the community level and both within and between communities. Popular/people's education emphasizes the importance of understanding how *historical events and oppression produced current-day realities*. Acknowledging that we learn with hearts, heads, and bodies and using arts, music, and drama *promotes healing*.

Given its emphasis on starting with what any group of learners already knows and does, and valuing their cultural wisdom and worldviews, when employed with skill and care, popular education is also inherently culturally centered. A group of CHWs interviewed for a 2009 study were asked whether and how they had to adapt popular education to fit the needs of their urban, African American community (Wiggins et al., 2009). They responded that they didn't have to adapt the methodology given its inherently flexible nature. In a 2015 study, Bridgeman-Bunyoli and colleagues explored the role of an Afrocentric, popular education-based curriculum in the empowerment of African and African American CHWs in Oregon. Results suggested that CHW participants experienced four types of awakening, in addition to changes in their interaction with their family members and increased community involvement. Similar to the synergy created by using popular education with the CHW model, intentional combination of popular education with a culturally centered curriculum can produce positive changes for both CHWs and communities.

Popular education arose out of a post-colonial context and shares many of the attributes and a similar epistemology with the decolonizing methodologies articulated by Indigenous scholars like Tuhiwai Smith (1999); Kawakami, Aton, Cram, Lai, and Porima (2007); and Morelli and Mataira (2010). Crucially, popular (people's) education decenters what has conventionally been deemed as knowledge by dominant communities and cultures and returns to marginalized communities the inherent right to define knowledge according to their own systems of value and verification (Rahman, 1991).

6.3.7   Capacitating CHWs to Use Popular (People's) Education

Generally, people teach as we were taught (Lortie, 1975). Most of us have a lot more experience with hierarchical, top-down approaches to education than with liberating approaches to education. This means that, if CHWs want to be able to use liberating educational methods in their work in communities, they need a variety of opportunities to develop those skills.

First, *popular (people's) education should be used in initial and ongoing capacitation (or training) programs for CHWs*. In fact, use of popular education in CHW training has been recognized as a best practice, for all the same reasons that PE is a best practice in community education (Calori, Hart, Tein, & Burres, 2010; Wiggins & Kaan et al., 2013). Evidence suggests that using popular education in CHW training results in increases in health knowledge that are at least as great as those achieved through formal education while producing even greater increases in empowerment (Wiggins et al., 2014). For specific examples of how popular education can be used in the capacitation of CHWs, see Wiggins & Kaan et al. (2013).

While using popular education carefully and consistently in CHW capacitation is important, this practice alone will not equip CHWs to become excellent and effective popular educators. Use of popular education in training must be accompanied by *inclusion of popular education as a discrete topic in CHW curricula* (taught using PE, of course!). PE practice should also be reinforced through *one-on-one mentoring* as CHWs begin to develop lesson plans and think through methods to share information with individual program participants. Often, this mentoring can be best done by other experienced CHWs.

Program administrators and CHW supervisors also need to *understand and support the use of popular education throughout the program*. This will usually require that the entire program staff participate together in learning about the theory and practice of popular education and the variety of ways it can be used, including use in staff meetings and in one-on-one interactions between program staff. Supervision consistent with popular education bears many similarities to reflective and trauma-informed supervision in that it emphasizes co-learning between supervisor and CHW; reflective listening and paraphrasing on the part of the supervisor; deep appreciation of the life experience, insights, and cultural worldviews that CHWs bring to their positions; and a strong emphasis on professional development (Damio, Ferraro, London, Pérez-Escamilla, & Wiggins, 2017).

By including coursework in popular education in CHW curricula, using popular education as the primary methodology for CHW capacitation, providing one-on-one mentoring for CHWs to develop their PE skills, and assuring that staff throughout the CHW program use and support PE, we can maximize the likelihood that CHWs will be able to use PE consistently and skillfully in their health education work in communities.

6.3.8   Case Studies of CHWs Sharing Health Education

In this section, we share three case studies of CHWs who use popular (people's) education to share health education and information in their work.

6.3.8.1   Case Study 1: Health Education at the Individual Level—Health Navigators of Community Health Centers of Benton and Linn Counties

Kelly Volkmann and Lizdaly Cancel Tirado
The Community Health Centers of Benton and Linn Counties ("CHC") in Benton County, Oregon, are the only comprehensive, primary healthcare service providers in the two-county area for the low-income, uninsured, underinsured, and migrant/seasonal agricultural workers (MSAW). Located in Oregon's agricultural Willamette Valley, CHC includes one dental clinic and six primary care clinics that have achieved "Tier 5 Patient-Centered Primary Care Home" status.

Meet "Maria" Maria,[3] a 67-year-old Latina woman, was diagnosed with diabetes in Mexico and came to live with her daughters in Corvallis, Oregon. Maria spoke only Spanish and established care at the Community Health Centers of Benton and Linn Counties (CHC), where her daughters had their primary care homes. When Maria was first seen at the CHC, her blood glucose readings were very unstable and were anywhere between 58 and 500 (normal is between 70 and 99). In addition, her long-term glucose test—her hemoglobin A1c, commonly known as "HbA1c or A1c"—was 9.7 (a "normal" HgA1c is below 5.7). In addition to feeling physically ill from her diabetes and unstable blood sugars, Maria said she

---

[3] Names and all identifying information have been changed to protect confidentiality.

felt like she was a burden to her children, indicating that she was at risk for depression.

Her provider took Maria's condition seriously, but did not speak Spanish. Using an interpreter, he recommended that Maria take the Diabetes Education class provided by the local hospital. Maria took the class, which was in English. There was telephonic interpretation available for the class, but Maria had difficulty hearing and understanding. The provider was also concerned about the communication challenges in her family; the daughter that brought Maria to her appointments and who spoke with the care team was not the daughter that Maria lived with, who provided Maria's meals and daily care. In spite of lengthy visits every 2 weeks, Maria was not making progress, and the provider referred Maria to Cristal, one of the bilingual, bicultural community health workers/health navigators (CHW/HN) who were part of Maria's care team.

The Health Navigation Program Beginning in 2008, the Health Navigation program at CHC has employed community health workers (CHWs) to provide culturally and linguistically appropriate outreach, referral, intake, care coordination, self-management, and follow-up services. Starting with 1 part-time, grant-funded CHW, we are now a team of 28 CHWs who function along the continuum of roles from the clinic to the community. CHWs, in the role of health navigators (CHW/HNs), work alongside the primary care team in the clinic setting, with primary care and social service agencies to provide health care and resource access, navigation, and support and with community members to provide advocacy, community capacitation, and leadership training (Fig. 6.3).

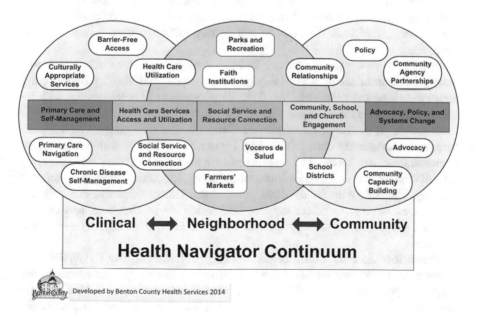

Fig. 6.3 Health navigator continuum

As CHWs, we participate in extensive training in a variety of subjects, with a special emphasis on popular education. Popular education is the foundation for the extensive self-management teaching that clinical CHWs do with our clients, both in groups and individually, and helps facilitate the personal empowerment and self-efficacy needed to make successful lifestyle changes.

As members of the primary care team, we help clients navigate the healthcare system, provide chronic disease self-management education and support, and facilitate referrals to social service and community resources. Clinical CHW/HNs work closely with registered nurse care coordinators (RNCCs) to ensure care coordination and self-management education and support for our clients. Working together, the CHWs/RNCCs are able to lace our skill sets together so that each is working at the "top half of our skills" and providing care, education, and interventions that are individually tailored for each client. This approach allows the CHW/HN, the RNCC, the client, and the client's family to work together as a unit, with the client in the middle, and increases the likelihood that the client will be engaged in the treatment plan and able to successfully implement changes.

Personalized Self-Management Education Using Popular Education Clients can participate in one-on-one chronic disease self-management education and continuous follow-ups with a CHW/HN in coordination with the certified diabetes educator, RNCC, and the rest of the primary care team: primary care providers (PCP), panel manager (PM), behaviorist (BH), and pharmacists. The level of care team involvement is based on the client's diagnoses and the number and type of factors affecting their ability to make healthy changes. Using popular education principles and strategies, we CHWs created our Chronic Disease Self-Management curriculum to uniquely adapt to the clinic population and to allow for use with different chronic conditions and cultural backgrounds. English and Spanish versions are available, and it is the base of self-management teaching across all CHC clinic sites.

In addition to the initial Chronic Disease Self-Management class, clients also have the option of taking a 2-h Diabetes Management and Healthy Eating group education class and "My Plate" cooking demonstration in collaboration with the Extension Program from Oregon State University and Las Comidas Latinas Oregon State University Nutrition Education and Outreach. The class consists of a 1-h diabetes self-management class followed by 1 h of a "My Plate" teaching and cooking demonstration. Any member of the primary care team can refer patients to the class. As CHW/HNs, we do the coordination, planning, marketing, outreach, delivery, tracking, and follow-up for the class participants. Our certified diabetes educator provides mentoring, technical support, and follow-up to clients as needed. The financial support comes directly from the CHC and the specific clinic site that hosts the class.

Remember Maria? Maria began working with Cristal, her CHW/HN, who provided care coordination and extended diabetes self-management education and support to Maria and her daughters. Cristal attended office visits with Maria and her daughter and had the time to sit with them after the visit to review the information they received. Using popular education and teach-back methods, Cristal could ensure that they understood and had input into the care plan. Cristal also met with Maria and her other daughter in their home and helped them develop some culturally and health literacy-appropriate methods of tracking blood sugar, exercise, and preparing meals.

With Cristal's assistance, Maria and her daughter attended a *Tomando Control de Su Salud* class—Stanford's chronic disease self-management class for Spanish speakers—which was such a success that the rest of the family signed up for a second workshop. In addition, Cristal made weekly follow-up phone calls with Maria, which reduced the need for frequent extended office visits and freed up the provider to see other patients.

Within 3 months of working with Cristal, Maria's blood sugar readings stabilized between 110 and 180, and her HbA1c dropped from 9.7 to 7.6. This is a level that indicates more consistent control and lower overall values of daily blood sugar and is a positive health metric. Maria's children knew more about her disease and were more understanding and supportive of her needs.

But perhaps the most important change was with Maria herself. She reported feeling healthier and having more confidence and told Cristal, her CHW/HN, that she was "enjoying her life now."

6.3.8.2 Case Study 2: Using Popular Education to Increase Health Knowledge and Leadership in the Latinx Community in Wood Village, Oregon

Teresa Campos Dominguez
Popular education is a form of education that encourages learners to examine their lives critically and take action to change their own health and social conditions. In my experience, popular education is a very effective way of increasing health knowledge at the community level.

In 2001, I started working with a Latinx faith community in Wood Village, a suburb of Portland, Oregon. Even though I come from the same culture, live in Wood Village, and have similar faith values, I was a CHW representing a governmental organization. This set me apart from the community. There was a powerful lack of trust in agencies, especially governmental organizations. The community did not access services because of their belief that governmental organizations took their information and reported it to the Immigration Department. Community members were very quiet; they did not want to know about available services nor receive information about health. They strongly believed that any help or information they might receive could be used to exterminate them or disappear them. My role was not to accept or reject this belief; instead, my role was to find out the causes of such distrust and share that information with my organization and others.

Teaching culturally appropriate health information is difficult or impossible if first we do not hear community members' concerns and build trust with the community. Community members began to tell me that in the past, many organizations came and did surveys or offered services and information but never came back to fulfill the promises they had made. Some people in the community were facing many health problems, hardships, and trauma caused by people migrating across long distances with the promise of jobs and income. Living away from your family, community, culture, and accustomed rhythms of life can make you feel lonely and homesick. Immigration issues create fear and insecurity and are related to experiences of human trafficking, crime, diabetes, kidney disease, heart disease, asthma, breast cancer, tobacco, alcoholism, stress, anxiety, panic attacks, etc.

In the Wood Village Latinx community, people are forced to work long hours at low pay and without human rights benefits because they need to earn money. When income is not certain, when unemployment threatens the survival or well-being of your whole family, this can create fear and stress for community members. When they work long hours, they do not feel motivated to attend any health education activities. Also, they can lose their connection with their families and communities and their own cultural values.

In 2002, the organization I work for was funded by the Centers for Disease Control and Prevention (CDC) to conduct a community-based participatory research project that we called Poder es Salud/Power for Health. By this time, we had already built trust. We had begun to prepare a group of Latinx faith leaders. Through the use of popular education philosophy and methodology, we were able to show faith leaders another way to really engage community to be part of their own learning process. During the Power for Health Project, we reinforced this practice even more.

In our health and leadership classes, we always started by using dinámicas. For example, we sat in a circle, and I asked participants to say their names, how many children they had or family members living here in this country, what is their state or country of origin, and how many years they have been living in this country. Sometimes I asked them to think about an animal that they remembered from their place of origin, and then we played the dinámica called "Sea, Land, and Air." In this dinámica, I throw the ball to someone, and if I say "sea," the person has to mention an animal that lives in the sea. I also applied the dinámica to their faith. For example, when I threw the ball, they had to mention something in the bible about health.

After playing the dinámica, I would always start by asking participants a question connected to their personal experiences or knowledge of the topic. If I was going to teach about diabetes, I might ask something like "Do you know someone who has experienced diabetes?" or "What would we like to know about diabetes?". Questions must be relevant for the participants. Many times educators fear that people do not know the correct information. However, one of the main ideas of popular education is that people know a lot based on their own experience. We have to believe in people's wisdom. On many occasions, there will be an opportunity to clarify information using questions and let the group discover the information or teach each other during the dialogue, instead of giving them the information. It is a powerful dance when a dialogue can happen between group participants, and the popular educator is just a facilitator during this dance. If the facilitator hears some information that is not accurate, it is an opportunity to clarify information.

After the brainstorm, I do an activity to share crucial information. I can do an educational game, a simulation, or a small sociodrama, where I can represent two or three main points that I want to emphasize so people can reflect and apply it to their own situation or their own communities. At the end of every class, I do a group evaluation, asking the group, "What did you like?" or "What did you learn?" and then "How can we improve the class?". When people say "I did not sleep in the class," that is a great sign that they were participating and engaging and felt that they learned something.

At the end of the Power for Health Program, we came back to the community to present the results of our work during the 3-year period; that helped us to continue building trust. Some of the ongoing issues that the community identified included domestic violence, teen pregnancy, youth violence and gangs, and the toxic stress that is a result of immigration raids. They believed that those were some of the reasons they were not able to control their physical health.

We tried to listen to the community concerns. So, we brought a program called "Striving to Reduce Youth Violence Everywhere" (STRYVE). STRYVE is a national initiative led by the CDC. STRYVE/Multnomah County was one of four demonstration sites in the nation. As one of its evidence-based interventions, STRYVE/Multnomah County chose Youth Empowerment Solutions (YES), a community-level violence prevention program that empowers youth to work with adults in making positive changes in their communities.

During this time, Immigration and Customs Enforcement (ICE) raids were becoming more common in our communities and that affected community participation in many activities. In order to decrease the stress and fear in the Latinx community, we wanted to work with the adolescent children of the parents we had worked with in the Power for Health Project.

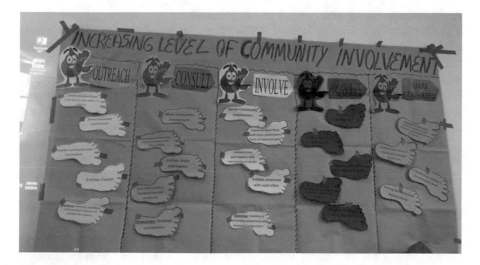

Fig. 6.4 An example of the popular education work conducted by the group in Wood Village

Originally, the parents said no, because they wanted to experience first the type of work that we were going to do with their youth. So, for about 2 years, we worked with the parents and some officers from the Multnomah County Sheriff's department who were ready and willing to be part of this process with the Latinx community. We brought together the Latinx community parents, youth, and officers. We used the same popular education methodology and philosophy (Fig. 6.4). To equalize the power among the group members, we used dinámicas. It is very powerful to see everyone playing and having fun, and the most wonderful result is building trust.

By listening we learned more about community concerns, and we assisted by finding resources and creating activities to release stress and tension. People are more willing and able to learn about their physical health when we connect physical health to all the dimension of wellness. People felt that we were listening in a holistic way. People many times feel divided if they have to learn about physical health in a way that is separate from other health dimensions, such as mental, emotional, and spiritual health. Especially in communities of faith, integrating knowledge about their faith-based values can make them commit more to their well-being.

Programs come and go, many times with communities still in the same place and sometimes with the same or more struggles. We have some community resources, but every year we are suffering budget cuts. So, for me, that is why building leadership very strategically all year long as we are teaching about health issues is important. Then when the program goes away, the leadership stays in the community to continue doing the work for the betterment of the communities.

6.3.8.3   Case Study 3: Using a Decolonizing Approach to Health and Wellness with Community Education Workers

Arika Makena Bridgeman-Bunyoli and Frances Kham
The Community Education Worker (CEW) Program began in 2014. The program emerged through the collaborative work of the Ready for Kindergarten Collaborative led by Social Venture Partners in Portland, Oregon. The purpose of the collaborative was to develop strategies for addressing the academic equity gap, commonly referred to as the achievement gap, so that low-income children of color would have an opportunity for success equal to white middle-class children. During one of these meetings, a Latina mother spoke up and mentioned that in her community *promotores* (CHWs) work with community members to address many issues in their lives. Wouldn't it be possible for *promotores* to also work with parents to help them prepare their children for kindergarten? From this point forward, the collaborative began to explore a strategy of having CHWs work with families to address the social determinants of health and educational equity. This eventually resulted in the Community Education Worker (CEW) Program.

In the first year of the pilot CEW Program, we only had enough funding to support 3.6 FTE in three cultural communities. The three original cultural communities were African American, Latinx, and Native American/Alaskan Native because these were large demographic groups in Portland that were currently and historically underserved in the local educational systems. They were experiencing egregious inequities in academic outcomes and disproportionate discipline within the schools. We believed that CHWs trained in early childhood development could work with families in our own communities to help them address the social determinants of health and educational inequities. CEWs were employed by a culturally specific organization, and all CEWs, supervisors, and community partners participated in a Steering Team that made key decisions about the project. This means that we provided culturally specific strategies and support for everything from nutrition and developmental screening, to how to advocate for your child and family with DHS or a child care provider, to how to do community organizing. We did this through home visits and parent groups in each community. While the curriculum for each culture is different, we agreed to cover some topics in every community, and we used popular education in all our efforts. Two years later, we added CEWs for the Somali/Somali Bantu communities as well as for the Zomi community and other communities from Myanmar (also called Burma). All CEWs became full time.

Since all CEWs started as CHWs, they were already grounded in the practices and principles of popular education, but the Steering Team felt it was important to fully develop a set of values for the Program as a whole. There were two reasons for this desire. The first was that many people from the community would come to the Steering Team with ideas about different projects. Core values were needed to help the Steering Team decide what to take on and not take on. The second reason was that one of the things that the Steering Team valued most highly was the opportunity to learn cross-culturally about each other's communities and devise strategies for our collective upliftment. Together, we decided that our values are parent-child engagement, popular education, equity, multiculturalism, decolonization, and systems change.

Values of the Community Education Worker Program
1. **Focus on Parent-Child Engagement**
Parent-child engagement promotes healthy bonds, positive learning opportunities, and the ability of families to work together to improve overall health.
2. **Utilization of Popular Education**
Parent-child groups and activities and socializations utilize culturally centered curriculum based in popular education.
3. **Emphasis on Equity**
Equity promotes healthy, inclusive, and culturally relevant practices to support the full integration and empowerment of refugees, immigrants, and communities of color.
4. **Promotion of Multiculturalism**
Culturally *specific* parent-child learning environments for families from the five cultural groups are complemented by the Steering Team's concurrent work to build influence *across* our communities.

5. **Support for Decolonization**
Decolonization facilitates interaction and learning in support of indigenous populations, to reclaim the value of their traditional ways and worldview.
6. **Activation for Systems Change**
Building partnerships within and across key sectors, including schools, housing, and health care, creates systems change to increase cultural responsiveness by providers serving diverse families.
7. **Kindergarten Readiness**
CEWs promote kindergarten readiness through parent-child learning activities, developmental screenings, and providing information about numeracy and literacy.

As part of this process, Alix Sanchez, who was a CEW supervisor at NAYA Family Center at the time, facilitated a "Decolonizing Parenting" training for the CEW Steering Team. At this training, all of us started to think deeply about what our communities were like before we experienced colonization, imperialism, and enslavement. In small groups we discussed how our ancestors parented before we had these experiences of oppression, how our parenting practices changed because of these experiences, what we learned from these experiences, how they helped our people survive, and whether these practices are still useful. During this first session, we were focused on exploring these questions for ourselves as CEWs, supervisors, and people in project management. This is not easy work. It takes courage to speak about the oppression that our people have endured. It took courage for the white people who were present to even remain in the room and listen to us speak of how our people used to be, the wounds that we feel, the beauty of our cultures which often goes uncelebrated, and how all of this is perpetuated onto the families that we serve. Some of us have come to think of some parenting practices as the way that things are done within our cultural communities, but often when we look at it more deeply, we recognize that these are practices that our people adopted to help our children survive war, colonization, Jim Crow, occupation, genocide, and more. We must ask ourselves "What is worth keeping and celebrating and what must be changed for our children to thrive in the generations to come?".

Decolonization became one of our core values, and as a Steering Team, we committed to pair decolonizing thought and methodology with popular education to guide our work. In our definition we say that "Decolonization facilitates interaction and learning in support of indigenous populations, to reclaim the value of their traditional ways and world view."

Then we decided to add a lesson on decolonizing parenting to the curriculum for every cultural group. During the first year that this was in place, our project manager visited with our culturally specific teams to support their lesson planning on this topic and to think with them about how to facilitate a session on decolonizing parenting using popular education. Sometimes this involved a lot of co-teaching. For example, our project manager is an African American woman, and when she met with the Zomi CEW, a man from Myanmar, both people had to ask a lot of questions to understand the history of their two communities in order to understand where to begin to plan activities around decolonization. There was no way for the project manager to be able to brainstorm potential dinámicas about this topic with the CEW without first understanding something about the history of colonization and oppression in Myanmar. Furthermore, it was important for the project manager to hear the story from the perspective of the CEW himself, not a story from the perspective of "experts" from the United States or Europe. This would not give her the information needed about where he and the parents in the program where starting from. Likewise, the CEW needed to understand something about what decolonization means in a US context and the positionalities of indigenous and Black people in the United States who are not immigrants, but do not have the status of people from dominant culture. Decolonization means separating ourselves from internalized messages about ourselves and our people that were given to us by people and systems that were designed to disenfranchise our communities and replacing those messages with values and beliefs that center the well-being of our communities and families. To do that we must first tell our stories; we must know ourselves.

After the launching of the Decolonizing Parenting lessons, we began to get many requests to facilitate this training with other home visitors who work with families in our communities. In addition, there were many discussions about how to create pathways for professional development for child care providers of color. We began to develop the idea of creating a CEW certification which would be a set of trainings that CHWs, home visitors, and/or parent educators could take to learn the CEW model. Latino Network, one of the culturally specific organizations in the collaborative, agreed to be the lead agency on a grant to create a CEW certification. We were able to secure funding from the Portland Children's Levy and planned a 60-h training. This training took place in January and February of 2019, and we are working to be able to offer this training again to early childhood educators in Oregon who want to learn this model. We hope that the training will provide a vehicle to bring CEW values—including the value of shared life experience—into other institutions in the early childhood education field.

6.3.9 Conclusion

In this section, we reviewed the spectrum of health education approaches and then provided an introduction to popular/people's education, which we view as the approach to education most consistent with the history and philosophy of the CHW model. As part of that introduction, we discussed how, when practiced intentionally, PE can be trauma-informed, culturally centered, and decolonizing. Next, we provided some recommendations for building CHWs' capacity to use PE, including providing coursework in popular education as part of CHW curricula, using popular education as the primary methodology for CHW capacitation, providing one-on-one mentoring for CHWs to develop their PE skills, and assuring that staff throughout the CHW program use and support PE. Through three case studies, we showed how CHWs and CEWs currently use popular education to increase knowledge about health and other topics at the individual, group, and community levels.

A central theme of all our case studies, and of the practice of CHWs and CEWs who use popular education, is the importance of truly valuing the knowledge that people, and especially people in marginalized communities, already possess, drawing it out, and using it as the basis for efforts to create change. This is equally true whether CHWs are helping an individual like Maria to control her diabetes, working with a community to gain more control over their own lives and health, or working with one another to understand experiences of colonization and oppression.

References

Calori, C., Hart, J., Tein, N., & Burres, S. (2010). *Exploring the integration of CHWs as integral team members of the public health workforce: A brief summary*. Washington, DC: National Heart, Lung, and Blood Institute, National Institutes of Health, US Department of Health and Human Services.

Chatterton, P. (2008). Using geography to teach freedom and defiance: Lessons in social change from 'autonomous geographies'. *Journal of Geography in Higher Education, 32*(3), 419–440.

Chilcoat, G. W., & Ligon, J. A. (1994). Developing democratic citizens: The Mississippi freedom schools as a model for social studies instruction. *Theory and Research in Social Education, 22*, 128–175.

Cochran, P. L., Marshall, C. A., Garcia-Downing, C., Kendell, E., Cook, D., McCubbin, L., et al. (2008). Indigenous ways of knowing: Implications for participatory research and community. *American Journal of Public Health, 98*, 22–27.

Crowther, J. (1999). Popular education and the struggle for democracy. In J. Crowther, I. Martin, & M. Shaw (Eds.), *Popular education and social movements in Scotland today* (pp. 29–40). Leicester: NIACE.

Damio, G., Ferraro, M., London, K., Pérez-Escamilla, R., & Wiggins, N. (2017). *Addressing social determinants of health through community health workers: A call to action*. Hartford, CT: Hispanic Health Council Policy Brief.

Delp, L., Outman-Kramer, M., Schurman, S. J., & Wong, K. (2002). *Teaching for a change: Popular education and the labor movement*. Los Angeles: Center for Labor Research and Education and the George Meany Center for Labor Studies.

Freire, P. (1973). *Education for critical consciousness*. New York: Continuum.

Freire, P. (2003). *Pedagogy of the oppressed*. New York: Continuum.

Gómez, M., & Puiggrós, A. (1986). *La educación popular en América Latina 1*. Mexico, D.F.: Secretaria de Educación Pública.

hooks, B. (2003). *Teaching community: A pedagogy of hope*. New York/London: Routledge.

Horton, M. (2003). In D. Jacobs (Ed.), *The Miles Horton reader: Education for social change*. Knoxville: The University of Tennessee Press.

Kawakami, A. J., Aton, K., Cram, F., Lai, M. K., & Porima, L. (2007). Improving the practice of evaluation through indigenous values and methods: Decolonizing evaluation practice returning the gaze from Hawai'i and Aotearoa. *Hūlili: Multidisciplinary Research on Hawaiian Well-Being, 4*(1), 319–348.

Knowles, M. (1988). *The modern practice of adult education: From pedagogy to andragogy*. Englewood Cliffs, NJ: Cambridge Adult Education.

Lortie, D. (1975). *Schoolteacher: A sociological study*. Chicago, IL: University of Chicago Press.

Morelli, P. T., & Mataira, P. J. (2010). Indigenizing evaluation research: A long-awaited paradigm shift. *Journal of Indigenous Voices in Social Work, 1*(2010), 1–12.

Rahman, M. A. (1991). The theoretical standpoint of PAR. In O. Fals-Borda & M. A. Rahman (Eds.), *Action and knowledge: Breaking monopoly with participatory action research* (pp. 3–12). New York: Apex Press.

Thomas, M. K. (2018). *Life through their lens: A photo collection by Amish and Mennonite communities* (Vol. I). Whipple, OH: Center for Appalachia Research in Cancer Education.

Tippett, K. (2013, March 28). *John Lewis—the art and discipline of non-violence [Interview]*. Retrieved from http://www.onbeing.org/program/john-lewis-on-the-art-and-discipline-of-nonviolence/5126.

Tuhiwai Smith, L. (1999). *Decolonizing methodologies: Research and indigenous peoples*. New York, NY: St. Martin's Press.

Wallerstein, N. (2006). *What is the evidence on effectiveness of empowerment to improve health?* Copenhagen: WHO Regional Office for Europe. Health Evidence Network Report: Retrieved February 01, 2006, from http://www.euro.who.int/Document/E88086.pdf.

Walters, S., & Manicom, L. (Eds.). (1996). *Gender in popular education: Methods for empowerment*. London: Zed Books.

Wang, Y., Chao, C. Y., & Liao, H. (2011). Poststructural feminist pedagogy in English instruction. *Higher Education, 61*, 109–139. https://doi.org/10.1007/s10734-010-9327-5

Wiggins, N. (2012). Popular education for health promotion and community empowerment: A review of the literature. *Health Promotion International, 27*, 356–371. https://doi.org/10.1093/heapro/dar046

Wiggins, N., Hughes, A., Rios-Campos, T., Rodriguez, A., & Potter, C. (2014). *La Palabra es Salud* (The Word is Health): Combining mixed methods and CBPR to understand the comparative effectiveness of popular and conventional education. *Journal of Mixed Methods Research, 8*, 278–298. https://doi.org/10.1177/1558689813510785

Wiggins, N., Johnson, D., Avila, M., Farquhar, S. A., Michael, Y. L., Rios, T., & López, A. (2009). Using popular education for community empowerment: perspectives of Community Health Workers in the Poder es Salud/Power for Health program. *Critical Public Health, 19*, 11–22.

Wiggins, N., Kaan, S., Rios-Campos, T., Gaonkar, R., Rees-Morgan, E., & Robinson, J. (2013). Preparing community health workers for their role as agents of social change: Experience of the community capacitation center. *Journal of Community Practice, 21*(3).

Chapter 7
Care Coordination, Case Management, and System Navigation

Caitlin G. Allen*, J. Nell Brownstein, S. Kim Bush*, Cecil H. Doggette, Durrell J. Fox, Paige Menking, Judith Palfrey, Kate Philley Starnes, Aubry D. Threlkeld*, and DelAnne Zeller

7.1 Introduction

Caitlin G. Allen, Durrell J. Fox, J. Nell Brownstein, and Paige Menking

The third core role, care coordination, case management, and systems navigation, was originally derived from the role "assuring people get the services they need." This role expanded to incorporate terms that are commonly used in

---

Authorship is organized alphabetically in ascending order by surname.

C. G. Allen (✉)
CGA Consulting, Charleston, SC, USA
e-mail: caitlin.gloeckner.allen@emory.edu

J. N. Brownstein
Texas Tech Health Sciences Center El Paso, El Paso, TX, USA

S. K. Bush (✉) · K. P. Starnes · D. A. Zeller
The University of Texas Health Science Center at Tyler, Tyler, TX, USA
e-mail: Sonja.Bush@uthct.edu

C. H. Doggette
Health Services for Children with Special Needs, Washington, DC, USA

D. J. Fox
JSI Research and Training, Inc, Atlanta, GA, USA

P. Menking
University of New Mexico Health Science Center, Albuquerque, NM, USA

J. Palfrey
Harvard Medical School and Boston Children's Hospital, Boston, MA, USA

A. D. Threlkeld (✉)
Endicott College, Beverly, MA, USA
e-mail: athrelke@endicott.edu

© Springer Nature Switzerland AG 2021
J. A. St. John et al. (eds.), *Promoting the Health of the Community*,
https://doi.org/10.1007/978-3-030-56375-2_7

healthcare and public health settings. The role expanded organically over the years based on changing client needs, changing systems of care, and workforce ability/capacity. Other major changes include the addition of two new sub-roles from the 1998 National Community Health Advisor Study.[i] The five sub-roles are participating in care coordination and/or case management; making referrals and providing follow-up; facilitating transportation; documentation and tracking of data; and informing people and systems about community assets and challenges.

Care coordination can be defined as, "the deliberate organization of patient care activities between two and more participants (including the patient) involved in patient's care to facilitate the appropriate delivery of healthcare services. Organizing care involves marshaling of personnel and other resources needed to carry out all required patient care activities and is often managed by the exchange of information among participants responsible for care."[ii] Care coordination is closely aligned with case management, which is defined as "a collaborative process of assessment, planning, and facilitation, care coordination, evaluation, and advocacy for opinions and services to meet a family's comprehensive health needs through communication and available resources to promote quality, cost-effective outcomes."[iii] Care coordination is also aligned with system navigation, which is a role focused on helping individuals and families who may have difficulty accessing and navigating the complex US healthcare and human service delivery systems.

Shifting toward formally defining "care coordination, case management, and system navigation" rather than the original role of "assuring people get the services they need" reflects a broader shift in health care via healthcare reform and transformation. The focus on value-based payments (rewarding providers for the quality of the care they provide) and patient-centered medical homes (a care delivery model in which primary care physicians coordinate patient treatment in a timely manner) has created incentives for systems to meet quality and cost targets. Additionally, accountable care and capitated payment models are allowing for the payment of nonclinical services (e.g., care coordination) via global and bundled payments. Overall, acknowledgement of the complexities of the healthcare system and the need to address broader issues (i.e., social determinants of health) have led to increased attention to the need for care coordination in healthcare systems—a role particularly well-suited for community health workers (CHWs).

This chapter highlights two examples of care coordination by describing the process of developing a patient care navigation system in a large healthcare organization and discussing the unique role CHWs play in assisting with care coordination for families with special healthcare needs.

---

[i] https://crh.arizona.edu/sites/default/files/pdf/publications/CAHsummaryALL.pdf

[ii] https://www.ahrq.gov/research/findings/evidence-based-reports/caregaptp.html

[iii] https://www.cmsa.org/who-we-are/what-is-a-case-manager/

7.2   Establishing a Patient Care Navigation System

S. Kim Bush, Kate Philley Starnes, and DelAnne Zeller

7.2.1   Introduction

The role of community health workers (CHWs) varies in different settings; however, when a group of CHWs was asked to describe in their own words what being a CHW means to them, several of them claimed, it's all about helping others. The group of CHWs described their work as making a difference by helping others. Family Practice Clinic CHW, Malinda Robertson, stated, "what I like about being a CHW is it is both challenging and rewarding. I get to assist people in need and that is what is meaningful to me." Another Family Practice Clinic CHW, Monica Johnigan, stated, "I love being a CHW, because I get to change lives for the better." As a CHW and a CHW instructor, it is important think about the role of CHWs and how we empower others and, more specifically, how to navigate the complex and ever-changing healthcare system. Completing various forms and applications for insurance, medication refills, or referrals to specialists can be extremely daunting for patients and families to access the care they need. In 2013, responding to the need, the University of Texas Health Science Center at Tyler (UTHSCT) invested in utilizing CHWs across the institution. UTHSCT placed CHWs in both specialty and primary care clinics along with the emergency department and hospital. In addition, UTHSCT utilized CHWs to promote and increase awareness for colon cancer screenings and chronic disease management within the community. UTHSCT implemented multiple models; however, this section will focus on the patient care navigation model of pre-visit planning. This section walks through how UTHSCT utilizes CHWs in this model and provides an overview of the system, successes, challenges, and lessons learned. Next, the section highlights how one CHW assists families as part of her role in helping children with asthma. The section ends with personal stories from UTHSCT CHWs and the impact a CHW has not only on patients but also on the CHW providing the service.

7.2.2   Description of Geographic Location/Population

UTHSCT is the sole academic hospital in Northeast Texas. An estimated 1.5 million people call Northeast Texas home, with 55% living in rural areas (Nehme et al., 2016). The majority of these rural areas have no primary care or, at the very least, they have limited healthcare access (University of Wisconsin Population Health Institute, 2017). For the last decade, key partners worked to assess the need of the

Northeast Texas population. Starting in 2007, the Texas Department of State Health Services (DSHS) undertook an East Texas Community Health Needs Assessment (ETCHNA) to document the scale of health issues in the region. This assessment, combined with an additional assessment in 2012 as part of the Texas 1115 Medicaid Waiver program, identified six distinct community needs (CNs) for Northeast Texas: (1) insufficient access to primary and specialty services; (2) insufficient access to mental/behavioral healthcare services; (3) high rates of chronic disease, including diabetes, heart disease, asthma, obesity, and cancer; (4) high costs due to potentially preventable hospital admissions/readmissions; (5) inappropriate emergency department utilization; and (6) efficiency in and effectiveness of healthcare delivery (Regional Healthcare Partnership [RHP] 1, 2012, updated 2018). Nehme et al. (2016) identifies Northeast Texas as outranking the entire state in the top five leading causes of death including heart disease, cancer, chronic lower respiratory diseases, stroke, and unintentional injuries such as motor vehicle accidents. Without proper access to care, self-management education, and efforts to improve health literacy, individuals will continue to utilize the emergency department (ED) as a source of primary care as opposed to establishing a medical home (DSHS, 2007; Kangovi et al., 2017). Based off the data and identified needs, UTHSCT designed and implemented a patient navigation system utilizing CHWs in primary care focusing on pre-visit planning.

7.2.3   Implementation from the Front Lines

DelAnne Zeller, RN, the Director of Cultural Development and Nursing Process at UTHSCT, served as the Internal Medicine Nurse Manager during the time the clinics first engaged CHWs. The following section outlines the implementation and development of pre-visit planning from DelAnne's experienced perspective from the front lines.

7.2.3.1   Phase 1: Can We Improve Quality of Care?

An experienced internist at UTHSCT posed the following question to me in 2012, "I want to improve the quality of care I provide by ensuring patients who are eligible have required colon and mammogram screening. Do you think a nurse can help with this?" Following this conversation, we developed an initial process whereby a registered nurse reviewed colon screening, mammograms, and pneumococcal vaccinations due to educated patients and solicited their authorization to enter orders on the day of the patient appointment. This process resulted in enhanced communication between patient and physician about preventive testing and immunizations recommended; however, this labor-intensive process sometimes impeded patient flow. To improve the clinic flow, we planned to perform this intervention and education *before the day of the visit*, which resulted in the concept of a "pre-visit planning team." Our inability to identify human resources, telephone the patient before their appointment, discuss care gaps, provide education, and seek the patient's approval to schedule follow-up testing/immunizations served as a barrier to this innovation.

In the fall of 2013, UTHSCT hired and trained individuals from the community as CHWs. Approximately 20 years ago, Texas passed legislation requiring individuals employed as a CHW to be a certified CHW. There are two ways to obtain certification: (1) complete a 160-h CHW certification course based on eight core competencies from a DSHS-approved CHW training site or (2) gain certification through previous work experience (1000 h within 6 years) verified and approved by DSHS. Furthermore, while in preparation of deployment to clinics, CHWs received additional training from physicians, nurses, human resources, and community resource agencies. Prior to clinic implementation, CHWs began to teach health education classes such as Diabetes Education Empowerment Program (DEEP) and heart health workshops. UTHSCT integrated CHW teams into designated clinics during early 2014. We assigned teams to specific clinics including (1) internal medicine clinic; (2) four family medicine clinics; and (3) two specialty clinics, pulmonary and cardiology. We designed an electronic template for CHWs to complete as part of the patient's electronic health record.

7.2.3.2   Phase 2: Introduction of the Community Health Workers

The CHW concept remained unclear to nurses and providers, and the lack of clarity and understanding resulted in a learning curve to truly understand how to utilize the CHW skill set. The idea that a CHW could provide support to help patients achieve good health practices and health improvement and facilitate health promotion intrigued clinic staff. With the new knowledge of the potential role of CHWs, the internal medicine leadership team created the first "pre-visit team" patient-centered care model consisting of an LVN and CHW medically directed by the physician and supervised by the nurse manager. We purposely opted to have CHWs and LVNs share an office to imbed them within the clinic so that they became members of a multidisciplinary team (Physician, RN, LVN, and CHW). We quickly identified the need for communication and collaboration among all members of the patient care team to effectively support, engage, and close care gaps. The following represents the basic framework for our model.

Pre-visit Workflow

1. Five to 7 days prior to the patient visit, the pre-visit LVN researches, reviews, and documents on a pre-visit worksheet on the current evidenced-based preventative patient care gaps using physician's standing delegation orders such as immunizations, colon screening, mammograms, etc.
2. The LVN passes the above information to the pre-visit CHW who contacts the patient regarding the appointment date and care gaps and provides education and seeks the patient's approval to schedule follow-up testing/immunizations. The CHW asks the patients about their history of any preventive testing/immuniza-

tions, recent hospitalizations, and ED visits, documents these items, and requests medical records from outside hospitals/clinics.

3. If the CHW requires assistance from the pre-visit LVN regarding patient's healthcare questions, they can immediately pass the telephone to the pre-visit LVN to provide more in-depth explanation about the need for preventive testing/immunizations. This is important as the CHW becomes even more skilled in educating the patients about the testing/immunizations. CHWs also explain to patients the option of speaking directly with their physician on the day of the visit.

4. Next the CHW reviews the payer source and provides assistance to patients that are self-paid or unfunded by explaining their options and assists them with signing up for programs. CHWs offer assistance with patient portal sign up, transportation, medical supply, and medications as needed.

5. CHWs reach out within 72 h of discharge to patients who have been hospitalized or had an emergency room visit to ensure they have a follow-up appointment with their primary care provider and have transportation to their visit. This improves continuity of care.

6. Utilizing the patient preferences and history gleaned from the CHW interaction above, the pre-visit LVN enters orders and medical information into the electronic health record.

7. On the day of the visit, the CHW delivers the pre-visit worksheets to the physician and nurse team at the beginning of the day. The team initiates a patient safety huddle and reviews the pre-visit worksheet (daily schedule review), noting follow-up patient needs, gaps in care, recent hospitalizations, hospital readmissions, and ED visits.

7.2.4 Pilot Results

Development of this pre-visit planning process in the internal medicine clinic has led to improvement compliance in preventive services and closing the care gaps. For example:

1. Mammogram screening quality measures improvement from 63.79% in 2015 to 81.26% as of May 2017.

2. Pneumococcal vaccination quality measures improvement from 85.68%, in 2015 to 97.81% as of May 2017.

3. Colon screening quality measures improvement from 27.39% in June 2016 to 73.67% as of May 2017.

At completion of the pilot project and after quality data review, the chief nursing officer congratulated the pre-visit team and the frontline staff for their success: "This is great confirmation of the hard work you and your team are doing. Great job. Thank you!"

7.2.4.1   Phase 3: Scaling Up to Other Primary Care Sites

In June 2016, the Department of Healthcare Quality noted the scores for the internal medicine clinic was 18.25% higher on average than other primary care practices. Due to the success of the pre-visit planning program's pilot, the chief medical officer and chief nursing officer championed the expansion of the model and recommended the institution to implement the internal medicine clinic pre-visit model in five other primary care practices.

7.2.5   Successes

Success has truly been an effort of relationship building. We continue to remind ourselves that open communication serves as a key factor in achieving success in general. Communication must remain fluid with all stakeholders involved such as clinical leadership, nursing management, administrative staff, and community partners. Furthermore, collaboration with others provides additional resources and networking creating an environment of knowledge and resources. In addition, appropriate team member recruitment is essential to retention and overall performance. Since inauguration of this program, improved communication resulted in an increase of referrals to CHW teams as illustrated in the chart below. Figure 7.1 depicts each year referrals have grown exponentially from 113 during 2013 to over 5000 in 2017.

Providers send referrals to CHW teams in an electronic format; however, a warm hand-off may be necessary from provider to CHW to mitigate time. CHWs document their assessment and work in an electronic template that stores information in the patient's electronic medical record. UTHSCT's information technology team

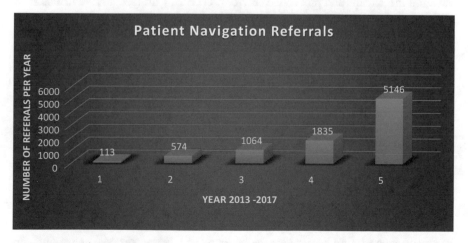

Fig. 7.1 Patient navigation referrals

built a report to track referrals and types of assistance CHW teams provide. This report also links the type of assistance provided by each referral with specific target population criteria such as poor health literacy skills, poor self-management skills, lack of resources, and identified barriers to care, for example, medication assistance. During 2017, approximately 800 patients received application assistance for Medicaid, Medicare Savings Programs, Health Insurance, and local grants that cover primary care services.

Comments the CHWs received from patients during the pre-visit calls included:

1. "It makes me feel good to know someone is looking out for me. I am getting older and I need all the help I can get!"
2. "Oh, I didn't realize it was time for my mammogram. I guess I got busy and forgot. Thank you for reminding me."
3. "Thank you so much for reminding me it is time for my flu shot! I have to stay healthy because I take care of my husband who has Alzheimer's. Can my husband get a flu shot when I come for my appointment also?"

7.2.6 Challenges

Change often presents challenges in a clinical environment. Since the CHW concept was new to medical providers, educating and obtaining buy-in of the nurses and physicians regarding the potential role of the CHW proved difficult. Clinical staff failed to grasp how CHWs offered an extension of the provider and nurse and could save providers time by communicating with patients. Over time concerns were alleviated through routine communication and supporting data. Clinical teams fully supported the CHW role and its impact on clinic flow and patient care.

Another challenge came in scripting for and educating patients in the need to have routine screens and preventive services. UTHSCT utilized CHWs in a clinical setting, where previously CHWs had often served in the community and were accustomed to spending hours with patients. The pre-visit planning offered a new opportunity for CHWs to assist patients, but the need for education existed. Finally, the last challenge was accessing real-time accurate data showing progress in achieving the goal of patient-centered care gap closures.

7.2.7 Lessons Learned

As with all new programs, sharing lessons learned throughout the process is important. First and foremost, having the involvement and support from senior leadership is vital to the success of this type of a program. Equally important, the clinical team must believe in and value quality improvement. The team needs to agree that there is always opportunity to provide better care and better service to patients. In speaking of "team," the clinical staff must work as a team. This strategy requires all players for the clinic to operate efficiently and effectively.

Further, we learned having a CHW available for consult and warm hand-off from a nurse/physician team regarding transportation, medication assistance, insurance eligibility, etc. is the best strategy. This further builds the rapport between a CHW and his or her patient. Cross-training of other members on the team to assist when the primary CHW is not available is another key lesson learned.

7.2.8 CHW Highlight

The reach of a CHW knows no boundaries, and time is not a factor since most CHWs are not driven by volume or service provided. More often than not, assisting one patient with a very specific need will open the door to opportunities to assist in other areas. Furthermore, opportunities for additional assistance often occur when CHWs work with pediatric populations. Moreover, UTHSCT deploys a mobile pediatric asthma clinic that travels to schools to help diagnose and treat children with asthma. After a short period of time, we found this clinic team needed someone who could assist patients with reducing barriers to care. Even though the mobile clinic eliminated the transportation and cost barrier, significant barriers remained that impacted the patients' abilities to self-manage their chronic disease.

Imagine a young mother and father with four children—all who attend the same school. For years, the children had breathing problems, often waking up at night coughing and unable to breathe. The young family could not afford to take their children to the doctor due to lack of insurance. One day, the young mother receives a flyer in her child's backpack asking three questions about asthma screenings. After answering "yes" to all three questions, the mother signs the form and schedules all four of her children for appointments on the free mobile clinic.

The mobile clinic arrived one early February morning at the small, rural school in a town with a population less than 1000 people. Due to the cold, the children seemed to be sicker than usual. The mom, with four young children in tow, arrived at the mobile clinic for 2 h of scheduled appointments. The clinic team quickly went to work taking health histories and performing spirometry on each child. As the appointments came to an end, the young mother now had two children with an asthma diagnosis. While grateful for the service, the mother was at a loss on what to do next. The nurse practitioner began to order medications for the children but quickly informed by the CHW of the family's uninsured status. This is often a common occurrence, so the provider tried to find free "samples," but did not have any the children could use. The CHW spoke with the mother at length and felt the children would qualify for Medicaid. Unfortunately, the family had no access to Internet to apply nor did they fully understand the forms or the requisite information needed to complete the forms. The CHW advised the mom of the documentation and said she would help complete the forms. The mom returned to the mobile clinic that afternoon and, with full assistance from the CHW, applied for Medicaid. After 2 weeks, the mom called the CHW with the great news that all children qualified for Medicaid, and she picked up the needed medications for her children.

While assistance in insurance enrollment is vital to a child receiving medication, there are other services that greatly impact quality of life for an asthmatic. What if mold is an asthma trigger and a child's bedroom is covered in mold? What if a home is infested with cockroaches? How do families on a fixed income afford the cost to exterminate or remove mold?

One day in late May, a mother brought her child to an appointment on the mobile clinic. The last 2 months had been unbearably hot, causing her electric bill to sky-rocket. What was she going to do with summer ahead? She confided to the CHW that she could not afford to pay her electric bill, and the CHW immediately thought about an available assistance program. The CHW helped the mother complete the application and faxed the application to the appropriate office. The CHW acted dili-gently and called to confirm receipt of the application at which point she received notification a key piece was missing from the application. The CHW relayed the missing information to the mom who sent the information immediately to complete the application. By early June, the mother received notice of qualifying for $400 toward her electric bill, which automatically enrolled her in the current bill program allowing assistance to help pay any extra fees if the electric bill is over a certain amount. Money saved allowed the family to make minor repairs around their home to help improve their child's asthma.

In addition to supporting families, the *Breath of Life* program CHW provides education to patients focused on self-management. She is in routine contact with the provider and nurse to ensure the patient is compliant and to assist in helping with medication adherence or simply a follow-up call to check on the patient's well-being.

7.2.9   Personal Stories

7.2.9.1   Zoila Morales, CHW, Breath of Life Mobile Pediatric Asthma Clinic

My personal life experiences and working in the community influenced my decision to become a CHW. At the age of 28, I acquired a new role as a single mother of four. I faced many challenges such as not being able to pay bills, purchase groceries for my family, and transportation. I never knew that life could get so difficult, even for the necessities that we need to live daily. Because of this, I was forced to let go of my pride and search for any assistance I could find. Luckily, my daughter Lissette qualified for the Head Start program, and we were assigned a Family Service Worker. This Family Service Worker impacted my life in many different ways. Her outlook on life and positive attitude quickly rubbed off on me. She was well-known in the community and earned the trust of everyone that she came in contact with. She empowered me to be the person I am today. Not only did she help me to initiate goals for myself and family, she supported me through them. As a result of this, I became a Family Service Worker for Tyler ISD Head Start in 2004.

I was able to work with over 2000 families in Tyler, Texas. This was one of the most rewarding jobs that I've ever had. This position helped me learn that these families needed compassion, patience, and guidance through their difficult times in their lives, which it quickly reminded me that I once walked in those same shoes. Doing home visits, family partnership agreements with my families raised awareness of the many needs in our community. Because of this, I became informed of many resources that are available to underserved individuals.

After 8 years with Tyler ISD, I was offered a career opportunity with Region 7 ESC Head Start. I accepted the position as a Program Compliance Interpreter. This opportunity opened many doors for me in many more counties. However, this job was more challenging because I was able to provide a voice to families but not able to assist them with the services they needed.

In 2013, I read an article about CHWs and that it was a growing career in Texas. It really inspired me to learn more. I knew it was the perfect career for me because it was doing what I personally love to do, which is to help people. I applied for the CHW position with UTHSCT Pediatric Asthma Mobile Clinic, and I was offered the position and accepted it. I completed the CHW certification course and officially became certified in December 2013. I am still a CHW today. I absolutely love my job. Not many people believe me when I tell them that, but it's the honest truth. It has brought many satisfactions to my life.

The people that I work with are also inspirations to me. I learn from them every day. Being able to work with people that have the same values and ambitions as myself makes my job even better. Also my supervisor supports me in everything that is needed to assist our families. I would not be able to do what I do without her. She is a great leader.

I honestly feel that God has given me a special gift to help others in my native language, Spanish and English. I am so blessed to be able to serve His people.

7.2.9.2 Jennifer Berry, CHW, Primary Care Clinic

I have worked as a CHW for almost 2 years; during this time, I have been blessed to help several individuals. Some patients I may only have one or two interactions with, but there have been some that I work with for months or years.

Previously I worked in a private preschool as a teacher, so in some ways, I have always had the heart of a CHW.

My very first home visit was with an older gentleman who lived all alone and didn't have any family who lived in the state. I was told he was cranky and noncompliant. The patient and I were able to form a great relationship and he allowed me to help him. He would call me sometimes weekly, especially when he was particularly confused. I was able to find a home health provider that showed him respect and helped him to live out his final days at home. I was his advocate when they took away his liquid oxygen, and he was miserable on a concentrator. With the help of his nurse, we found a company that could supply him with liquid oxygen. I would talk to his sons with his permission and keep them informed on his status. He was cranky, but he will always hold a special place in my memory.

Another patient I was able to help was a husband and wife. They are your average middle class retired couple—having to choose between medication and paying bills. No one had ever told him about Medicare Savings Program or extra help with medication. We filled out every application. They were approved for extra help; he came back to the office so very thankful. He said if they had been anywhere else, they wouldn't have received that kind of help.

7.2.9.3 Pam Thurman-Ford, CHW, Primary Care Clinic

Every day in the life of a CHW comes with different types of situations, and each day is driven by the patients' needs. There are routine events such as transportation, food, and medication referrals and then you get the one referral that kicks you in gear and makes your adrenalin flow. November 2017, I received a referral from the provider I work with requesting support for her patient that had been diagnosed with a very aggressive breast cancer. The referral was submitted because the patient had canceled several appointments that her provider had ordered for follow-up. These appointments included a biopsy to confirm the findings from her routine mammogram and stage the cancer diagnosis.

I reviewed the patient's file and noticed that she had insurance coverage but did not quite understand why the patient was not seeking the follow-up that was needed to ensure a successful outcome for her diagnosis. I called the patient but she was not available. I left her a message, and she did not return my call by the close of business day. The next day I tried to contact the patient and received her voicemail. My assumption was I was either dealing with someone in denial or the financial burden was too much for the patient to handle. Either way I had a job to convince this person to make this a priority without crossing the line of telling the patient that death is imminent if the care is not received. Knowing this situation could go very badly if I did not get in touch with the patient soon, I began to review and call all numbers we had on file for the patient and finally received an answer at her employer. I asked to speak to the patient and the lady on the phone stated that she was out of the office. She asked if I would leave a message for the patient and I responded, "Please have her contact her doctor's office as soon as she gets this message; ask for Pam." The lady continued to state that the patient had gotten a diagnosis, and she was not sure of how to pay for the procedures. Concerned for HIPPA, I hesitated to discuss any aspect of the diagnosis with this person; however, I told the lady to tell the patient that I could possibly help her with this situation, but I need to speak to her to discuss services needed. Later in my shift, I received a call from the patient, and the relationship was established.

The conversation began with me trying to get an understanding of her diagnosis. During this process, the patient expressed understanding that the follow-up was a vital part of her treatment and wanted to pursue the treatment, but she would not be able to pay the $1800.00 co-pay and deductible until after the beginning of the year. I explained that we might be able to get assistance for her if she would be willing to fill out paperwork and contact the locations to see if she would qualify for their programs. The patient took the information and assured me she would follow-up on the leads.

Understanding a patient always has the right to refuse to seek help is important, and I always give them time to think about the resources offered because they are dealing with the shock of the diagnosis, what is next, and not knowing what tomorrow holds. One week later, I called the patient to follow up on the progress of the assistance. She informed me that she applied for assistance through the program I provided her and she did not qualify because she was over the income limit due to approximately a $200 Christmas bonus she received from her employer. She also shared that she used the bonus to provide Christmas for her family not knowing she would be facing this situation. The organization told her to come back next month, and they will review her finances to see if she could qualify with a different check stub reflecting the change in income. In the meantime, I advised the patient to go to a local health clinic that provided basic care and access to more advanced care for people that work at least 20 h/week to see if they offer assistance since she was considered underinsured. I also advised her to reach out to Ross Breast Center and the Cancer Society to see if these agencies had any assistance programs that might be able to help her gain the needed assistance.

February 2018, I called the patient to pre-visit for her return to clinic visit. We discussed her pre-visits items, and I followed up on the breast cancer care. She informed me that she was off work with a knot under her arm which was hurting so bad she could not wear a bra. I began to question if the knot was on the same side that the breast issue was, and she stated it was. I put the patient on hold and consulted with her primary care provider. The provider advised me to get patient scheduled for evaluation visit the next day. Unsure if the cancer had spread or metastasized, I worked with our scheduling team to get her scheduled to see the provider. The patient kept the appointment, and I did not hear anything from her after this visit. I found that I was praying in my personal life for this patient and other patients that I encountered with difficult situations. I always asked God to provide me with the tools I needed to assist anyone that come in contact with me.

March 2018, I was making pre-visit phone calls when I noticed that the patient's biopsy appointments were rescheduled. I was so excited, as if I had gotten news on a family member. I called the patient to discuss pre-visit items for her primary care office visit, and I utilized this call to have discussions with the patient about other appointments that have been recommended by the provider and other referring physicians. The patient stated that she only had $700.00 dollars and that she was going to seek care at another agency in our area. Knowing this could result in lost revenue, I encouraged her to do so even though I knew I had a responsibility to represent my agency. The patient's life is as important to me as the reputation of our agency. What would I expect if it was me or my family member in this situation? I evaluated the situation and assured the patient that her provider would support any decision that she made and would be glad to send any referrals and documentation that is needed to expedite the process to the provider of her choice. "Our concern is that you get the follow-up care that is needed to ensure you have a long and healthy life." At that moment, the outcome was more important than the ownership of the patient's care. I knew the patient needed our support rather than our need to be the one providing the care. Knowing the role and when to transition the role helped this patient to receive the immediate help that was needed. The patient was able to seek care and completed her biopsy to get the cancer staged, and now the cancer providers would be able to create a plan of care to address the diagnosis.

The patient informed me that she planned to seek her treatment at UT MD Anderson clinic, and I know she feels very confident in the care that her primary care provider has given her. Some might say that my decision to support this patient's decision took revenue from our agency; however, this actually increased our revenue over the long term because the patient had the confidence in knowing that our agency is willing to put the patient's needs first. The lesson to take away from this story is that caring for patients is first and foremost the reason we are in this business. If we allow the bottom line to overshadow caring for the patient, our actions could be detrimental to our patients and ultimately harm our agency through increased morbidity rates in areas that can be prevented. This story is only one of the many rewarding stories that I have experienced as a patient service coordinator/ CHW. Always remember that we must make caring our goal in every patient encounter!

7.2.10　Conclusion

Working with clinical leadership, the role of CHWs has dramatically improved efficiency and compliance with delivery of evidence-based preventive and quality measures. Physicians and nurses throughout the institution now embrace CHWs. Dr. Shafer met his original goal of making strides to improve the quality of patient care; however, quality care is a journey toward population health. Evidence continues to confirm the physicians working with the pre-visit CHW, and the LVN team deliver a higher quality of care, helping to close some of our preventive service gaps leading to lower costs, improved patient experience, and better health outcomes. Although reaction to change may be resistance when first introduced, change is not always bad. A healthy change leads to new and better circumstances such as with the integration of CHWs into clinics at UTHSCT. As demonstrated in the stories above, CHWs have led to healthy changes for patients and their families as well as the institution.

References

Kangovi, S., Mitra, N., Grande, D., Huo, H., Smith, R. A., & Long, J. A. (2017). Community health worker support for disadvantaged patients with multiple chronic diseases: A randomized clinical trial. *American Journal of Public Health, 107*(10), 1660–1667. https://doi.org/10.2105/AJPH.2017.303985

Nehme, E., Elerian, N., Morrow, J., Mandell, D., Puga, E., & Lakey, D. (2016). *The health status of Northeast Texas 2016*. Austin, TX: UT Health Northeast/University of Texas System Office of Population Health.

Regional Healthcare Partnership (RHP) 1. (2012). *Community needs assessment*. Tyler, TX: UT Health Northeast.

Texas Department of State Health Services (DSHS). (2007). *East Texas community health needs assessment (ETCHNA)*. Retrieved from https://www.dshs.texas.gov/easttexas/reports.shtm

University of Wisconsin Population Health Institute. (2017). *County health rankings 2012*. Retrieved from https://www.countyhealthrankings.org/

7.3   Special Connections: CHWs Engaged with CSHCN and Their Families

Cecil H. Doggette, Aubry D. Threlkeld, and Judith Palfrey

7.3.1   Special Children, Special Families, and Special Communities

In the United States, an estimated 15% of children have a special healthcare need. These children and youth meet the US Bureau of Maternal and Child Health's definition of children and youth with special healthcare needs (CSHCN) because they "have or are at increased risk for a chronic physical, developmental, behavioral, or emotional condition and who also require health and related services of a type or amount beyond that required by children generally." Of these children, roughly a third to a half have problems that are severe enough to interfere with their daily life functioning. A small subgroup of CSCHN (estimated at about 3% of the US child population) has very severe and complicated conditions—often referred to as children with medical complexity (CMC).

CSHCN have a wide range of disabling conditions including physical, sensory, cognitive, social, emotional, and behavioral disorders. They may be diagnosed with conditions such as cerebral palsy, spina bifida, hydrocephalus, muscular dystrophy, or other disabilities that may require the use of wheelchairs, walkers, and standers. The children may have cognitive delays or sensory impairments that obligate their parents' learning new ways of interacting and communicating. The children may demonstrate unusual or even challenging behaviors that affect their daily interactions with family members, schoolmates, and the larger community.

Over the past 50 years, through major advances in medical, surgical, and educational technology, these CSHCN and their families have benefited in terms of overall health, development, and function. However, these benefits have not been shared equally. National surveys that are conducted every few years have documented unequal access to medical, educational, recreational, and vocational services for traditionally underserved groups. In particular, CSHCN of color or those who speak a language other than English have a hard time taking advantage of services. Sometimes this is because professionals have not made sure that their families are aware of programs. Sometimes it is because the services are offered at times and in places that are not convenient for the families of CSHCN from minority and non-English speaking populations. Often, the families have pressing priorities (paying rent, keeping food on the table, applying for citizenship), and they are juggling many competing demands at once—making it particularly hard to fit into inflexibly designed service structures.

Communities have within them many of the resources that can assist families who have children with special medical, developmental, and educational needs.

Neighborhood clinics, schools, and religious and cultural centers can serve as bulwarks of support for families who newly learn that their child has a special healthcare need. This may happen right at birth or be the sudden outcome of an injury or the long-term consequence of a chronic illness. In each of these cases, the new information affects all the members of the family. Strong communities buffer these impacts through outreach and through direct actions that bring comfort and alleviate stress. Community health workers (CHWs) can galvanize the special strengths of communities so that families do not feel alone when they are faced with unexpected medical and developmental situations.

CHWs who are aware of the resources in medical and educational institutions can also be of tremendous benefit to families in guiding them to clinical resources and helping them find needed equipment for feeding, bathing, and transporting their children. They can help to coordinate rides and improve physical access to services for CSHCN. They can also help families decode medical and educational jargon and learn to advocate for their children and themselves by speaking about what is most important to them, their child, and the rest of the family.

Recently healthcare institutions have explicitly begun to address family and community issues in a systematic fashion. The emergence of interest in social determinants of disease has been a healthy stimulus pushing healthcare and educational institutions to broaden their perspectives about both the causes of poor health and the resources that can ease some burdens. One of the contributions of the Affordable Care Act has been the addition of payment mechanisms for alternative providers including CHWs. In addition, as a number of states are experimenting with Accountable Care Organizations (ACOs), there is increasing interest in augmenting the traditional workforce with CHWs who can expand the reach of the clinical programs and make connections with some of the natural supports that reside in the communities.

While there clearly are not enough CHWs in our US communities now as interest in the roles that CHWs can play. In May of 2015, the HSC Foundation in Washington, DC, pulled together a national meeting of CHWs, families, professionals, and agency officials to discuss ways to promote the expanded role of CHW to include specific work with CSHCN. The outcome of the groups' deliberation was the recommendation that a specific curriculum be developed to prepare CHWs to work with CSHCN. The group defined the core competencies of CHWs engaging with CSHCN and called for the development of training and monitoring materials. Special Connections has grown up in response to this call to action.

7.3.2   CHWs as Trailblazers

Despite the fact that there is a critically important role that CHWs can play for CSHCN and their families, currently very few programs around the country bring CHWs together with CSHCN and their families. This is largely a reflection of the fact that there are relatively few CHWs in general. Most of these CHWs work with adults on disease-specific programs. Our group carried out an environmental scan to find CHWs working directly with CSHCN and found six such groups that stood out and accounted for the success of the programs. The common elements of the CHW programs that were serving CSHCN were:

- Community Outreach
- Integration across Service Sectors
- Family Engagement
- Care Coordination and Accompaniment

The HSCSN was one of the early adopters of the CHW model and incorporated CHW work into every aspect of the work of the healthcare program. The HSCSN CHWs spent their time visiting families in their home. They presented the various benefits of Managed Health Care to the CSHCN in DC who were eligible for SSI and Medicaid. CHWs joined the corps at HSCSN for a variety of reasons including their desire to work with children with disabilities and their interest in developing strategies to engage families in the community. CHWs also began to work at HSCSN because of their own personal experiences with children in their own families who had multiple disabilities. The original CHWs were pioneers who knew the value of having concerned and compassionate individuals who were also comfortable in the community setting.

As they reached out to families of CSHCN, they learned that many families had experienced failed promises made by healthcare providers. They encountered a deep mistrust of the healthcare establishment within the special needs/disability community. Few of the families had a regular source of care (or medical home) and often had to rely on emergency rooms as their only source of health care. Because the CHWs lived in the community, they understood firsthand the barriers to high-quality care that the families faced. It was exciting to be in the position of offering a real change for families. For the first time for some families, the HSCSN program would be ensuring that each family had a primary care physician. The success began when families began to realize having one individual (PCP) coordinate their care created better outcomes. Realizing there was more to clinical care than seeing a physician, the HSCSN CHWs also began to see the need for family support. Families wanting to meet and hear from others who were like them, children needing activities that were not provided in traditional settings and men of children with special needs who were a long lost and undervalued resource for their child. The CHWs were able to create a platform for each of these activities. The success from these experiences built on itself and led to experiences that the CHWs would cherish throughout their lives.

The lessons from the original experiences of CHWs who worked in the communities were formed by trial and error, surprising encounters, unanticipated occurrences, and good and not so good outcomes, but they were not written down. At best during ad hoc gatherings, they passed orally from one CHW to the next. We set out to capture these stories and this narrative learning to truly prepare CHWs for the work they would encounter. So, we listened and recorded the stories and lessons that veteran CHWs had to offer and weaved this knowledge throughout all aspects of the curriculum.

7.3.3   Veteran CHW Voices Shape Learning

Narratives often form the basis for adult learning because they follow a learned, predictable pattern, can be relayed easily to others, and serve as a basis for rich discussion.

The process of writing the Special Connections curriculum involved a deep commitment to deriving the fundamental lessons from the lived experience of CHWs. The Special Connections team wanted to impart specific information about working with CHSCN and general knowledge and useful tips from CHWs working in a variety of settings and systems. As a result, the first year of curriculum development involved meeting with CHWs to hear their stories and to learn about their successes and challenges. The CHWs involved in the project were extremely generous with their time and the contributions they made to the written curriculum and to a series of video tapes that explored relevant topics such as early childhood education, communication with CSHCN, transition planning, housing resources, and active listening.

The meetings and focus groups with CHWs helped the Special Connections team select and develop the curriculum modules. The CHWs validated or rejected ideas about what would be of value in a curriculum to train new CHWs. What we all learned in this process was that becoming and being a CHW entails lifelong learning in the same way that professional athletes, doctors, nurses, and teachers continue to learn and grow throughout their careers. Every one of the meetings with the CHWs who helped to create the Special Connections curriculum was rich with interaction, insight, and innovation. The team tried to capture the process that allowed for this active learning throughout all of the modules.

7.3.4   Aims of the Curriculum

The curriculum uses common questions to structure discussion and learning:

1. What does it mean to be a community health worker (CHW) working with children and youth with special healthcare needs (CSHCN)?
2. What are special healthcare needs?
3. How do I advocate for a patient and my community?
4. How do we conduct a home visit? How do I participate in evaluating services?
5. How do I communicate with CSHCN?
6. How do I help families understand and plan for life transitions?
7. How do we support children and youth with behavioral health needs?
8. How do we maintain a healthy balance between work and life?
9. How do we know what information to share with our communities?
10. How do we take what we have learned back to our communities?

The overall aim of the curriculum is to introduce the CHWs to the unique characteristics of children with special healthcare needs and their families and to point out the ways CHW involvement can help the families and children. Community health workers have the opportunity to work with children with a wide range of disabilities. In the Special Connections curriculum, we provide details about the most common health, developmental, and behavioral conditions that the CHWs will encounter through some didactic teaching, a set of tools that detail the conditions and a series of videos where young people and their parents tell about their conditions and offer suggestions for the ways CHWs can be most helpful. The stories that come from the CHWs' own experiences augment this other material and deepen the understanding that the CHWs can have of common disabilities and special healthcare needs.

As an example, the story of Felix[1] who is a 12-year-old boy with learning and behavioral challenges depicts some serious dilemmas that the school and family face. The story allows the CHWs to consider how they would handle the situation and what resources they would turn to in order to be of the greatest aid to Felix. The crux of the story is that Felix struggles in school because of his learning disabilities and becomes very frustrated in both the school and home settings. This is quite typical for children in middle school because the increasing amount of written material and homework requirements tax a child with learning and attention problems more than they do a typically developing child. The consequence is often that the child stops doing assignments and becomes angry and even rebellious when asked to do school work.

Felix followed this pattern with an increasing amount of problematic behavior just around the time of his birthday. Three days before Felix's birthday, his teacher sent a letter to the parents saying that if these behaviors continued, she would have no choice but to suspend him. The parents were shocked and distressed. They took the stance that they must punish Felix by canceling his much-anticipated 12th birthday party.

The scenario of Felix and his family brings up for CHWs many of the aspects of the impact of chronic developmental conditions on the child and on the family. Often it seems to families that nothing is "just normal." Why can't they get through the week or the holiday season or a child's birthday without something erupting that causes them distress? CHWs getting to know the families and the school situations can be enormously helpful in guiding the families to a place of balance that gets them back on kilter to a kind of "normal" that accommodates the expected ups and downs. CHWs with an unbiased perspective can provide common sense solutions to situations like the one that Felix's family faces. They can also serve as a liaison from the family to the school in order to get more educational attention and intervention for Felix at a time when his behavior signals a clear "cry for help" from his school, his family, and his larger community.

---

[1] With the exception of the authors' names, all other names have been changed to protect privacy and confidentiality.

Our experience with using this story in the curriculum is that the CHWs appreciate learning how the child's disability itself is the underlying cause for all of the behavioral consequences as well as the teachers and parents' reactions. They often have "Aha!" moments during the discussion of the case and want to learn more about cognitive impairment, learning disabilities, attention disorders and the special education, and medical and community interventions that can be most beneficial in assisting the children.

7.3.4.1 What Impact Does Learning That a Child Has a Disability Have on the Family?

A community health worker may be one of the first people that a family shares their thoughts and fears with when they learn that their child has a disability. To illustrate this and to stimulate discussion about the expected emotional reactions that families have when they learn their child has a lifelong disabling condition, a number of the stories play out typical scenarios. The story of Baby Alexandria depicts the experience of a young family whose baby is born extremely premature at 26 weeks postconception. Children who are born so early have the potential for lifelong health and developmental concerns including serious lung disease, poor growth, impaired functioning of their gastrointestinal tract and developmental delay, motor problems, seizures, and other neurological complications. The family is scared about the future but also is continually questioning, "Why did the happen? What did we do that was wrong? They also wonder what they can do to protect Alexandria and how they should take care of her. This scenario brings up all the issues that surround the realization that a child has special medical and developmental needs and puts forward the areas where community health workers can have a very positive role in alleviating much of the stress that the family is experiencing. While the CHWs cannot directly answer all the questions the families have about the child's medical condition, they can help the families form a list of questions for the medical team so that the family can have up to date and accurate information about the current situation, possible diagnoses, and likely interventions that will be carried out for the baby.

Families like Alexandria's feel isolated and sometimes stigmatized. They have to spend weeks in the unfamiliar environment of a neonatal intensive care unit, surrounded by beeping machines and scurrying health professionals. They hear and see the emergency responses that are necessary for their child and the other babies. They are exposed to a whole new culture and language with words like "intubation," "catheterization," "sepsis," etc. CHWs can be a welcoming and calming presence who reminds them that their own community is nearby and eager to help and support the new baby. CHWs have resources that they can introduce to families that bring them together with families like themselves—families from their own community who speak their same language and have gone through similar experiences. Neonatal support groups are a major boon for families like Alexandria's. Through her story, we introduce new CHWs to the situation that the family faces and provide them strategies they can employ to be of great assistance to the families at a time of great need.

7.3.4.2   What Are the Challenges Families Face When Interacting with the Health Sector?

The voices of CHWs help us to understand a great deal about the complex interplay of health condition, service sector availability, culture, and language. A story we use about a child named Jabril points out how the condition of epilepsy affects children with the condition and how cultural and language miscommunication can seriously interfere with the optimal care for a common condition. Jabril's story focuses on a series of unfortunate interactions where there was inadequate transmission of critical medical information by the doctors that resulted in the family administering the incorrect medication to the child for his seizures. The child had to be rushed to the emergency services for the episode. The fortunate outcome of the story was that the family transferred their care to a community health center where there was a CHW from their community who was able to assist them in feeling comfortable with the healthcare providers. They also gained an advocate who understood their language and culture and who was an expert at communicating their needs and desires to the new healthcare providers. This powerful story underscores how a language and culture play a key role in the lives of children with common special healthcare needs.

A second story about a child with autism further illustrates the complex struggles that families with children with special healthcare needs face when they are trying to learn about their child's condition and find services for the child. The little boy's mother Maria knew that her son was not developing typically and that he had serious developmental concerns, but every doctor she approached had a different interpretation and sent her on to another service or simply did not answer her questions. Through the process of looking for answers, Maria was given over four different diagnoses. When she eventually learned that her son had autism, she began seeking appropriate services for him to help with his social interactions and his language development. Unfortunately, she found that there were few services that met her son's needs in the area where she lived. And, almost no materials were available in Spanish, which is her native language. Maria realized that many other parents were experiencing the same difficulties as she was, and she took steps to form a local support group for Hispanic families with children with autism. People flocked to the support group, and Maria was ultimately able to work with her state Autism Chapter to create programs and materials for Hispanic families.

The issues raised by this story are ones that CHWs hear over and over again. In discussion during our Special Connections training, the trainees often begin to think of approaching the situation using the type of advocacy and creativity that Maria employed to improve her community's situation. Using stories that combine a discussion of the condition, its effects on the family and community, and a series of possible solutions has stimulated rich conversation, reflection, and action on the part of the newly trained CHWs and their supervisors.

7.3.4.3   What Innovations Are Community Health Workers Making in the Field?

Our stories highlight inspirational and positive experiences of fellow community health workers who have been working with children and youth with special health-care needs and their families. Each story is centered on a common experience or value among community health workers. Exploration requires community health workers to discuss and practice implementing something that they could use in their fieldwork. This is an opportunity for community health workers to walk away with a clear and practical tool or set of questions. This is intended to mirror the kinds of tools that may be shared with them via medical facilities—not to replace them. Exploration tools were developed using the best available general and practical knowledge about the range of possible situations in which community health workers may be placed by sponsoring organizations.

By definition, community health workers are service providers who are embedded in the community where they can both identify needs and resources. They are the "joiners" who tie everything together. They are also the "promoters" who assist families in learning to use their own voices and to find the resources and power they need to move forward with their lives in balance. One of the first tasks CHWs are often assigned by the agencies that employ them is to make their presence visible in the community so that community members begin to trust them and turn to them when they need help.

The story about Darryl and Portia is instructive about how CHWs can introduce themselves in the community. Darryl routinely set up a table for his agency at local healthcare fairs and provided "assessments" for families to determine if their children could benefit from the sponsorship by his agency that served CSHCN. Portia had heard about the agency and recognized its logo on Darryl's jacket and the materials. She had a level of trust about the agency because a friend had a child who had benefited from the services provided by the group. Portia was especially hoping to find some respite care for her family since caring 24/7 for a child with significant special healthcare needs can be exhausting. She was impressed that Darryl was responsive to her specific needs and although he clearly had many other things to offer, he listened to her carefully and zeroed in on what has her top priority.

In discussing stories like this one about community outreach, new CHWs can learn that even though the situations of families with CSHCN can sometimes appear overwhelming, a systematic family-centered approach like the one Darryl took can get a family started in the process of finding the range of services that can benefit them by addressing many of their concerns.

7.3.5   *The Value of Continuous Learning*

A story that emphasizes how much being a CHW is an art that draws on a CHW's strong listening skills but also stretches the creative side of the CHW is that of Tony. In the voice of a veteran CHW, Tony, the learners hear about how Tony at first found that there were so many gaps on health, education, housing, recreation, and financial and social services for families that he felt a bit overwhelmed, but as he began to tackle the problems of the families he met, he gained the confidence and skill to meet the individual needs of the families. His first encounters with families were often difficult because many of the families had had bad experiences with representatives from each separate social service agency with the complex rules and regulations that the families found hard to comprehend. He found that teaching himself about each "different story" he became more and more confident that he had something he could offer and that he personally derived great satisfaction at solving the unique puzzles and problems that others had avoided because they did not fit neatly into one set of rules and expectations.

As the CHWs in the Special Connections training hear the story of Tony, it reinforces what they are experiencing. They talk about how important it is to persist, to try a variety of approaches, and most importantly to find people in the local health, education, recreation, and financial and social agencies who have the same "can do" attitude that they have and that are proud when they resolve a problem for a family and give them the resources to turn to if the problem reemerges.

7.3.5.1 How Do I Coordinate Services?

A major innovation that veteran CHWs have instituted as they have worked over many years in the community is that coordination of services is a key element. Successful CHWs have realized that many families had experienced failed promises made by healthcare providers leading to mistrust. For many families it was a challenge to understand the benefits of having a primary care physician vs. the standard practice of using the emergency room. CHWs who were from or lived in the community understood those barriers. The success began when families began to realize having one individual (PCP) coordinate their care created better outcomes. Realizing there was more to clinical care than seeing a physician, CHWs also began to see the need for family support. Families wanted to meet and hear from others who were like them, and children needed activities that were not provided in traditional settings.

Because of CHWs, there are more families aware of their healthcare benefits, able to understand and comfortably meet the daily challenges of providing the appropriate care for themselves and their family. To continue to meet those needs, CHWs must strive to beat the challenges of social determinants and be creative in developing better outcomes. CHWs can be champions for those in need and can advocate on their behalf.

There are many components of being a successful CHW. The development of community partnerships helps families obtain additional resources, support, and advocacy through the development of a relationship with others. This effort also leads to more families having better outcomes for their children, family, and community.

7.3.6   Advice for the Future

From our initial piloting of the Special Connections curriculum, we have learned that expert CHWs have a lot of advice for recently hired CHWs working with children with special healthcare needs and that prior to this curriculum, there were no formal mechanisms for capturing this advice and sharing it with new professionals in the field and that what opportunities did exist operated outside of traditional professional learning environments in hospitals and other community organizations.

The fields of medical education and public health continue to need ways to engage best practices outside of medical facilities and in communities disproportionately affected by social determinants of health. The stories, tools, and practices of culturally embedded CHWs can influence the ways in which we support families that have children with special healthcare needs and, ultimately, make care coordination more effective.

Furthermore, for CHWs themselves, we need more opportunities to bring people together and build communities of practice.

Chapter 8
Providing Coaching and Social Support

Caitlin G. Allen*, Alexandra Anderson, Melinda Banks, Gabriela Bustos, Maria C. Cole, Carolyn Dixon, Princess Fortin*, Almitra Gasper, Kim Jay*, Stephanie Jordan, Rhonda M. Lay, Javier Lopez, Helen Margellos-Anast, Fatima Padron, Michael Perry, Floribella Redondo-Martinez, Carl H. Rush, Jessica Sunshine, and Madeline Woodberry

Authorship is organized alphabetically in ascending order by surname.

C. G. Allen (✉)
CGA Consulting, Charleston, SC, USA
e-mail: caitlin.gloeckner.allen@emory.edu

A. Anderson · P. Fortin (✉) · A. Gasper · J. Sunshine
New York City Department of Health and Mental Hygiene, New York City, NY, USA
e-mail: pfortin@health.nyc.gov

M. Banks · G. Bustos · K. Jay (✉) · R. M. Lay · H. Margellos-Anast · F. Padron ·
M. Woodberry
Sinai Urban Health Institute, Chicago, IL, USA
e-mail: kim.jay@sinai.org

M. C. Cole
Baylor Scott & White Research Institute, Dallas, TX, USA

C. Dixon
Where Do We Go from Here, Inc (formerly from Life Camp, Inc.), Queens, NY, USA

S. Jordan
Sinai Urban Health Institute, Munster, IN, USA

J. Lopez
Red Hook Initiative, Brooklyn, NY, USA

M. Perry
True 2 Life, Central Family Life Center, Stapleton, Staten Island, NY, USA

F. Redondo-Martinez
Arizona Community Health Workers Association, Douglas, AR, USA

C. H. Rush
Community Resources, LLC, San Antonio, TX, USA

© Springer Nature Switzerland AG 2021
J. A. St. John et al. (eds.), *Promoting the Health of the Community*,
https://doi.org/10.1007/978-3-030-56375-2_8

8.1   Introduction

Caitlin G. Allen, Maria C. Cole, Floribella Redondo-Martinez, and Carl H. Rush

The fourth core role, providing coaching and social support, includes four sub-roles: providing individual support and coaching; motivating and encouraging people to obtain care and other services; supporting self-management of disease prevention and management of health conditions (including chronic disease); and planning and/or leading support groups. Originally, this role included "informal counseling," but the language in the updated role shifted away from informal counseling to "coaching." The role of informal counseling was deemed to be encroaching on other health-related fields, and the term coaching and social support was substituted.

Social support is vital to building and maintaining healthy social relationships, expanding social capital, and increasing individual and community resilience. There are four commonly identified types of social support behaviors, all of which may be demonstrated by community health workers (CHWs). The four behaviors include emotional, instrumental, information, and appraisal support. While social support can be provided by people other than CHWs, CHWs as a profession are unique in their ability to provide all four types of social support to their patients or clients, whom are often their peers and/or neighbors. CHWs may also coach their clients to identify additional resources for each type of social support. For example, a CHW may help provide an individual who is newly diagnosed with diabetes informational support by offering the client advice and health education materials about the disease. Additionally, the CHW may further work with the client to identify sources of emotional support (e.g., close friends and family members) that may be helpful as the individual learns to cope with and manage the new diagnosis.

Noting the distinct features of coaching and social support that CHWs can enact, along with how they can help clients to build long-term social support, remains important. This CHW role is unique from—but complementary to—clinical counseling that may occur from other professionals in healthcare and public health settings (e.g., social workers), as it primarily occurs in the context of self-management and disease prevention.

The following two sections provide examples of how CHWs engage in coaching and social support. Specifically, the sections detail how CHWs can use their unique life experience to provide culturally relevant social support and coaching to encourage violence prevention and assist with challenges outside of medicine.

8.2   Community Health Workers Extend Solutions to Violence Prevention

Princess Fortin, Jessica Sunshine, Alexandra Anderson, Michael Perry, Carolyn Dixon, Almitra Gasper, and Javier Lopez

8.2.1   Introduction[1]

Community health workers (CHWs) add a rich social perspective to persistent gun violence in communities and influence how organizations and agencies respond to the problem. To illustrate this specific contribution to the health field, this section provides personal accounts of CHWs in New York City (NYC) extending solutions to gun violence prevention and highlights the support and coaching inherent in their work. Hundreds of CHWs across NYC leverage their lived experience to address gun violence in their communities through Cure Violence (CV) programming, conflict mediation, resource coordination, and provision of holistic services. This section profiles two extraordinary NYC-based CHWs doing this important work and provides a narrative on the role they and many other CHWs play.

> Growing up in Richmond Terrace Houses on Staten Island, I've seen a lot of violence. I've seen people shot, stabbed, I've seen drug disputes gone bad. I've seen it often and it kind of affected me in a way where I grew up thinking that it was cool to be violent. It was cool to gain a reputation for being violent. So I [was] asked to do this work, and I struggled with that initially because I thought, *'I have a reputation of being violent and just being a particular type of guy. Would coming back on the streets promoting peace strip away all of [my] so-called 'popularity'?* So when I was propositioned to do the work, I was struggling but that thought changed quickly. I said, *'Wait a minute, let's think about this Iron Mike guy. How he was almost killed twice; he almost killed somebody; he's seen death, jail, destruction his whole life. He was looking at thirteen years in prison. I didn't want to be a part of that no more, I want to rewrite my narrative.'*   - Mike

This is a quote from Michael Perry, known to his community as Iron Mike. Mike, a Black man who lost his father to gun violence at an early age, started working for True 2 Life[2] in Stapleton, Staten Island, in 2013 as a Violence Interrupter and has since been promoted to Program Manager. Mike is a CHW with an unmatched ability to intervene when interpersonal conflicts are brewing. He is able to connect with individuals and shift mindsets away from using violence as a way of dealing with disputes. Mike's daily work is changing the narrative that accepts violence as a normal occurrence, especially in a historically disinvested neighborhood.

Similar to Iron Mike, Carolyn Dixon is a CHW. She is a Hospital Responder at LIFE Camp[3], in South Jamaica, Queens. She began working with the program in 2014 as a volunteer, following the death of her son from gun violence. Carolyn supports families impacted by gun violence while promoting peace and community healing. She speaks of her personal loss and works tirelessly to prevent other families from experiencing similar trauma. She provides informal counseling with both participants and community members.

> As a mother, I can talk to [youth] and explain that even though you have difficult times with your parents, you are loved. I explain my story and the death of my son, and I let them know that whatever action they take and do, reflects on your family. Picking up a gun and killing someone, if you go to jail, your mom and dad are doing time with you. Your family will die with you. It's difficult to go to the cemetery and visit your child – I try to explain what it is like to lose a child and having thoughts of suicide. Their action affects everyone, even the community. A lot of kids are loved by many. But some want revenge of a death, you have some that become mentally disconnected through death. [These are the] circle of events that happen through the death of a loved one.   - Carolyn

Mike and Carolyn utilize their experiential knowledge and their shared lived experience with the communities they serve to prevent gun violence and change community norms. This section offers personal accounts from Mike and Carolyn about how their firsthand insight and relationship with the communities they serve make them uniquely equipped to provide support and coaching to the individuals they work with as they strive to reduce gun violence in their communities (Fig. 8.1). This section describes CHW contributions to building community resilience and how their efforts have spearheaded a shift in how local government agencies work to prevent violence in afflicted communities. The section closes with a summary of considerations for elevating the reach and impact of CHW work, particularly the important role of CHWs to provide coaching and social support.

8.2.2   Disparities in Community Gun Violence in NYC

New York City (NYC) has been cited as one of the safest big cities in the country, with historically low incidents of firearm-related homicides (New York City, Mayor's Office of Criminal Justice, 2017). Although NYC has seen downward trends in gun violence, those most affected by the burden tell a story of great disparity in violent outcomes. What is clear is that select neighborhoods face a disproportionate amount of health inequities and disproportionate access to fundamental needs and resources like quality health care, housing, education, public transportation, and employment (Lander, 2018). We also see that racist and discriminatory practices have intentionally and systematically created and maintained residential segregation within NYC neighborhoods (Bailey et al., 2017) which is linked to adverse birth outcomes (Acevedo-Garcia, Lochner, Osypuk, & Subramanian, 2003; Bailey et al., 2017), increased exposure to air pollutants (Bravo, Anthopolos, Bell, & Miranda, 2016), decreased longevity (Williams & Collins, 2001), increased risk of chronic disease (Acevedo-Garcia et al., 2003; Bailey et al., 2017; Kershaw et al., 2011; Williams & Collins, 2001), and increased rates of homicide and other crime (Krivo et al., 2015). Given these conditions, the fact that gun-related homicides in NYC disproportionately impact

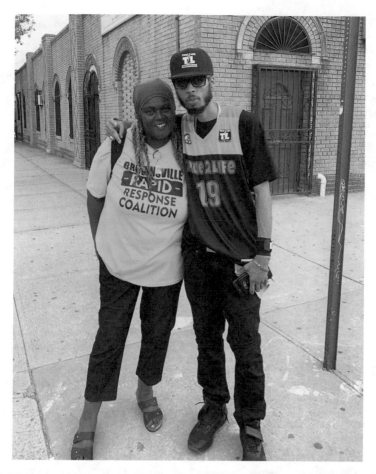

Fig. 8.1 Pictured are Carolyn Dixon, left, and Michael Perry, right, at a community rally that was organized in response to the mass shooting that occurred during the annual Brownsville Old Timer's event on Saturday, July 27, 2019. CV CHWs frequently attend events outside of their own target area in order to support local coalitions and denounce violence

certain neighborhoods and communities comes as no surprise (Fig. 8.2). In NYC, one-quarter of neighborhoods account for nearly 50% of gun-related homicides (Li et al., 2016). These data show us that select neighborhoods are situated in ways that lead to much higher rates of gun violence than others. These are the conditions under which CHWs do their work, bringing in support and resources, and taking part in changing norms and increased advocacy alongside the community.

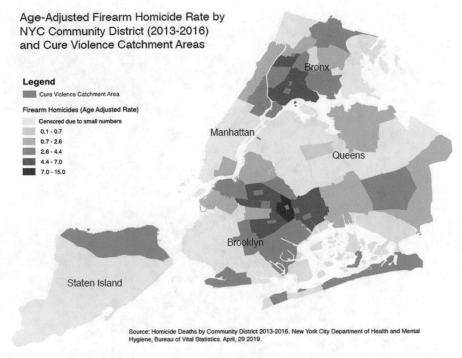

Fig. 8.2 Age-adjusted firearm homicide rate by New York City Community District (2013–2016) with Cure Violence catchment areas. (Source: Homicide Deaths by Community District 2013–2016. New York City Department of Health and Mental Hygiene, Bureau of Vital Statistics. April, 29, 2019. Retrieved from https://a816-healthpsi.nyc.gov/epiquery/VS/index.html, New York City, Department of Health and Mental Hygiene n.d.)

8.2.2.1 Community Health Workers Preventing Gun Violence in NYC

Historically, interventions aimed at reducing gun violence have been informed through criminal justice and public safety frameworks. Such interventions center on punishing misbehavior and criminal offenses with arrests and detainments and typically only have a short-term effect on behavior change. Many in the criminal justice reform space have called for systemic change in how neighborhood safety is enforced in neighborhoods consisted primarily of people of color (e.g., American Public Health Association [APHA], 2018; Slutkin, 2017). As an alternative to the criminal justice and public safety framework, Figure 8.3 illustrates a health system that prevents violence (Lovelidge, 2017). This system includes various settings in which CHWs can be positioned to address detrimental inequities in health and to improve outcomes for all communities.

Given increasing acknowledgment of gun violence as a public health issue, interventions have begun to take a harm reduction approach with attention to the social determinants of health (e.g., APHA, 2018; Slutkin, 2017). Public health ideology promotes prevention approaches that help build community resilience and enhance

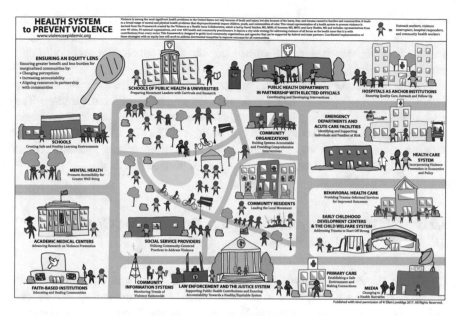

Fig. 8.3 Health system to prevent violence. (Published with kind permission of © Ellen Lovelidge 2017. All Rights Reserved. Retrieved from http://violenceepidemic.com/, E. Lovelidge 2017)

protective factors that help individuals and communities overcome social and environmental stressors (Cunningham et al., 2009).

Gun violence is a public health issue because of the physical and emotional harm, psychological trauma, and persistent fear gun violence causes individuals and communities. Entire lifespans are damaged by violence causing inequities in birth outcomes, childhood development and health behavior, the onset of physical and mental illness, and premature death. Gun violence tears apart families and communities; the collective and individual trauma resulting from it is passed down from generation to generation ("End the Violence Epidemic," n.d.). This framing has contributed to NYC's municipal investment in public health-driven and community-centered approaches for reducing the burden of gun violence. One approach being implemented is Cure Violence (CV).

CV is a neighborhood-centered, evidence-based approach to gun violence reduction (Slutkin, 2017). The program relies on the efforts of community-based *outreach workers* and *violence interrupters* in neighborhoods that are the most vulnerable to gun violence. These staff assume the health worker role and leverage their personal relationships, social networks, and knowledge of their communities to dissuade specific individuals and neighborhood residents in general from engaging in violence (Delgado et al., 2017). The CV outreach workers and violence interrupters embody the term "credible messenger"; in this case, they are trusted community members with similar backgrounds to the high-risk individuals they are serving. These credible messengers are CHWs by every sense of the definition. They are direct care workers that have an intimate understanding of the community that they serve. They promote physical and mental wellness. They also appreciate and integrate the experience, language, culture, and socioeconomic reality of the neighborhood in which they are embedded into their mentoring and community mobilizing.

CV CHWs preempt violence and mitigate retaliatory violence by building trust with high-risk individuals, conflict de-escalation, and conflict mediation. They assess the risk of engaging in violence, provide referrals for services, and bring awareness to the issue of community gun violence. The CV CHWs are a key link between social services and the community, facilitating access to resources and informing the quality and cultural competency of service delivery.

8.2.3   CHW Support and Coaching: Essential for Gun Violence Prevention

CV CHWs provide the people they work with the social and emotional support needed to heal and take agency in redefining what health and safety looks like in their own lives and the lives of people in their community. The coaching and support that they provide program participants has linked some of the most vulnerable and marginalized individuals and communities to critical services that are often stigmatized, underutilized, unavailable, or inaccessible. CV CHWs receive extensive training on conflict mediation, detecting and interrupting violent events, providing ongoing behavior change support to individuals at risk for engaging in violence, and changing community norms that exacerbate gun violence. They can successfully translate their training, experiential knowledge, and connection to the communities they serve to motivate and encourage individuals, communities, and systems to take a stand against violence.

8.2.3.1   Providing Individual Support and Coaching

CV CHWs work to mitigate the impact of generational disinvestment and oppression that has contributed to the disproportionate rates of gun violence in their communities. The relationships and trust they have built in the community speak to their credibility and allow for a more flexible, culturally appropriate service delivery system (Cosgrove et al., 2014). In addition to conflict mediation, they help quell brewing interpersonal issues that may escalate to violence. They coordinate wrap-around services, referrals to additional resources (e.g., legal services, housing, job readiness, and education programs), and access to opportunities. They also create connections to professional mental health resources and help individuals navigate systems to decrease the barriers that impede participants from seeking the services they need to progress. For example, in 2017, the 18 New York City-based CV programs worked with 876 program participants and issued 4000 participant referrals for service—referrals including 541 for education-related services, 252 for substance abuse treatment, 653 for job readiness training, 538 for legal aid, 345 for therapeutic services, and 797 for employment opportunities.

This uniquely skilled and positioned workforce provides support and coaching to the people they work with, even among the backdrop of unfair opportunities and disadvantages due to race, income, or other social determinants that they themselves have also experienced in the neighborhoods they serve. CHWs link participants—including people overexposed to the criminal and family courts systems, people previously shuffled through education and foster care systems, and people experiencing gentrification—to services they might not otherwise pursue. Support is offered to help change the mindset of youth facing the highest risk of victimization and perpetration of gun violence within the focus neighborhood in order to promote peace and reduce violence.

Examples of their support and coaching are listed below. CV CHWs:

1. Create a space for clients to *explore their unmet needs* and help with concrete tasks to *reduce barriers to access* (e.g., supporting clients in health insurance enrollment, housing applications, accessing birth certificates, social security numbers, etc.).
2. Build trust and model what a *healthy relationship* can look like. CHWs have ongoing check-ins and engagement opportunities with participants. A positive role model can buffer exposure to negative influences and experiences, acting as a protective factor and promoting resiliency (Hurd, Zimmerman, & Xue, 2008). When faced with resistance from participants, CHWs are trained to maintain ongoing contact in order to demonstrate that their relationship is non-conditional. Even if a participant engages in high-risk activities, the CHW will continue to support and care for this individual. CV CHWs have been exposed to similar historical traumas as their participants and are able to connect to participants on a different level of care than perhaps a case worker or social worker. This level of support helps the individuals they serve to stay on track, as they feel supported by and accountable to someone other than just themselves.
3. Coach participants through the *behavior change* process. There is a myriad of risk factors that contribute to individual- and community-level violence (Slutkin, 2017). CV CHWs work directly with program participants to develop personalized risk reduction plans. They take a client-centered approach and look to the participant as the expert of their own lives—touching on issues like adverse childhood experiences, exposure to trauma, drug use, poor social support, and education. The ultimate goal is to change the mindset of high-risk youth from thinking that violence is the only solution to their conflicts to seeing that there are alternate, nonviolent options that are safe and socially acceptable. CV CHWs:

   (a) Utilize motivational interviewing techniques to coach participants to explore and identify their own strengths, challenges, and priorities
   (b) Facilitate the identification of emotional and behavioral triggers, underlying emotions, and coping strategies
   (c) Strengthen problem-solving skills by exploring choices and consequences

(d) Promote alternative, nonviolent responses for productive conflict resolution
(e) Coach participants to engage in supportive, healthy relationships and surround themselves with positive influences

In order to effectively engage a participant, the CV CHW will initiate smaller, more attainable risk-reduction goals. For example, if a participant is unemployed and wants to get a job, the CHW will break this down into multiple short-term, actionable items. These smaller goals may include creating a resume, practicing interview skills, and completing a job search. Successfully completing these steps contributes directly to the larger goal, while simultaneously fostering a sense of control, confidence, and self-efficacy in the participant.

4. Lastly, CV CHWs actively work to *limit re-traumatization* of the people they work with by taking a *trauma-informed* approach. This approach allows for nonjudgmental engagement with participants and community members and helps to reframe the conversation from what is wrong with this individual to what happened to this individual.

> So much of our youth has been exposed to so much trauma like I did when I was ten, whether it be death, violence in the home, drugs, arguments … any type of physical violence, verbal abuse. All of the youth grew up under that. And it's never been treated. So now you've got these fifteen, sixteen, seventeen-year olds in the communities [who are] untreated and super emotional … So, you can blame them, but you don't really want to blame them when they react emotionally. Something happens in the street and they go get a gun, all they know is emotions and [reacting].　　　　　　　　　　　　　　- Mike

Removing the blame and taking the onus off the individual can empower the participant and build resiliency. By recognizing the signs and symptoms of trauma in people's lives and its impact, CHWs are able to respond by integrating this knowledge into their practice.

8.2.3.2　CHW Skills

CHWs doing this work understand that to get to a place where individuals and the community are engaged in support and coaching, they must be able to:

Extend Motivation and Encouragement for Seeking Services

Available and accessible services do not always lead to service utilization. Individuals targeted for CV program participation tend to have a history of criminal activity or high-risk street activity, may have been a victim of a shooting, or previously incarcerated. When working with these individuals who have been surrounded by violence their entire lives, CV CHWs are often met with tremendous resistance by the high-risk youth when it comes to participating in the program. Therefore, motivating and encouraging participation is typically a slow process. Staff spend hours canvassing the neighborhood in order to build strong relationships with youth, adults, faith leaders, businesses, and other community groups. Program and staff visibility provide significant opportunities for engagement with potential participants.

> We are constantly in the schools and street – we talk about the program and the different activities that we offer – we ask them to come to movie night and tell them about employment opportunities such as the Anti-Gun Violence Youth Employment Program. Once they come and mingle and see other kids their age, they become part of the program. It's about having a safe space. A safe haven.   - Carolyn

Be Mindful to Timing of Engagement

CHWs effectively reframe negative experiences into teachable moments, changing the entire trajectory of an individual's life. The most opportune moments for participant recruitment are immediately following involvement in a mediation, in the aftermath of a shooting incident in the community, or during the "golden hour" in the hospital after personally experiencing violence. High-risk youth are sometimes hesitant to change and need an adjustment period before fully engaging with the program. CV CHWs have mastered their ability to exemplify patience and persistence, keeping the lines of communication open, networking with friends and family, all the while demonstrating the positive support system the program can provide. CHWs are key to motivating participation and encouraging service utilization.

> Well there is this one participant, he was always very rough around the edges. [At first], we engaged him to do other things, to work, to volunteer. Anything to keep him out of trouble and lead him towards the positive. He is now the senior ambassador to [the program], and he shows hope to the youth that are now recruited. He shows them how they can go this positive way. He's working and volunteering and doing other things within the community. He has been with the program for almost 5 years. He just received the community impact award from the NYC Health Department.   - Carolyn

Draw from Their Own Experiences Using Similar Services

One way that CHWs encourage use of services is by *referencing their own utilization of that service*. A major barrier to engagement with therapeutic services, for example, is stigma surrounding mental health and trauma. As stated throughout this section, identity and reputation are paramount, particularly for youth and young adults.

> It's so hard to [promote] mental health services because nobody wants to be labeled as crazy. The way I create buy-in is I tell them, 'Look I need somebody to talk to as well. I'm talking to you so I can be the start of your mental health [care].'   - Mike

Fear of being stigmatized for seeking mental health services often acts as a deterrent, so when a person who is looked up to and respected indicates that they needed help, the impact can be significant. This again highlights the importance of relationship building.

… what happens is, [if they are not ready,] we don't just push people away and tell them to go somewhere else. We start [the process] because we are our best wrap around service. We are the best because we are the start. We can provide mental health [support], not on the clinical level but we can start it.   - Mike

Speak on Their Own Transformation

Another frequently utilized strategy for motivating and connecting with at-risk youth is *storytelling*. CHWs speak about their own transformation by engaging in transparent conversations pertaining to past experiences. Hearing stories of change and success can instill feelings of hope for the future.

I pull out my phone and I go to a NY1 clip of me being on the news for something not so good. I pull up a Daily News post and I show the youth because they could be in the same position. And they may be on their way to a newspaper or a television broadcast for doing something stupid. So I use that. And then I fast forward to two and a half years later when I was on NY1 news doing an interview about my [violence prevention] work. It blows them away, they're like, 'are you kidding me, Bro?' So, they have me on NY1 waving pistols in a rap video for something negative, and then sitting down with a suit jacket on, comfortable, in the studio, speaking about being a credible messenger, speaking about pushing peace in the neighborhood where I'm from. So that's one of my biggest go to [examples] that I use to create buy-in. Especially for the younger guys.   - Mike

8.2.3.3   Building Neighborhood Resilience and Changing the Narrative

The support and coaching that CV CHWs provide is building individual and community resilience to reject and reduce gun violence. Evaluation of CV shows declines in acts of gun violence and increased expression of pro-social norms in neighborhoods compared with similar neighborhoods not operating CV programs (Delgado et al., 2017). Several CV programs have experienced decreases in shooting incidents in their target areas and increases in the number of days without shootings. The impact of the CHW work in this area is laudable and deserving of attention.

The numbers speak to what we've been able to do. You've never seen 500+ days without a homicide in Stapleton/Park Hill in I don't know how long. But since I've been doing the work, that's our number now, we're inside of 500 days without a homicide. We've seen stretches of 365 days without a shooting in a specific area twice since I've been doing the work. The men and women that do the work are the actual reason why it's changed because you gotta have particular people in place doing the work. You can't just send anyone out there to talk about peace and change. That's not going to work. You absolutely have to have the right people to do the work and to spread the message, to push the Cure Violence model. We've been able to do that, and we are the trailblazers of it. When it's all said and done the story is going to read, there is a group of men and women who absolutely changed the mentality and the whole dynamic on Staten Island in terms of violence.   - Mike

The public narrative around how to prevent gun violence has also changed—CV CHWs in NYC have been a catalyst for how local government agencies work to prevent violence in inflicted communities, positively impacting community, and agency investment in residents. For example, the NYC Mayor's Office to Prevent Gun Violence (OPGV)[4] serves as the lead oversight of a citywide network, called the Crisis Management System (CMS), that is strategically aligned to deploy violence intervention and trauma services in communities that experience high incidents of gun violence (NYC Office to Prevent Gun Violence, n.d.-a, n.d.-b). The NYC Department of Health and Mental Hygiene[5] has also been instrumental in CV's promising results in gun violence reduction and efforts to elevate community health and wellness (NYC Department of Health and Mental Hygiene, n.d.). These local government entities have invested in the CV CHW workforce as one strategy to prevent gun violence and to create safe, empowered, and interconnected communities.

Conversations around gun violence were previously limited to the traditional criminal justice and public safety frameworks and interventions. However, over the last decade in NYC, the CV CHW community has successfully illustrated the need for having a comprehensive coordinated response to community gun violence. In NYC, planning tables across all five boroughs (counties), government agencies (like those listed above), and elected officials have begun to welcome citizen-led and neighborhood-based prevention perspectives on what it means to have resilient and violence free neighborhoods.

> The Cure Violence program and the Crisis Management System have seen incredible success in the East Flatbush community and around the city, saving lives and completely transforming the way that we address gun violence. Years of efforts by members of the Council, administration, and community advocates have seen the Crisis Management System grow and our city at its safest in over 60 years. The expansion of the program into new communities and with new resources is a testament to the effectiveness of an approach that we were told was impossible, and I plan to continue to work with the administration and the City Council to implement a system that addresses the public health crisis of gun violence in this revolutionary way (New York City, Mayor's Office of Criminal Justice, 2018). - New York City Council Member Jumaane Williams[6]

This approach to violence prevention is a departure from the conventional criminal justice and public safety problem-solving strategies. However, CV CHWs have shown to be an effective vehicle for reducing gun violence in neighborhoods by advancing a new prevention discourse and by reframing gun violence as a public health issue.

> To really be dedicated to [the work], to really understand the nuances, understand the mentalities [related to conflict and violence] that we're dealing with, I think you have to have been through something … I have been that kid so I understand. I understand when people say 'These kids have lost their damn minds.' I understand and know what that's like. I know what that is, they didn't lose their mind, they are just dealing with trauma that's never been dealt with … They are out here, emotional because of all of the trauma, so this is what the youth are doing right now … We [CHW's] talk the talk, we walk the walk, and we really have that gift to be able to reach our youth. - Mike

Many have also spearheaded a shift in the narrative that gun violence is not the result of an individual's moral failing but instead shaped by environmental factors and historic municipal disinvestment. Reframing the conversation to consider a more holistic approach where gun violence needs to be seen not as a result of a moral shortcoming but rather a symptom of a much larger, systemic issue that has impacted entire neighborhoods.

There are not enough people getting out and reaching out to the youth. Because [if you sit them down and talk to them] a lot will say, 'I want to change, I want to work, I don't want to get in trouble, I don't want to die, I don't want to go to jail'. [The youth are] growing up untreated and [unheard]. We [as CHWs] want to change that narrative of what [youth experience] in our neighborhoods. - Mike

8.2.4   Conclusion

This section highlighted the multifaceted and invaluable support and coaching inherent in CHW work and the application of these skills in gun violence prevention. Violence provides a good example of a complex issue requiring both localized and systemic solutions and highlights the unique capabilities, tenacity, eminence, and diversity of the only workforce equipped to address this issue: CHWs. The credibility, experience, and incomparable skillsets of CHWs like Mike and Carolyn enable them to use transformative approaches to change the landscape of street- and youth-related gun violence. These credible messengers have contributed to the current record low numbers of homicides and shootings and have done this by providing linkages to government, clinical, and social services, while also focusing on building individual and community resilience.

Violence is a crisis with roots in social-structural inequality, economic distress, trauma, and behavioral and public health. Law enforcement alone cannot address the gun violence epidemic. CV CHWs in NYC, in particular, have made considerable contributions to health service delivery, public safety, criminal justice, and overall public policies. This section shared accounts of how CHWs have impacted local government's response to gun violence and improved individual and neighborhood health. As such, we must elevate this work and emphasize the reach and impact of CHW work as a discipline. In closing, we present the following statements as considerations for acknowledgment and building support and security of the workforce.

- CHWs are seen and treated as experts as they are the best positioned to advocate for the complex needs of their communities because of their close relationship with the community and its history.
- Given their competence of community culture and experience, CHWs must be given the autonomy and platform to integrate their lessons and recommendations into program and policy.
- Use of CHWs in this way can potentially place less demand on the political and administrative resources of law enforcement and the larger criminal justice system.
- Sustainable streams of funding and Medicaid reimbursement for CHW services are adjusted to meet public health needs. Improved outcomes of priority populations, when identified, are rewarded and scaled.
- Support is offered for network building among the CHWs for sharing resources and opportunities. CHWs build networks across disciplines to foster added collaboration and the exchange of knowledge and best practices among peers.
- Employers ensure organizational infrastructure among employers to promote staff wellness and therapeutic supports for lived and vicarious trauma experi-

enced by CHWs. Also, employers are mindful of the triggers, re-traumatization, and potential for vicarious trauma that CHWs encounter.

- Employers ensure organizational infrastructure to support equitable compensation and benefits for CHWs and support their continuous learning.
- Professional development opportunities are continuous and accessible.

References

Acevedo-Garcia, D., Lochner, K. A., Osypuk, T. L., & Subramanian, S. V. (2003). Future directions in residential segregation and health research: A multilevel approach. *American journal of public health, 93*(2), 215–221.

American Public Health Association. (2018). *Violence is a public health issue: Public health is essential to understanding and treating violence in the U.S. (20185).* Retrieved from https://www.apha.org/policies-and-advocacy/public-health-policy-statements/policy-database/2019/01/28/violence-is-a-public-health-issue

Bailey, Z., Kieger, N., Agénor, M., Graves, J., Linos, N., & Bassett, M. (2017). Structural racism and health inequities in the USA: Evidence and interventions. *The Lancet, 389*(10077), 1453–1463. https://doi.org/10.1016/S0140-6736(17)30569-X

Bravo, M. A., Anthopolos, R., Bell, M. L., & Miranda, M. L. (2016). Racial isolation and exposure to airborne particulate matter and ozone in understudied US populations: Environmental justice applications of downscaled numerical model output. *Environmental International, 92-93*, 247–255. https://doi.org/10.1016/j.envint.2016.04.008

Central Family Life Center. (n.d.). *True 2 life.* Retrieved from http://www.centralfamilylifecenter.org/project/true2life/

Cosgrove, S., Monroy, M., Jenkins, C., Castillo, S. R., Williams, C., Parris, E., … Brownstein, J. N. (2014). Community health workers as an integral strategy in the REACH U.S. program to eliminate health disparities. *Health Promot Pract, 15*(6), 795–802. https://doi.org/10.1177/1524839914541442

Cunningham, R., Knox, L., Fein, J., Harrison, S., Frisch, K., Walton, M., … Hargarten, S. W. (2009). Before and after the trauma bay: The prevention of violent injury among youth. *Annals of Emergency Medicine, 53*(4), 490–500. https://doi.org/10.1016/j.annemergmed.2008.11.014

Delgado, S., Alsabahi, L., Wolff, K., Alexander, N., Cobar, P., & Butts, J. A. (2017, October 7). *The effects of cure violence in the South Bronx and East New York, Brooklyn.* Retrieved from John Jay College of Criminal Justice, Research and Evaluation Center: https://johnjayrec.nyc/wp-content/uploads/2017/10/CVinSoBronxEastNY.pdf

End the Violence Epidemic. (n.d.). Retrieved from http://violenceepidemic.com/

Hurd, N. M., Zimmerman, M. A., & Xue, Y. (2008). Negative adult influences and the protective effects of role models: A study with urban adolescents. *Journal of Youth and Adolescence, 38*(6), 777–789. https://doi.org/10.1007/s10964-008-9296-5

John Jay College of Criminal Justice, Research and Evaluation Center. (2015, April 15). *LIFE camp.* Retrieved from https://johnjayrec.nyc/2015/04/15/lifecamp/

Kershaw, K. N., Diez Roux, A. V., Burgard, S. A., Lisabeth, L. D., Mujahid, M. S., & Schulz, A. J. (2011). Metropolitan-level racial residential segregation and black-white disparities in hypertension. *American Journal of Epidemiology, 174*(5), 537–545. https://doi.org/10.1093/aje/kwr116

Krivo, L. J., Byron, R. A., Calder, C. A., Peterson, R. D., Browning, C. R., Kwan, M. P., & Lee, J. Y. (2015). *Social Science Research, 54*, 303–318. https://doi.org/10.1016/j.ssresearch.2015.08.005

Lander, B. (2018, April). *Desegregating NYC: Twelve steps toward a more inclusive city.* Retrieved from New York City Council: https://drive.google.com/file/d/17yqKmyjsVXJEezRc-Dxfiz08F8C3MW_n/view

Li W., Zheng P., Huynh M., Castro A., Falci L., Kennedy J., … Van Wye, G. (2016). *Summary of vital statistics, 2016*. Retrieved from New York City Department of Health and Mental Hygiene, Bureau of Vital Statistics: https://www1.nyc.gov/assets/doh/downloads/pdf/vs/2016sum.pdf

Lovelidge, E. (2017). *Health system to prevent violence*. Retrieved from http://violenceepidemic.com/

New York City, Department of Health and Mental Hygiene. (n.d.). *EpiQuery: Mortality module* [Data file]. Retrieved from https://a816healthpsi.nyc.gov/epiquery/VS/index.html

New York City, Mayor's Office of Criminal Justice. (2017, March 23). *Mayor de Blasio announces 18% drop in city jail population since taking office* [Press release]. Retrieved from https://criminaljustice.cityofnewyork.us/press-release/mayor-de-blasio-announces-18-drop-in-city-jail-population-since-taking-office/

New York City, Mayor's Office of Criminal Justice. (2018, July 10). *Mayor's office to prevent gun violence set to expand, launch major peacekeeping programs* [Press release]. Retrieved from https://criminaljustice.cityofnewyork.us/press-release/mayors-office-to-prevent-gun-violence-set-to-expand-launch-major-peacekeeping-programs/

New York City, Office to Prevent Gun Violence. (n.d.-a). *Interventions: Crisis management system*. Retrieved from https://www1.nyc.gov/site/peacenyc/interventions/crisis-management.page

New York City, Office to Prevent Gun Violence. (n.d.-b). Retrieved from https://www1.nyc.gov/site/peacenyc/index.page

NYC Department of Health and Mental Hygiene. (n.d.). *Violence: A health issue*. Retrieved from https://www1.nyc.gov/site/doh/health/neighborhood-health/anti-violence.page

Slutkin, G. (2017). Reducing violence as the next great public health achievement. *Nature Human Behaviour, 1*, 0025. https://doi.org/10.1038/s41562-016-0025

Williams, D. R., & Collins, C. (2001). Racial residential segregation: A fundamental cause of racial disparities in health. *Public Health Reports, 116*(5), 404–416. https://doi.org/10.1093/phr/116.5.404

8.3   CHWs: A Bridge to Wellness

Kim Jay, Fatima Padron, Helen Margellos-Anast, Madeline Woodberry,
Melinda Banks, Gabriela Bustos, Rhonda M. Lay, and Stephanie Jordan

8.3.1   Introduction

We begin our section with some profiles of the two communities that CHWs from
the Sinai Urban Health Institute (SUHI) predominantly serve, a history of the communities that explains the reasons behind the social challenges the communities
face and the story of how and why SUHI was created to support these communities
(Fig. 8.4).

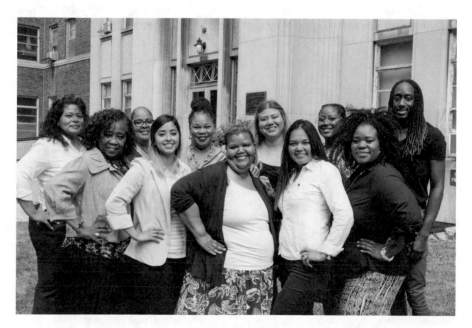

Fig. 8.4 SUHI's CHW team pictured from left to right: Melinda Banks, Madeline Woodberry,
Stephanie Jordan, Ana Diaz, Kim Jay, Rhonda Lay, Aidyn Ocon, Gabriela Bustos, Adlaide
Holloway, Faith Williams, and Jatavius Brown, in Chicago in July of 2018 (Rosman, 2018)

8.3.2   Community Profiles

SUHI is the community research arm of Sinai Health System (SHS). SHS is the largest, private safety net health system in Illinois, which via two campuses, one on the west side and one on the southwest side of Chicago, serves some of Chicago's poorest neighborhoods. Mount Sinai Hospital (Sinai), one of two ambulatory care hospitals of SHS, sits in an urban community on the west side of Chicago in between two neighborhoods named North Lawndale (NL) and South Lawndale (SL). South Lawndale is also known as Little Village (Fig. 8.5). These communities are disproportionately affected by illness, poverty, and social challenges. The Sinai Community Health Survey 2.0, one of the largest community-engaged, face-to-face health surveys ever conducted in Chicago, showed that in 2015–2016, the geographic areas served by Sinai have particularly high rates of food insecurity, obesity, and chronic disease (Hirschtick et al., 2017). The survey also showed that both communities are heavily affected by trauma and mental health issues. Results showed that 25% of adults in NL had symptoms of post-traumatic stress disorder (PTSD), which are higher than those of veterans returning home from active conflict situations (Hirschtick et al., 2017).

The majority of people who live in these two communities are non-Hispanic Black (in NL), are Mexican (in SL), and are poor. This is exemplified by the fact that in 2014, both NL and SL had a median income much lower than that of median income of $47,831 of Chicago as a whole (Hirschtick et al., 2017).

Little Village

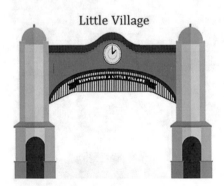

North Lawndale

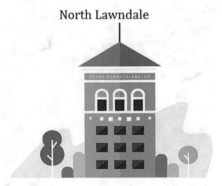

Median Household Income: $30,348

Percentage of Food Insecure Households: 45%

Percentage of Obese Adults: 33%

Percentage of Adults Screening Positive for PTSD Symptoms: 13%

Median Household Income: $21,763

Percentage of Food Insecure Households: 37%

Percentage of Obese Adults: 53%

Percentage of Adults Screening Positive for PTSD Symptoms: 25%

Fig. 8.5 A snapshot of community profiles (Hirschtick, Roesch, Monnard, & Mante, 2018a, 2018b) created for Little Village (left), also known as South Lawndale, and for North Lawndale (right), with information collected in the Sinai Survey 2.0 (Hirschtick, Benjamins, & Homan, 2017)

While poverty is prevalent in both NL and SL, there are distinct differences as well. In NL, green space is limited, and there is an abundance of empty lots and boarded up buildings interspersed between family homes, apartments, and businesses. In contrast, in SL there are thriving businesses, many of which are family-owned. There are also many well-kept homes with well-kept lawns and a much greater sense of community. However, violence and social disparities remain a common thread in both communities. While the blaring ambulance sirens are constant, they are not symbolic of the attitude of the communities where there is still so much compassion, vibrancy, and hope.

8.3.3   History

While an abundance of empty lots and boarded up buildings in NL is the current reality, it has not always been this way. Rhonda Lay, CHW, recalls:

> I've lived in North Lawndale since the early 1960's. I remember when children played jump rope on the sidewalk and rode their bikes up and down the streets freely, and jacks were the game of choice. I also remember when the blocks were filled with majestic Greystone houses and had perfectly manicured lawns and neighbors who looked out for each other. We kept each other safe and when there was a need, be it food or clothes, we as a community took care of each other. There were many mom and pop businesses in the community, from beauty salons to pharmacies. However, when Dr. King died and the riots happened, we lost a lot. We saw our community burn to the ground in protest. It was never rebuilt and many fled the neighborhood because there were only remnants left. This led to the scarcity of home owners and businesses. Those that remained were left with vacant lots as their landscape and income streams dried up. These events also contributed to one of the greatest public health tragedies we have seen, the 1995 Heat Wave of Chicago.

The population shifts experienced by North Lawndale between 1930 and today are as significant as they are a microcosm of US urban history. According to the US Census, North Lawndale residents numbered over 112,000 people in 1930, about 125,000 in 1960, and dropped to a low of about 35,600 in 2010. Between 1950 and 1960, the predominantly White (Russian, Jewish, Polish, and Czechoslovakian) population began migrating out of the community as NL became a point of entry for Black people migrating from the South. Within 10 years, the population went from being predominantly White to predominantly Black. The precipitous decline in population that occurred between 1960 and 2010 has its roots in several concurrent economic losses, including the flight of businesses after the 1968 riots which followed the assassination of Dr. Martin Luther King, Jr. Several large industrial and commercial companies left the area following the riots, including the Sears headquarters and the Western Electric plant, leaving a lack of viable employment opportunities for residents. In 2010, 90% of the population was non-Hispanic Black, 7% was Hispanic, and 2% was non-Hispanic White. The dramatic shifts in the racial composition of North Lawndale and many other Chicago communities have been detailed in several excellent books.[2]

The communities we serve have endured difficult historical tragedies, but they are also areas of great historical significance, have many cultural landmarks, and have experienced some economic success, realities which are less often talked about. In 1966 Dr. Martin Luther King lived in NL with his family in order to bring attention to the poor living conditions. At the time, it was Dr. King's belief that if things could change in Chicago, it could catapult change everywhere. Little Village, or SL, is known as the "Mexico of the Midwest" and has the second highest grossing shopping district in Chicago, second only to the "Magnificent Mile"—an area known for its high-end stores, posh hotels, and trendy restaurants. This historical context is a great reminder that people, not statistics, live in these communities and call it home. Madeline Woodberry, CHW recalls:

> North Lawndale has been my home for over 50 years. I remember when the community thrived with outdoor activities, families, and friendships. The beauty of our community with its landscapes and history makes me believe that we can revive our community to its previous greatness. I see hope and potential in North Lawndale ... I come to work every day to be a part of that revival."

SUHI's CHWs are deeply connected and committed to the members of the communities in North and South Lawndale. As Madeline stated above, we come to work every day to support our neighbors, one at a time, in order to be a part of the revival of these communities.

8.3.4 Sinai Urban Health Institute (SUHI)

Sinai Urban Health Institute (SUHI), the research arm of SHS, has employed CHWs since its inception in 2000. Daily, SUHI's CHWs do a job that reaches beyond the four walls of the hospital. SUHI's CHWs live in the communities served by SHS and bridge gaps between the health system, community organizations, and the clients they serve. SUHI and its CHWs work toward the mission of achieving health equity in Chicago communities through data-driven research, interventions, evaluation, and collaboration. The majority of SUHI's health interventions have utilized the CHW model, with effective approaches developed and tested in asthma management (pediatric and adult), breast cancer screening and navigation through treatment, and diabetes management, among others. SUHI is continuously innovating with the CHW model, with new CHW initiatives being developed and tested in the areas of oral health, visual lead-based paint assessments, and in holistically addressing the complex health and social needs of clients/community members. CHWs address community issues by engaging clients in their homes, at clinics, or other designated places, assisting them to deal with not only their health issues but also with the social factors that are often hindering optimal health of body and mind.

SUHI's CHW interventions were born out of need, compassion, and a desire for health equity through the vision of SUHI's founder, Steve Whitman, Ph.D. (1943–2014). As one example, Dr. Whitman noted that mortality rates between White and Black women in Chicago were similar throughout the 1980s and into the early 1990s. However, beginning in the early 1990s, White mortality rates began to decline, while Black rates remained steady, ultimately resulting in significant disparities in breast cancer mortality rates. By 2005, Black women in Chicago were nearly two times more likely to die of breast cancer than White women (Whitman, Ansell, Orsi, & Francois, 2010). Advances in early diagnosis and treatment seemed not to be translating effectively to Black women in Chicago. Furthermore, SUHI studies assessing disparities for Chicago and the USA more broadly for 17 health status indicators (birth outcomes and mortality rates) found that disparities between non-Hispanic Black and non-Hispanic White people since the early 1990s have generally been widening both for Chicago and the USA, but to a greater extent in Chicago (Hunt & Whitman, 2014). The associated mortality gap is responsible for more than 60,000 excess Black deaths per year in the USA. Dr. Whitman passed onto us his motivation and vision of moving toward health equity in the form of CHWs bringing personalized care and support to people's doorsteps. SUHI was founded on the principle of identifying evidence-based solutions to health inequities; over our history we have identified CHWs as a key element to achieving health equity and their role as providers of social support as one that is fundamental and vital.

8.3.5   CHWs: Providers of Social Support

While there are various formal definitions for and some debate regarding the exact constructs that go into social support, social support is essentially the belief that one is cared for, combined with the availability of family, friends, neighbors, and others who offer emotional and tangible support, companionship, and advice. Social support is critical to health and well-being; yet, supportive social networks are often lacking in the communities we serve. As you have already seen, there are profound historical reasons behind the relatively recent breakdown of social support networks. This part will focus on the importance of how and why we as CHWs provide social support and one of the primary reasons we provide it, social isolation.

8.3.5.1   How We Provide Social Support

As CHWs, we know that there is more to a person than meets the eye in terms of overall health. Health, as defined by the World Health Organization (WHO), is "a state of complete physical, mental, and social well-being." Given this broad definition, improving health necessitates a focus, which includes the social determinants of health—for example, having transportation to a doctor's appointment, having food for one's family, or having support when going through a challenging diagnosis. As CHWs, we help clients overcome barriers to well-being by identifying the most urgent among their competing priorities and creating a realistic and time-targeted plan together to deal with the issues at hand. This process requires mutual trust and respect. One of the ways we connect and foster trust with clients is by prioritizing what is most important for the client and listening to their concerns, rather than pushing our own program agenda. Kim Jay, CHW, illustrates this well:

> My reason for being in a home, whether it is to check in on a client's asthma or diabetes, sometimes has to take a back seat. I may have to handle the matter of greatest urgency to the client before I can get to that. First and foremost, I have to build trust and what matters most to them matters most to me. That's how we as CHWs build trust.

We find that most clients are not purposely ignoring what a doctor or caregiver recommends, but rather, their life's challenges dictate their priorities. For example, if we arrive at a client's home and they are worried about putting food on the table, they likely are not prioritizing taking their diabetes medication as prescribed. Instead, they are going to be focused on how they are going to feed their families. Clients have competing priorities, and their attention becomes a game of "whack the mole," as they jump around to where the current urgency is greatest. Many times things such as managing their diseases properly with medication or regular primary or specialty care appointments ranks low on that list of priorities.

Across programs, SUHI's CHWs assess the social factors that potentially influence their clients' health and then provide linkages to community resources. Despite the "door" through which we enter a client's life, more times than not, the individual is dealing with multiple illnesses and multiple social challenges. One of our primary roles across our programs is to partner with our clients to guide them through their health journey which often means putting our own agenda aside to provide social support in areas outside of the primary goal of our program. This principle is necessary in being a successful CHW because we show clients that we actually care, which is vital to their willingness to ultimately allow us into their private space. Being allowed in their private space is essential in working with clients in a compassionate and effective manner and in developing the trust needed to later coach clients toward that goal of thriving in health.

8.3.5.2 Social Isolation

Sometimes when we are making home visits, we stay and talk with clients over our allotted time because people just want someone to listen to them, and we are sometimes the only company they have. Listening to the client's life concerns allows us to foster a relationship of trust and openness. Social support is the feeling and reality that one is being cared for. Some of the ways we provide social support include listening, asking about the client's family, giving clients a number where they know they can reach us, going to community events, and sometimes even going to personal events. Having a lack of social support produces poor health outcomes, contributes to loneliness, and heightens a feeling of low self-esteem. The consequences of social isolation on health can be devastating. Having someone support you in times of urgency could be the deciding factor between life and death as exemplified in the heat wave that occurred in July of 1995 (Klinenberg, 1999).

During the heat wave, the temperature in Chicago reached a high of 106° and remained elevated for five consecutive days. Many NL residents died because there was no one to come and check on them. The vibrant, beautiful homes of previous years had been replaced by vacant lots; instead of open windows and fans to catch a breeze, there was rampant crime and fear. Therefore, neighbors were afraid, and windows were often nailed shut for safety purposes. Instead of families living together, adult children and other family members moved out and away from older family members. Seniors and those less fortunate who could not afford to leave were often left alone. Unable to help themselves and with no support from the community, many died. Tragically, there were 739 heat-related deaths in Chicago over that 5-day period. Most of the victims were from the most vulnerable populations, including the poor and elderly residents of the city, who could not afford air conditioning and did not have effective social networks in place, meaning no one was around to check on them. NL was one of the most affected communities; conversely SL, with its stronger social ties and more connected community, experienced very few deaths. The effects of social isolation on health and well-being are vast and are something we as CHWs still see a lot.

An example of the positive impact that having social support can make can be seen in the experience of Stephanie Jordan, one of SUHI's CHWs who works in breast health. Stephanie recalls:

> I learned that one of my clients, "Ms. Jackson", needed to have a biopsy. Ms. Jackson was very afraid and refused to have the biopsy. I finally persuaded her to schedule and to attend her biopsy appointment by agreeing to go with her when no one else could. When Ms. Jackson arrived at the appointment, she refused to go forward with the procedure unless I was allowed to stay in the room with her. The doctor tried to convince the client that everything would be okay and that I would be waiting for her afterwards. Ms. Jackson insisted that I be present in the room and, that if I could be in the room that she would stay and calm down. The doctor recognized the bond and allowed me in the room. Ms. Jackson said my presence gave her a sense of calmness. Everything went well with the procedure and she was immensely grateful that I had cared enough to hold her hand through her fears. I believe Community Health Workers are not only the bridges between patients and doctors, but we are the calm in the midst of someone's storm.

Stephanie's presence allowed Ms. Jackson to overcome her fear of having the necessary follow-up she needed. In this client's case, the biopsy came back negative, but in many cases, the results don't happen that way. People go through years without the necessary procedures because of fear and lack of social support which can be life-threatening especially with things such as breast cancer and diabetes. This client's daughter called Stephanie to thank her for being there for her mom and for being her mom's "stand-in daughter."

As CHWs, we are often a client's stand-in daughter, stand-in friend, and stand-in neighbor. We provide the social support that clients do not have in moments of need to help them reach their goals and improve health outcomes.

8.3.6   CHWs as Coaches

In this section we will cover the history of why our communities mistrust the medical system and why CHWs make effective coaches.

8.3.6.1   History and Mistrust

For many people of color, historical (and current) atrocities have severely damaged their trust of the medical community. For example, in 1932, Black men were asked to participate in a study to treat "bad blood" also known as the Tuskegee study. At the start of the study, a cure for syphilis was not available. The purpose of the study was to assess the progression of untreated syphilis and its effects on the body, even unto death. In 1947, penicillin was identified as a cure for syphilis. However, participants in the Tuskegee study were given ineffective treatments and hindered from obtaining penicillin. This practice went on for 40 years. Many needlessly suffered, passed on the condition to others, and even died as a result of this study. As another example, in 1936, under the Eugenical Sterilization Law of the early 1900s, Puerto Rican women who needed to work to support their families were forced into sterilization as a condition for work, preventing them from ever having children. They were never offered the alternative of birth control even when available. These atrocities may not have happened directly to our clients, but the legacy of mistreatment and mistrust lingers, affecting current client's willingness to appropriately access health care. Establishing and regaining trust between clients and the medical system is a major part of a CHW's role, which at times means we must apologize for previous mistreatment and for the past experiences of clients with the medical system.

The lingering legacy of mistrust can be seen in many common challenges in effective healthcare delivery, two of which are honest, transparent communication between patient and physician and compliance with the set treatment plan. The people in the communities we serve are not completely honest with their physicians for a variety of reasons including that lingering feeling of mistrust. They also may be embarrassed or ashamed of their life challenges and struggles and think the physician will not be able to relate, or fear judgment or mistreatment. As CHWs, we make great coaches because we can address these challenges.

A CHW inherently comes from, is a part of, or has a close understanding of the community being served. Because we often look and sound like the community we are serving, the people in the community are more likely to trust us. This is because they know we can relate to their experience, and they are therefore more likely to be open and transparent with us about their situation and their struggles. We can often anticipate what some of their barriers to achieving their goals or overcoming their struggles will be because we have either lived them or know someone who has. We can share our own personal story of overcoming the same struggles or share the story of someone we know. We can therefore better coach them to overcome those barriers.

In this coaching role, our job is not to diagnose or treat medical conditions but rather to understand and work together with the client to help them follow their healthcare provider's recommendations to improve their health. Because we can relate to clients and the clients trust us, we can give them honest advice and work with them as a team to find solutions. Working as a team is imperative to maintaining trust with the client because while patient-centered care is trending, this is not what our clients are used to receiving when interacting with the medical system.

Perhaps due to lack of time, or a doctor's training to diagnose and treat, doctors often do not have time or the ability to effectively dig deeper to identify the root cause of an issue or learn why patients are not following their medical advice. We often encounter clients whose providers are not aware of their life circumstances, are uncomfortable discussing such matters, or do not account for those circumstances when providing medical advice and treatment. As a result of these interactions, clients leave their appointments feeling unheard, hopeless, disempowered, and sometimes worse than before their appointment. Our role as CHWs is to bridge that gap between the patient and provider.

CHWs serve as a bridge by offering the extra time, support, and coaching that the client needs and then by helping to communicate the information they collect back to the healthcare team. When we empower clients to make decisions and to be part of the plan, we get their buy-in, and therefore they are more likely to follow the plan. We do this by figuring out the root of what's going on and then coming up with a customized plan together with the client on how to address the issue. Making sure the plan is customized and fits the needs and ability of the client is key to setting the client up for success.

8.3.7 Social Support and Coaching Strategies

Like any great coach, we need to know our players' strengths and weaknesses in order to understand how to help them be successful. At SUHI, we are all trained by SUHI's Center for CHW Research, Outcomes, and Workforce Development (CROWD). The adverse childhood experiences (ACEs) and social support modules within this training provide us with foundational knowledge necessary to provide effective social support, while the motivational interviewing, stages of change, and goal-setting modules prepare CHWs to coach clients effectively.

As mentioned previously, social support is vital to gaining a client's trust. In order to provide great social support, we must understand the client's experience. ACEs help to explain how the trauma people experience growing up between the ages of birth and 18 years manifests as health and emotional challenges. Establishing an understanding as to why people are who they are allows us as CHWs to connect to people from a place of understanding rather than a place of judgment. One story of how ACEs training came into play is relayed by Kim Jay, CHW:

I remember working with a single mother of three with asthma; she was a bit reluctant to allow me in her home because she didn't feel her home was up to par. She was a 27-year-old African American woman and her children's ages ranged from 3 to 12. As I made my visits to her home, we addressed her asthma and we would talk more and more about why she had children at an early age. She expressed that she had been molested as a young girl and was very promiscuous and ashamed. My training in ACEs prepared me to share with her how who she was as an adult could be in part due to the sexual abuse she experienced as a child. I assured her that the emotion she was feeling was nothing to be ashamed of and who she is now was the most important part of her journey. Knowing that traumatic life experiences before the age of 18 often lead to risky health behaviors and therefore poorer health allowed me to be a better support to her.

Once we have provided the needed social support and built trust with the clients, we assess a client's readiness to change. Some clients can make immediate and drastic healthy changes, while others need to take baby steps toward their goals. As CHWs and coaches, we meet people where they are in their readiness to change. For one person that might mean committing to drinking two glasses of water a day, while to another this may mean cutting all sugary beverages and only drinking water. When a client is not ready to change, we address the underlying challenges such as literacy, lack of trust and understanding, or other social needs that are of priority to the client in order to move forward. Once other priority needs are addressed, if a client is still feeling ambivalent to change, we use motivational interviewing (MI) and the "change talk" to help them overcome that ambivalence.

MI is used when a client acknowledges that there is a change they need to make but is feeling ambivalent, uncertain, or unsure about taking steps toward making that change. There are stages of change (Prochaska & DiClemente, 1983) that we all go through when deciding whether we need to make a change: pre-contemplation, contemplation, preparation, action, and maintenance. The state of ambivalence described above happens when someone is in the contemplation stage. Being trained in MI teaches CHWs how to listen actively, ask open-ended questions, make affirmative statements, make reflective statements, and make summary statements. These types of questions and statements help us to get deeper insight into what is causing the ambivalence and allow the client to do most of the talking. To take things a step further, we use the "change talk" which involves asking the client open-ended questions to allow them to vocalize their need or desire to change, their ability to change, and their own commitment to change. The training we receive helps us learn and practice the types of questions to ask to help our clients talk through these various topics. Most importantly, MI allows the client to come up with their own solution and plan. The utility of MI can be seen in the following example, told from the perspective of Melinda Banks, CHW:

Mr. O is a 51-year-old Mexican male with diabetes who works for a landscaping company. Getting ready for work one day, he quickly put on his work boots. He came home after a long day and took off his boots only to discover that there was a lot of blood in one of his boots; a small piece of wood had found its way into Mr. O's boot and cut his foot. His wife attempted to care for his injury but over time it got infected.

He was admitted to the emergency department (ED) because of an infection on his big toe. During my first session with Mr. O, he explained to me that though he had been diagnosed with diabetes in 2011, he did not have a primary care physician or any supplies such

as a glucometer to check his sugar levels. Mr. O did not have any medication for his diabe-
tes either. He also shared that his father, as well as ten of his uncles on his father's side, had
passed away due to diabetes complications. Each one of them had lost at least one limb as
a result of their diabetes before dying.

That same day after our meeting, I reached out to Sinai's clinical diabetes team to make
him an appointment as well as to obtain a glucometer so that he could check his sugar read-
ings at home. Mr. O's Hemoglobin A1C (A1C) was at a 14.7. An A1C is a common blood
test done every three months and is used to diagnose type 1 and type 2 diabetes as well as
to gauge how well an individual is managing their diabetes. Ideally, one's A1C should be
no higher than 6.

Since Mr. O did not understand the seriousness of his diabetes, he continued to eat and
drink whatever he pleased. He loved apple and cranberry juice. After we began meeting,
one of his first goals was to slowly stop drinking so much juice. It wasn't easy for him to
give up his juice at first. He thought that he could just switch from one juice to another, but
I showed him by looking at the label that it was the same thing. He was able to accomplish
this goal through our conversations and by recognizing for himself what he was doing to
raise his sugar levels, and by setting a couple SMART goals for himself which included
slowly transitioning from regular fruit drinks to sugar free fruit drinks as well as diluting
his juice so it was half juice and half water. By the end of the program, his number one drink
was water and an occasional 7-up.

My training in MI helped me ask Mr. O the right questions and move him toward getting
ready to make a change. Through the questions I learned to ask, we were able to uncover
his desire to live a long life and not lose any of his limbs. He was also able to recognize how
eating balanced meals, exercising, and taking his medications would help him accomplish
his goal of living a long healthy life. Mr. O now checks his blood sugar regularly and stays
active. He takes walks every chance he gets with his dog Oreo. He stated that he now feels
more energetic and does not feel sleepy like he used to. He even tries to convince his
20-year-old daughter to walk instead of drive to the neighborhood grocery store which is
two blocks away. From diluting his juice to his new regimen of walking rather than driving
to the neighborhood grocery store, we made sure the decisions were his. Noticeably, as his
confidence grew so did his goals.

Thanks to her training in ACEs, Melinda was able to recognize that experiencing his father's and uncles' deaths so early in his life affected Mr. O's behaviors today. By providing a listening ear to his story and being a social support for him, she was able to learn more about his family history and garner his trust. Then using MI technique, Melinda was able to ask Mr. O questions to uncover his desire to live a long and healthy life, effectively helping him overcome the ambivalence to make the necessary changes to manage his diabetes. Asking clients questions such as "what would need to be different in order to make that change?" and "if you were able to make all the changes you'd like to, what would your life look like?" helps clients uncover their desires and their needs. When we have the client's trust, we are also able to ask harder questions such as "suppose you don't change, what is the worst thing that might happen?". Having the client's trust, especially when asking the harder questions is vital because they know that we care and we are trying to help them. MI is a powerful tool that helps us help the client overcome their own ambivalence to change. Once we are able to help them do that, we can move on to helping them tailor a plan to make that change.

As a coach, effective goal setting is an essential part of that custom game plan. If the goals in the plan are not tailored for the needs and challenges of the client, we are doing the client a disservice and setting them up for failure. Our team is trained and practices creating these custom plans during our core skills training. We start by asking the client what they would like to focus on. Usually they say something broad such as, "I want to lose weight." These tend to be the bigger goals that we work toward. In a conversational manner, we ask questions to help the client create smaller, SMART (Specific, Measurable, Attainable, Relevant, and Time-targeted) goals to help them reach that bigger goal. SMART goals target things that are relevant to the person's overall goal. Importantly, these goals need to be measurable so progress can be monitored and goals can be adjusted as necessary. Equally important is that the goals be attainable and have a deadline or time frame in which to be completed. Having SMART goals allows us to measure progress and allows for adjustments where needed. So if someone starts by saying they'd like to lose weight, we might follow-up with, "That's a great goal to have. What is one thing you can focus on this week to move you toward that goal?" We would then ask follow-up questions to make sure the smaller goal fits all of the criteria of a SMART goal. Once the goal is created, we assess their confidence in reaching that goal on a scale of 1–10. If their confidence is low, we readjust the goal to make it more attainable. Even if this means starting with something small, setting clients up for success is important in building the client's confidence and motivation in their ability to achieve and tackle even bigger goals. Finally, we help clients learn to problem solve how they will overcome barriers they may face in meeting their SMART goals. Through all of the social support and coaching, we are always trying to build self-efficacy so that the clients learn how to do these things for themselves.

The "I do, we do, you do" strategy is fundamental in building a client's self-efficacy. We start by showing the client how something is done while they observe and start learning, then we do it together, and finally they do it on their own while we cheer them on. The goal is always to get a client to be self-sufficient so that when we as CHWs are no longer there, they know how to do things themselves. For example, when in a home, we may need to schedule an appointment and the client has not done that before or has given up on scheduling appointments because they can never get through to anyone. The first time, we allow them to listen to us go through the process using speaker phone so they can hear the questions being asked and how to answer them. On the next call, we make the call together on speaker phone. Finally, we let the client take the lead on talking while we standby cheering them on and providing support. This process builds the client's confidence and empowers them so that when it's time for the next appointment to be made, they can do this on their own.

8.3.8 Summary: Coaching and Social Support

Our goal as CHWs is to identify with a person's truest needs, gain their trust, and to coach them to an effective solution. As our approach is always individualized to a specific person's needs, the door we walk through originally is not always the one we need to address first. The following story told by Kim Jay, CHW, exemplifies how gaining trust, getting to the root of an issue, and effectively coaching toward a solution can make a large impact to a person's overall physical and mental well-being:

> I was working with a single mom, "Ms. Jones", and her three daughters living in an apartment on the west side of Chicago. I had called her the day before to confirm our Asthma Program visit and remind her of the time I would be there. When I got to the door the next day she appeared relieved that I was there. Being a CHW doing frequent home visits, you immediately become aware of odors, furniture conditions, walls, floors, and other environmental factors, and in this case, there was a distinct odor that I noted upon entering her apartment. A standard part of our asthma healthy homes visits is to do a comprehensive walkthrough and environmental assessment. So I asked if I had her permission to do the walkthrough of her home to assess if there was anything that could be causing her daughter's asthma to flare up so frequently. I had already noticed an abundance of air fresheners and candles. In addition, I noticed an area rug over the carpeted floor. Ms. Jones began to look a bit worried as I asked questions and her face turned red when I asked about the rug. She said there was some flooding and she couldn't get the carpet clean enough so she covered the floor. When I looked under the rug, I could smell a strong musty odor and saw that there was black mold. She told me that management knew about the flooding but that they hadn't done anything about it in over six months. I knew that in order to get her daughter healthier, and for the sake of everyone living in the house, that we had to address the mold.
>
> With her permission I spoke with her management office and informed them of who I was and of my role in the tenant's life. I described the severity of the situation, and they promised they would take care of it. I promised her I would follow up by our next visit which was three weeks later. To both of our delight, the very next day someone was out looking at the floor, and they were shocked at how extensive the water damage was. In the next two weeks, contractors were there removing and replacing the floor because the mold had eaten the floor boards.

As a CHW, seeing the difference our effort and hard work can make is amazing. Seeing our efforts pay off in improved client outcomes validates our work and is a motivator for us to continue to do the work. We get a lot of feedback from our clients that show us how important the work we do is and how much of an impact we make. In the case of Ms. Jones above, she wrote to us saying:

> I appreciate that you acted fast and were willing to diligently assist my family and I to obtain better living conditions. As this was definitely something that stressed me out and posed health risks to us. I cannot express how happy I was that day in July of this year when the contractors arrived to pull out the old carpet and tile the entire apartment. We are so happy that we now have better living conditions, and I no longer have to explain the condition of my carpet to visitors. I can now proudly open the door and host a dinner without feeling embarrassed about the condition.

Even though Kim did not go into Ms. Jones' home intending to get the floor replaced, she saw this as her duty by the time she left. Ms. Jones further shared that she was actually depressed and did everything she could to stay away from her "four walls," but now she is proud of where she lives and elated at the better condition and health of her daughters. Ms. Jones leaned on Kim for emotional support, sharing things with her that she was not comfortable sharing with family for fear of being judged. Kim listened and offered her hope; she assured Ms. Jones that the situation was not her fault, allowing the guilt she felt because of her child's illness to be released. Kim coached Ms. Jones through the necessary steps for remediation of the mold, and together, they achieved a positive outcome.

As CHWs, our role in coaching is to empower our clients in the process. We must be reactive to the needs of the clients, allowing them to prioritize what is most important to them. Importantly, our clients must feel that the decisions made are their own. Historically, many individuals we work with have not had a say in their treatment plan, so changing the narrative using these coaching strategies is key in erasing the stigma of mistrust and in leading people to better health outcomes.

8.3.9 Successes

SUHI rigorously evaluates all our CHW programs; thus, we know that when CHWs work with clients to better manage their chronic disease, improve their home environment, or more appropriately access the health system and community resources, we impact outcomes in ways that ultimately lead to improved health and well-being. Through our asthma initiatives, which involve CHWs working with children and adults who have evidence of poorly controlled asthma over multiple home visits (usually four to six), we have significantly reduced emergency room visits and increased quality of life (Gutierrez Kapheim, Ramsay, Schwindt, Hunt, & Margellos-Anast, 2015; Karnick et al., 2007; Margellos-Anast, Gutierrez, & Whitman, 2012). As one example, evaluation findings from our CHW-led, healthy homes asthma interventions, which have been in the field for nearly 20 years, have indicated that emergency department visits and hospitalizations decrease by about 70% in the year following the intervention and that quality of life is significantly improved (Gutierrez Kapheim et al., 2015; Karnick et al., 2007; Margellos-Anast et al., 2012). Notably, cost savings have been substantial across asthma initiatives, ranging from $2.33 to $7.79 per dollar spent (Gutierrez Kapheim et al., 2015; Karnick et al., 2007; Margellos-Anast et al., 2012).

The Helping Her Live program is SUHI's community-based CHW program that educates women on the importance of screening mammograms and navigates them through the process of completing mammograms and if needed additional diagnostic tests and treatment. The Helping Her Live program has educated over 15,000 women since 2007 and has navigated over 4000 women to mammograms.

A SUHI intervention that added CHW-led community outreach and home-based intervention (based on the National Diabetes Education Program) to Sinai's standard clinical diabetes services (which include a diabetes clinic, an 8-week Diabetes Learning Circle led by clinical dieticians, walking clubs, and cooking classes) found that participants who also worked with a CHW were significantly more likely to achieve diabetes control and that HbA1c levels decreased by 0.5% (Hughes, Yang, Ramanathan, & Benjamins, 2016).

Due to the breadth of experience amassed over nearly two decades, SUHI is a recognized leader in the training, hiring, and supervision of CHWs and in developing, implementing, and translating impactful CHW health interventions to a variety of populations and organizations. In 2014, with funding from the Lloyd A. Fry Foundation, SUHI developed a report putting forth best practices for implementing and evaluating CHW programs in healthcare settings (Gutierrez Kapheim & Campbell, 2014). Stemming from this experience, in 2017 SUHI launched CROWD (Center for CHW Research, Outcomes, and Workforce Development), our CHW consulting, training, and technical support center. CROWD works to advance the CHW workforce by working with organizations interested in utilizing CHWs to identify, hire, and train CHWs, along with doing quality assurance, and process and outcome evaluation for a variety of interventions. This would not have been possible without involving CHWs in the process. Kim Jay, CHW, knows this well:

> When I was first hired as a CHW, I received all the necessary training in house to educate on the chronic condition I was to address. However; the "real life" of the intervention wasn't inserted to really prepare me for the field work. A lot of visits were missed around the 1st of the month and our program managers didn't understand why this was happening. As a CHW from the community, I know that government assistance funds are issues on the 1st of the month and that people are busy paying bills and buying groceries. Therefore, seeing clients in the home or in the clinic during that time is nearly impossible because other things take priority. To most healthcare providers, this underlying reason for missed visits would never cross their minds, but it is a well-known fact of life in the neighborhood. As a CHW at SUHI I have been able to incorporate this, and many other invaluable pieces of community knowledge, into our program processes and training modules.

The SUHI CHW team has been instrumental in the success, development, and evaluation of SUHI's program intervention and training. The stories shared throughout this section further testify to the success we have had with CHW interventions at SUHI.

8.3.10   Lessons Learned and Challenges

There's an adage that says: "It takes a village to raise a child," and we have learned and believe that similarly, a team is needed to foster good health. While Chicago is a far cry from a village, a team-based approach that includes the client, healthcare providers, social service agencies, and community resources is needed to assist our population effectively. In order to achieve health, some people may need a little help, while others may need a lot. This is a matter of equity (each person receiving the level of support that they need), not equality (each person receiving the same support). As CHWs, we are able to help provide that additional support that people need in order to help level the playing field in a client's journey to better health.

There are many challenges we face as CHWs in Illinois. Specifically, there is no credentialing agency in our state to allow CHWs to be compensated directly by Medicaid, Medicare, or other health plans, thus limiting many organizations' ability to afford and sustain CHWs. More generally, we struggle with a lack of understanding of the unique role CHWs play on the healthcare team and the value we can bring to the healthcare team. Importantly, as CHWs, we must be confident in our understanding of the value we bring to the team and that we can speak to that value when questioned. We as CHWs are an extension of the healthcare team and a bridge to the community that is second to none. We are not, nor do we pretend to be, doctors, nurses, or social workers, but there are invaluable contributions we make to a patient's care. We modify our approach based on the person in front of us, providing more patient-centered care. Despite this, healthcare professionals sometimes feel threatened and resistant to the change that CHWs bring to a long-standing health-care system and the way things have been done for so long. We know the way things have been done is not working. When patients go into the doctor's office, they won't tell the doctor or nurse: "I have mold, roaches, or smokers in my home which affects my health." However, as CHWs, we can get that information when we are in the home and that can allow for a course of treatment that does not inevitably involve an increase in medication or more services but rather addresses the root cause of the problem at hand. The ability to uncover information the medical team otherwise could not can be seen in many of our team's stories.

One example of how CHWs can contribute to the healthcare team by bringing otherwise unknown information to the attention of the healthcare team comes from Kim Jay's experience working with a client who had poorly controlled asthma:

> I remember when I enrolled a client, "Mr. Eddie", into our adult asthma intervention program. My position on this intervention was to see what was keeping this client from being well. At my first visit I noticed some medication technique issues that were addressed and corrected. I also noticed that Mr. Eddie had a cat which can be a barrier for asthma management, so I knew that had to be addressed also. From experience, I know those who have animals love them like their children, and I observed from the freedom the cat had in the home, he was loved in that way. I asked Mr. Eddie if he knew that pets can be a trigger for asthma, and he stated he did not. I went on to ask more questions on the cat, including where the pet slept to determine the best course of action. We discussed some options such as keeping the cat out of his room or off the bed to keep his room dander free, as well as perhaps housing the cat elsewhere. Mr. Eddie listened but was not sure what he could commit to doing in order to better manage his asthma. He also shared that he was just released from prison and that the cat was his 'buddy'. I left the visit knowing I would have to work at getting this addressed in a way that would work for him. This young man had already lost so much, and I didn't want to have to take the comfort the cat brought him as well.
>
> Two days later Mr. Eddie was in the ED with an asthma exacerbation, and I was able to go to the ED and speak with the doctor while the patient was still there. I introduced myself as his CHW, and I was then able to ask what the plan was for his care. The doctor informed me that he was increasing the dosage of his asthma medication. I then asked if the patient told him he had a cat. The doctor stopped mid key stroke and said 'a cat?' I said 'yes and we are working on the best solution to address it'. He then got up and went to the exam room and told Mr. Eddie that he needed to get rid of the cat because of his asthma. Mr. Eddie looked at me because I had sort of told on him and then turning to the doctor said, 'We are working on it.' Of course, the doctor was adamant about getting rid of the pet, but I knew the approach would have to be gentler because of his connection to the pet. At the end of this ED experience, I was able to keep Mr. Eddie from receiving an increased dose of medication because of what I had seen in the home and because of my ability to relay that information to the doctor.
>
> I made my next visit to Mr. Eddie's home soon after. I asked if he decided how he wanted to deal with the cat situation. At first, the patient said he was going to keep the cat and take more medicine because he couldn't get rid of his buddy. But he remembered our conversation about at least keeping the cat out of his bedroom. Ultimately, he allowed the cat to live upstairs with his aunt where he could still visit. He said, 'I just didn't want anyone to take anything else from me.' Because it was his solution, he felt empowered and included in making a decision that was best for him and as a result, our outcome was favorable. Mr. Eddie

went from using his inhaler three times a day to twice per month. He indicated that his energy level was better because he didn't feel out of breath all the time. He also kept his sense of security because he didn't have to totally disconnect himself from his pet. He got to keep his cat and his asthma improved dramatically.

Situations like this often result in increased medications, increased hospital visits, and missed appointments. However, having someone like a CHW to explain, listen, and help with solutions proves to be very effective in bettering outcomes.

Another example, this one from the work of Gabriela Bustos, a bilingual breast health CHW navigating a 41-year-old patient named "Angela" shows how CHWs can eliminate barriers clients face in navigating the health system:

Angela was first diagnosed with breast cancer in 2017. In 2018, she found more lumps in her breast, and a biopsy revealed a malignant tumor. Angela expressed to me that she was feeling sad, worried, and anxious about the diagnosis because she had been on the waiting list for her chemotherapy treatment and did not believe she would ever get better. Angela did not speak English and indicated to me that she felt lost when trying to find out the status of her appointment due to the language barrier. As her CHW, I went to the physician's office on Angela's behalf and spoke with the primary care doctor's assistant. I learned that the doctor was not aware that Angela had been waiting all this time for her chemotherapy. By connecting with Angela's doctor and bridging the language barrier, I was able to support the patient in getting the treatment she needed. I am happy to report that as of June 2018, Angela is now receiving her treatment and continues to be thankful for the support I provided and that her faith in the health care system has been renewed. By earning Angela's trust, I was able to be the bridge between her and the medical system that no one else had stepped up to be. Being the voice for someone who feels they don't have one is a small act that affects a larger outcome. This experience reinforced the fact that our presence makes a difference.

CHWs often break down communication barriers between a provider and diabetic patients in relation to obstacles and appropriately managing blood sugar levels. In one case, the doctor could not understand what was going on because the patient was very compliant with her medication and kept all her appointments, yet her blood sugar levels were still high. When Kim visited her in her home, she found that she was running a candy store out of her home. She was also eating a lot of the candy. The patient also shared with Kim that she had the candy store because she was trying to raise enough money to purchase a headstone for her mother and her brother who had passed away and that she did not know any other way to raise the money. Kim was able to share that information with the doctor who was then able to modify her care plan. Rather than simply increasing medication, the doctor was able to create a better care plan for her diabetes and even connected the client with a counselor for her underlying depression.

Clients do not often share that their pets are flaring up their asthma or that they have roaches or mold in their home or that they are eating way too much sugar during a doctor's appointment. As CHWs, we play an invaluable role in obtaining that information and bringing the information back to the healthcare team. We need to own that and know what our role is in order to be confident and speak when presented the opportunity. Equally as important is for our supervisors, managers, and directors to intervene as needed and to speak to our role and to the value we bring to the healthcare team. Oftentimes, once a physician sees that we are capable and the value we bring, they come to us for everything. Finally, we have learned that identifying respected physician and/or nurse champions for CHWs can be particularly helpful in breaking down barriers we encounter when being integrated into healthcare team as those champions can support, promote, and validate our role to the larger team.

8.3.11 Conclusion

As CHWs, we are a priceless bridge to reaching a community that might otherwise seem beyond help. We are effective because of who we are. Our identity and qualities help create trust and rapport with our clients. We come from the communities we serve, we share some of the same concerns and experiences, and we understand the client's struggle because oftentimes we have the same struggles.

We know we must consider the person in a holistic manner considering the context of their life. We approach our work in a nonjudgmental manner, knowing that every situation is complex and striving to understand our client's personal situation. We take the time that doctors and nurses often do not have to look at the root causes of a person's ill health and then to provide the social support and coaching a client needs to work toward better health together. As demonstrated numerous times, both by our team of CHWs and others, properly trained CHWs can improve health knowledge, behaviors, and access to the health system in ways that meaningfully improve health outcomes. The integration of CHWs into all medical teams should be a no brainer. Our role is invaluable and second to none.

Our training in effective social support helps us meet clients where they are by prioritizing the needs of greatest urgency to the client. We are a pillar of social support to many clients who have no other support systems in place. Our training in coaching allows us to help our clients overcome their ambivalence and fear of change. Through effective coaching that includes working together, goal setting, and empowerment, we support our clients in striving to "thrive in health."

References

Gutierrez Kapheim, M., & Campbell, J. (2014). *Best practice guidelines for implementing and evaluating community health worker programs in health care settings* (Tech.). Chicago, IL: Sinai Urban Health Institute.

Gutierrez Kapheim, M., Ramsay, J., Schwindt, T., Hunt, B. R., & Margellos-Anast, H. (2015). Utilizing the Community Health Worker Model to communicate strategies for asthma self-management and self-advocacy among public housing residents. *Journal of Communication in Healthcare, 8*(2), 95–105. https://doi.org/10.1179/1753807615y.0000000011

Hirschtick, J., Benjamins, M. R., & Homan, S. (2017). *Community health counts: Sinai Community Health Survey 2.0* (Tech.). Chicago, IL: Sinai Urban Health Institute.

Hirschtick, J., Roesch, P., Monnard, K., & Mante, A. (2018a). *Sinai Community Survey 2.0: Community health profiles, Little Village*. Chicago, IL: Sinai Urban Health Institute, Sinai Health System. Retrieved from https://www.sinaisurvey.org/community-health-profiles

Hirschtick, J., Roesch, P., Monnard, K., & Mante, A. (2018b). *Sinai Community Survey 2.0: Community health profiles, North Lawndale*. Chicago, IL: Sinai Urban Health Institute, Sinai Health System. Retrieved from https://www.sinaisurvey.org/community-health-profiles

Hughes, M. M., Yang, E., Ramanathan, D., & Benjamins, M. R. (2016). Community-based diabetes community health worker intervention in an underserved Chicago population. *Journal of Community Health, 41*(6), 1249–1256. https://doi.org/10.1007/s10900-016-0212-8

Hunt, B., & Whitman, S. (2014). Black:White health disparities in the United States and Chicago: 1990–2010. *Journal of Racial and Ethnic Health Disparities, 2*(1), 93–100. https://doi.org/10.1007/s40615-014-0052-0

Karnick, P., Margellos-Anast, H., Seals, G., Whitman, S., Aljadeff, G., & Johnson, D. (2007). The pediatric asthma intervention: A comprehensive cost-effective approach to asthma management in a disadvantaged inner-city community. *Journal of Asthma, 44*(1), 39–44. https://doi.org/10.1080/02770900601125391

Klinenberg, E. (1999). Denaturalizing disaster: A social autopsy of the 1995 Chicago heat wave. *Theory and Society, 28*(2), 239–295.

Klinenberg, E. (2002). *Heat wave: A social autopsy of disaster in Chicago*. Chicago, IL: The University of Chicago Press.

Lemann, N. (1992). *The promised land: The great black migration and how it changed America*. New York, NY: Vintage Books.

Margellos-Anast, H., Gutierrez, M. A., & Whitman, S. (2012). Improving asthma management among African-American children via a community health worker model: Findings from a Chicago-based pilot intervention. *Journal of Asthma, 49*(4), 380–389. https://doi.org/10.3109/02770903.2012.660295

Mendicino, L. (n.d.). [Photograph found in Chicago Tribune, Chicago, IL]. Retrieved from http://graphics.chicagotribune.com/riots-chicago-1968-mlk/ (Originally photographed 1968, April 7)

Prochaska, J. O., & Diclemente, C. C. (1983). Stages and processes of self-change of smoking: Toward an integrative model of change. *Journal of Consulting and Clinical Psychology, 51*(3), 390–395. https://doi.org/10.1037/0022-006x.51.3.390

Rosman, A. (Photographer). (2018, July 12). *The SUHI CHW team [Photograph]*. Chicago, IL: Sinai Health System.

Whitman, S., Ansell, D., Orsi, J., & Francois, T. (2010). The racial disparity in breast cancer mortality. *Journal of Community Health, 36*(4), 588–596. https://doi.org/10.1007/s10900-010-9346-2

Chapter 9
Advocating for Individuals and Communities

Caitlin G. Allen*, Brook Bender, Heather Carter, Jill Guernsey de Zapien, Maria Lourdes Fernandez, Wandy D. Hernández-Gordon, Gail R. Hirsch, Ilda Hernández, Maia Ingram, Sahida Martínez, Floribella Redondo-Martinez*, E. Lee Rosenthal, Samantha Sabo, Yanitza Soto, Julie Ann St. John*, Kathryn Tucker, Maria M. Velazco, and Lorena Verdugo

9.1 Introduction

Caitlin G. Allen, Floribella Redondo-Martinez, Gail R. Hirsch, and
E. Lee Rosenthal

Advocacy refers to act or process of supporting some cause and includes both individual and community advocacy. The three sub-roles related to advocacy include advocating for the needs and perspectives of communities; connecting to resources

---

Authorship is organized alphabetically in ascending order by surname.

C. G. Allen (✉)
CGA Consulting, Charleston, SC, USA
e-mail: caitlin.gloeckner.allen@emory.edu

B. Bender
Hualapai Tribe, Peach Springs, AZ, USA

H. Carter
Arizona House of Representatives, Arizona Center for Rural Health, Mel and Enid
Zuckerman College of Public Health, The University of Arizona, Phoenix, AZ, USA

J. G. de Zapien · M. Ingram · K. Tucker
University of Arizona Prevention Research Center, Mel and Enid Zuckerman College of
Public Health, Tucson, AZ, USA

M. L. Fernandez · F. Redondo-Martinez (✉)
Arizona Community Health Workers Association, Inc., Douglas, AZ, USA
e-mail: floribella@azchow.org

W. D. Hernández-Gordon
HealthConnect One, Chicago, IL, USA

G. R. Hirsch
Massachusetts Department of Public Health, Boston, MA, USA

© Springer Nature Switzerland AG 2021
J. A. St. John et al. (eds.), *Promoting the Health of the Community*,
https://doi.org/10.1007/978-3-030-56375-2_9

and advocating for basic needs; and conducting policy advocacy. Noting and distinguishing between the multiple levels of advocacy community health workers (CHWs) may be engaged in remains important: advocacy may be for individuals and families, or advocacy may be for groups of individuals in communities, or even for the CHW workforce itself. At these different levels, CHWs need to understand available resources and how to leverage these directly. CHWs may also need to understand private and public sector rules and regulations in order to advocate for changes in access to resources and/or in practices in order to benefit the individuals and communities they serve, or at times, the CHW workforce. The advocacy role may also incorporate or overlap with other roles, such as cultural mediation. For example, a CHW may advocate for an individual within a healthcare system by educating providers within the system about the cultural or religious beliefs of individual clients or communities.

Compared to the original advocacy role from the National Community Health Advisory Study in 1998 study, the definition and sub-roles for advocacy have largely stayed the same.[1] Similar to other roles, the current version of advocacy incorporates examples and nuances in the sub-roles. Of note, there was one sub-role added: policy advocacy, which was missing from the 1998 set of roles. As you will see in the following sections, policy advocacy has become an important element of CHWs' work. Further support for this role and policy-specific advocacy sub-role comes from the National Community Health Worker Advocacy Survey (NCHWAS), which was led by the University of Arizona.[2] The 2014 study was the largest online survey

---

[1] https://crh.arizona.edu/sites/default/files/pdf/publications/CAHsummaryALL.pdf

[2] https://azprc.arizona.edu/2014-national-community-health-worker-advocacy-survey-reports

---

I. Hernández · S. Martínez
Enlace Chicago, Chicago, IL, USA

E. L. Rosenthal
Texas Tech University Health Sciences Center, El Paso, TX, USA

S. Sabo
Department of Health Sciences, Center for Health Equity Research, Flagstaff, AZ, USA

Y. Soto
Arizona Department of Health Services, Phoenix, AZ, USA

J. A. St. John (✉)
Department of Public Health, Texas Tech University Health Sciences Center,
Abilene, TX, USA
e-mail: julie.st-john@ttuhsc.edu

M. M. Velazco
El Pueblo Clinic, El Rio Community Health Center, Tucson, AZ, USA

L. Verdugo
El Rio Community Health Center, Ventanilla de Salud Consulado de Mexico,
Tucson, AZ, USA

of CHWs to date, representing nearly 2000 CHWs from 45 states. The study specifically aimed to describe advocacy and community engagement efforts CHWs undertook by gathering national-level workforce data. Data from this survey found that nearly 75% of CHW respondents engaged in some form of advocacy: advocating within their agency (77%), civic (57%), and political (46%) domains.[3] Clearly, advocacy continues to be an essential role for CHWs and deserves further attention to parse out the types of advocacy CHWs are engaged in, how they are engaged, and ways that they can be best supported in pursuing advocacy-related activities.

The following two sections expand upon the role of advocacy by presenting examples of CHWs advocating for themselves as a CHW profession and CHWs advocating on behalf of their clients and communities during the COVID-19 pandemic.

---

[3] https://www.ncbi.nlm.nih.gov/pmc/articles/PMC3682609/

9.2 CHWs' Collective Voice: CHWs Advocate for Their Profession

Floribella Redondo-Martinez, Maia Ingram, Kathryn Tucker, Heather Carter, Jill Guernsey de Zapien, Samantha Sabo, Yanitza Soto, Lorena Verdugo, Brook Bender, Maria M. Velazco, and Maria Lourdes Fernandez

9.2.1 Introduction

9.2.1.1 Floribella's Story

Floribella Redondo-Martinez is the President of the Arizona Community Health Workers Association.

Do you ever stop and think about what it means to be a community health worker?

I didn't. I just knew that I enjoyed doing the work. I had just began working as a promotora de salud providing health education to migrant farm workers living and working along the U.S.-Mexico border of Yuma County. I knew that helping our clients get an appointment at the clinic or helping them understand what diabetes really means felt good. Sometimes supporting them even felt like we were creating something that was missing in our community, as if we were discovering a different way of helping our clients and their families. During my first years as promotora, I did not think about positive health outcomes, health measurements, or even who cared about those things besides the client and family.

We were successful because we could bring together the services and resources we had in our community. The best way I can describe this is, "it was as if we were putting together a recipe that would not only be good for one client, but also for others with the same need."

My new role within my community was magical; not only did I help our clients in this role, but being a promotora also helped me to understand that I had so much knowledge that I had learned from my life experiences. Being a promotora made me believe that people did not need to have a bachelor or advanced degree in order to be knowledgeable and help others. But that was not the end of my learning process! A few years later, I began to truly "hear" other words such as advocating, environmental change, health equity and policy change. Again, this meant that we had to learn what these words really meant for my Promotora/CHW work. I never would have imagined advocating for myself. At that time, personal advocacy was a dream beyond my knowledge.

A story comes to mind. One day, a while back, my aunt from Mexico was visiting and she asked "Y tu, ¿que haces en tu trabajo?" ("and what do you do at your work?"). To tell you the truth, I had to stop for a second, and I responded to the best of my ability, since at that time I did not recognize the importance of my work. So, I told her, "Well, I provide education on certain health topics, help people learn how to manage their chronic conditions and connect them to resources they need". My aunt responded, "Ah, that sounds like a nice job," and moved to another conversation. I sat there and thought about all the things that I could have said--asking myself why I had responded with just those three things when my job is really so much more than that? This was the first time that I realized that I did not know how to talk about the important role that we have in a community's health. Now when people asked me what I do at my work, I often still stop to think a bit about this question before responding because this is a very important question. I want to make sure that I know how to respond; after all, the response is not what I do but what our CHW workforce does collectively.

Throughout this chapter on advocacy, you will read stories that will seem familiar to many of you. You may identify yourself within many of the stories presented here. Advocacy is a core competency of our workforce, and we all have done some type of advocacy for our participants, clients, patients, our family, and, hopefully, ourselves. You might identify with stories about our supervisors, directors, managers, or providers who do not recognize our value. We hear the pain and disappointment in the voices of the CHWs sharing their personal experiences about not having the recognition or respect from their own organization's leadership.

9.2.1.2 What Is Professional Advocacy?

When we think of advocacy and community health workers, we immediately envision all the wonderful advocacy work that CHWs have always done with the communities they work with—whether they are advocating for patient rights, helping patients to navigate health and social services system, or helping clients become better advocates for themselves. We can also easily envision the community advocacy CHWs have done to support the health and well-being of their clients. In Arizona, for example, CHWs have brought community members together to advocate for better transportation systems, longer clinic hours, safer streets, community facilities, community gardens, and safer working conditions. However, we do not often think about what advocating for our CHW workforce means. Advocating for our workforce means working to gain recognition and respect from other professions, understanding and being able to articulate our unique skills and roles to others, and ensuring that our important work has sustainable funding mechanisms. Advocating for our workforce is vitally important because this allows us to put the other core competencies into practice. CHWs have been working for years to create a strong, sustainable, and competent CHW workforce. In Arizona, our recent legislative victories were built upon more than a decade of advocacy by CHWs and those who support the CHW workforce.

9.2.1.3 Why Is Professional (Workforce) Advocacy Important?

CHWs improve the cultural competency, quality, and cost-effectiveness of health services for medically underserved through education, outreach, and advocacy (Kim, Choi, Choi, et al., 2016; Ingram, Sabo, Rothers, Wennerstrom, & De Zapien, 2008; Rolan, Milikin, Rohan, et al., 2017). Our work is invaluable in improving the health and well-being of vulnerable populations; however, significant obstacles prevent the CHW workforce from gaining recognition, improving their professional identity, and receiving adequate training and compensation. These obstacles include the lack of professional recognition of CHWs and their work, lack of financial sustainability, and lack of dissemination of information and best practices for CHWs (Pittman, Sunderland, Broderick, & Barnett, 2014). While numerous organizations incorporate CHWs into their programs, employers do not always have the capacity to train CHWs adequately or ensure they have received quality or standardized training. Many employers do not themselves have a comprehensive understanding of the workforce and have few resources to describe scope of work and training needs of CHWs in a uniform manner, which makes ensuring a competent and pre-pared workforce difficult. Many CHWs work from grant to grant addressing spe-cific health topics within specific programs but are not integrated into organizations in a holistic way. Limited mechanisms for health plan reimbursement through pri-vate and public means also prevent CHWs from being integrated fully into health-care programs in a way that optimizes the unique capabilities of this workforce (Pittman, Sunderland, Broderick, & Barnett, 2014).

CHWs work under several different job titles across numerous organizations. A CHW might work as a "community health educator" or "clinical care coordinator" in a community health center, a "behavioral health specialist" or "case worker" in a nonprofit organization, a "volunteer health advocate" at a community center or community-based organization, or a "housing aide" at a group home. The list is exhaustive. The individuals fulfilling these different job titles may have various job responsibilities, but they are united by their close relationship with the community served, as well as by a common set of skills and competencies. However, many CHWs do not recognize themselves as part of the broader CHW workforce. They may not understand their scope of practice, core competencies, and essential roles, even if they have worked as a CHW for decades.

Advocating for yourself or for your profession is difficult. As CHWs, we are used to putting the needs of others before our own, and we work with professionals who often have a lot of education, experience, and authority. However, we must recognize that advocating for our workforce is a way to improve the health of our community. If the CHW workforce is respected, has sustainable financing mecha-nisms, and is well-trained, the whole community benefits from our work and experience!

There are many ways to advocate for our CHW workforce. Some CHWs advo-cate for the workforce in their organization by ensuring that other professionals understand and value the unique roles and competencies of CHWs. Some CHWs advocate for their workforce on a community level. For example, community health representatives in Arizona have worked to pass tribal resolutions in support of the CHW workforce because they were concerned that the community health represen-tatives' voice was not being heard.

There is also advocacy on a state level. For example, the Arizona Community Health Workers Association (AzCHOW) brings together the CHW workforce and CHW supporters for an annual training conference which allows CHWs to network and understand their roles and competencies. On a national level, the Community Health Worker Core Consensus Project (C3) has worked since 2014 to examine CHW skills, roles, and qualities in order to create a standardized set of core compe-tencies for the workforce (Rosenthal, Rush, & Allen, 2016). Several states, including Arizona, have adopted the C3 competencies, roles, and qualities as the national standard for the CHW workforce. All of these efforts help decrease barriers and increase the professional recognition of the CHW workforce.

This section will focus on an effort to advocate for the integrity and sustainability of the CHW workforce on a state level. Many states are moving toward increased recognition of CHWs through legislation and advocacy efforts. The Centers for Disease Control and Prevention (CDC) released a report in 2016 documenting voluntary certification policies in the United States. According to that report, 15 states had statutes defining the scope of practice and functions of CHWs, 6 states had authorized a certification process, and 7 states have laws that authorize Medicaid disbursement or other insurer reimbursement for services provided by a CHW. Some states offer certification through approved community and technical college training programs, through a certifying agency, or through verified experience as a CHW. Several states have been able to navigate Medicaid rules to allow for CHW reimbursement, and the Affordable Care Act provides opportunities for integrated payment models and prevention efforts for wider integration of CHWs into health services (Burton, Chang, & Gratale, 2013).

In Arizona in 2018, CHWs' advocacy resulted in the State Legislature passed voluntary certification for the CHW workforce. This legislation is one step toward increased recognition and sustainability of the CHW workforce, and this section will discuss the journey of CHWs and CHW allies in passing this important legislation.

9.2.2 A Brief History of the Community Health Worker Workforce in Arizona

CHWs have a long and rich history in Arizona. Our CHW story in Arizona goes back to the late 1960s when the Gila River Indian Tribe, along with other tribal nations and the Indian Health Service (IHS), established the Community Health Representative (CHR) Program. CHRs bridged the healthcare system and the community. CHRs had many roles, including advocating for their patients and connecting them to health and social services, as well as focusing on broader community issues including access to care, transportation systems, water issues, and many others. This model became an integral part of the healthcare systems of approximately 17 tribes in Arizona.

Beginning in 1986, the University of Arizona Rural Health Office began working with the farm worker community in Yuma, Arizona. They collaborated with the local Federally Qualified Community Health Center (FQHC) and University of Arizona medical students to increase access to prenatal care and address the high incidence of low birth weight. Several of university researchers were familiar with the community health worker model that was widely used throughout Latin America, where CHWs are called *promotoras de salud* or *promotoras*. Armed with a small grant from the Mailman Foundation, they set forth to identify and train community health workers to deliver prenatal education classes, connect pregnant women with the healthcare system, advocate for quality non-discriminatory care at the local hospital, and, above all, provide a mechanism for farm worker women to become in charge of their health.

The program was tremendously successful. Within 10 years, the Arizona Department of Health Services regularly funded CHW programs for prenatal care throughout the state. Beyond this effort, the researchers and community health workers established a collaboration focused on breast and cervical cancer, cardiovascular disease, diabetes, and HIV/AIDS among other community health issue.

In 1998, the University of Arizona received funding from the Centers for Disease Control and Prevention for the Arizona Prevention Research Center. Since that time, the AzPRC's main focus has been to support the CHW model and advocate for the workforce. The Center provided many opportunities for CHWs and academia to partner to develop programs, trainings, and research and evaluation efforts, which resulted a strong evidence base for CHW effectiveness in Arizona.

9.2.2.1 Maria's Story: CHWs as Patient Advocates

Maria M. Velazco is a Community Health Advisor at El Rio Community Health Center in Tucson, Arizona.

> As a Patient Advocate and a Community Health Advisor, I have learned how vital my role has been in creating a trusting relationship with my patients so that I can be an advocate and a second voice for them. I work as a Community Health Advisor at a large FQHC located on the far south west side of Tucson, Arizona. Every day I help my clients navigate the health and social service systems in our state.
>
> The individual advocacy is coupled with healthcare advocacy at a policy level. I serve on the Community Advisory Board for the Arizona Prevention Research Center at the University of Arizona. Through this role, I meet with advocacy committee team members, and we learn about the latest issues that relate to healthcare policy changes. We discuss how we can educate our coworkers and get involved in letter writing meeting with our representatives and social media campaigns. Recently, a law was passed that would cause childless adults to lose their healthcare coverage through Medicaid if they did not renew on time. I called clients to advocate and educate them about how to renew and the consequences if they did not renew on time. I was instrumental in saving thousands of childless adults from dropping off Medicaid. This illustrates the importance of advocacy at a policy level.

9.2.3   History of Advocacy in Arizona

9.2.3.1 Moving Beyond Individual and Policy Advocacy Toward Workforce Advocacy

Community health workers take on many roles. Like Maria M. Velazco, we use our unique strengths to advocate for our clients and our community. But what happens when CHWs advocate for themselves? How can CHWs translate our unique skills and experience into action that strengthens our profession? How do we build alliances and foster broad community support for our workforce, when many CHWs don't even recognize themselves as part of a workforce? CHWs spend their lives helping others, and sometimes in order to do the work we love, we must continue to fight for professional respect, recognition, and sustainability.

In Arizona, AzCHOW, the professional organization representing CHWs, worked with our allies to form a coalition of CHWs and CHW supporters to pass a law in the state legislature to create a voluntary certification mechanism for CHWs. We will discuss our process and share insights into the skills, challenges, and reward of advocating for our workforce on the state level.

The Arizona Community Health Workers Association (AzCHOW)

The CHW workforce in Arizona grew with the support of academic institutions and healthcare organizations. However, the CHW voice was still missing. In 2001, graduates from Project Jump Start, a community college basic certificate training program for individuals working in the area of health education, outreach, or advocacy, founded the Arizona Community Health Outreach Worker Association (AzCHOW). The organization grew with support from the University of Arizona's Area Health Education Centers (AzAHEC) and the AzPRC. AzCHOW became Arizona's CHW professional network designed to unite, connect, and support the growing CHW workforce in Arizona.

Since then, AzCHOW has led Arizona's grassroots movement to unite and strengthen the CHW workforce through training opportunities, advocacy, partnership building, and policy development. Today, AzCHOW's membership includes community health workers, *promotoras de salud*, community health representatives, lay health workers, community health advisors, and several other job titles.

9.2.3.2 Lorena's Story: Realizing the Need for Voluntary Certification

Lorena Verdugo is a Community Health Coordinator at El Rio Community Health Center in Tucson, Arizona.

> *Advocacy is crucial within the CHW workforce since we are the voice for many of those who are unable to defend their rights. Our clients deal with issues of health disparities, human rights violations, environmental issues, fair housing, equal work opportunities, and other social aspects affecting the community we serve.*
>
> *My realization for a need of a voluntary certification came when I noticed that our work load had increased and that the need for CHWs was greater and greater each day. Seemingly, all health plans, community organizations, community health centers, schools, and even early childhood learning programs needed CHWs. However, these organizations did not necessarily know what a CHW was or what special qualities and skills CHWs brought to their work. We were being asked to solve big health problems, but we were not necessarily being given the support and recognition we needed to do so.*

9.2.4　Uniting the Workforce

If we want to create a strong and sustainable workforce, the first step is to unify CHWs in the recognition that we are one workforce and that we must work together. CHWs might have different titles and job responsibilities, but we are united by our skills, roles, and unique competencies.

Arizona is a diverse state and over 1000 CHWs work throughout the 15 counties of the state. CHWs work with Native American communities as community health representatives (CHRs), in US-Mexico border communities as *promotoras de salud*, with migrant farm workers and refugee populations, from inner-city neighborhoods to rural mining towns. However, until recently, all of these CHWs completed their work with different job titles and varying responsibilities, and there was little to no recognition of a CHW workforce. CHWs worked in their communities and clinics without recognizing that they were part of something larger. In Arizona, our first step was to unify the workforce under the umbrella term of "community health workers."

In order to accomplish this task, AzCHOW teamed up with the CHW manager at the Arizona Department of Health Services to conduct listening sessions throughout the state. We talked to CHWs and CHRs from all over Arizona, and they told us about their view of the workforce and how they wanted the CHW workforce to grow. These listening sessions helped us build unity and consensus as a workforce. A few important themes came out of these listening sessions. The workforce wanted increased recognition and respect for the invaluable work that they do in their communities. They also wanted more sustainable financing mechanisms so that they could work according to the needs of the community, not according to a specific grant.

Through these listening sessions, AzCHOW determined that the creation of a voluntary certification mechanism would best promote the CHW workforce in Arizona. Voluntary certification would provide recognition for the unique roles and competencies of the CHW workforce and promote continued training and education for the CHW workforce—providing valid career pathways for CHWs. A voluntary certification would also create the possibility of reimbursement through insurance companies, which would help the workforce become more financially sustainable.

Voluntary certification would not happen on its own; we would need to pass a law in the state legislature so that the Arizona Department of Health Services (ADHS) would create and recognize a voluntary certification of community health workers.

9.2.4.1　Brook's Story: Community Health Representatives Joining the CHW State Efforts

Brook Bender is the CHR Program Manager for the Hualapai Tribe in Arizona.

> *I understood that the CHW Voluntary Certification bill was out there, and I knew it had very little input from Tribal Governments. I knew there was some opposition to the certification bill. I thought having a tribal organization and government to support this bill wouldn't hurt. I truly felt that having the CHRs perspective and voice be heard during this process. I knew at some point this bill could have some adverse effect on the CHR Workforce but*

didn't know how. I wanted to energies that CHRs as a whole would be a part of the process. I decided to present a resolution to the council for support of CHRs in Indian country. Not just CHRs on their reservation but CHRs throughout the state. The information from the fiat CHR Summit was focused on the certification and its potential to lead to third party billing was a major reason to support this bill. CHR program are supported and funded by IHS like all IHS programs they are seriously underfunded. Community and community's needs are increasing and the demand for services are high but staffing is limited and resources are slim. So assisting in passing the bill was in the best interest in the CHR workforce and the CHW as a whole in the state.

9.2.5   Creating a Coalition

Movements require many people with diverse backgrounds, skills, and connections; great work is rarely done in isolation. In Arizona, we recognized the need for a coalition of supporters in order to make our dream of voluntary certification a reality. CHWs had worked for years to cultivate support in the Arizona Department of Health Services, state universities, clinics, health departments, health plans, and community-based organizations. Our allies in these organizations understood the importance and value of CHWs, and they joined us in the effort to gain professional recognition through voluntary certification.

9.2.5.1   Jill's Story: Coalition-Building

Jill Guernsey de Zapien is the former Associate Dean for Community Programs at the University of Arizona Mel and Enid Zuckerman College of Public Health. Jill was one of the founding members of the Arizona CHW Workforce Coalition.

We began our Coalition with 13 members and quickly realized that in many ways we were starting at ground zero as key stakeholders beginning with legislators did not even know what a community health worker was and even less how important they were to both the health care system and community change. Five years later, our Coalition includes an incredibly diverse set of stakeholders including community health workers, health plan executives, hospital and clinical staffs, community activists, health educators, local, tribal and state health departments, and academic institutions. But more importantly almost all of our legislators understand the dynamic role of community health workers in the health care system and the community! As folks testified for legislation, we would hear legislative committee members tell us that community health workers are an inspiration to us all! We knew we were on the right track and had built a strong voice in Arizona.

The Arizona CHW Workforce Coalition

Building a coalition takes time and dedication and does not happen overnight. In 2013, the Arizona Department of Health Services funded a CHW workforce coalition convened by AzCHOW and the AzPRC. The first meeting in Tucson in Southern

Arizona included about 20 individuals, mainly individuals who had worked as or with CHWs in US-Mexico border communities for decades. The coalition quickly grew and expanded its geographical and organizational representation as coalition members connected their network to the Coalition's work.

Since this initial meeting, the CHW Workforce Coalition has grown to include over 200 academic, public health, healthcare, tribal, and nonprofit organizations throughout the state. We meet each quarter and work together to set and meet goals. In June 2014, ADHS hired a CHW program manager in the Bureau of Tobacco and Chronic Disease, signaling their ongoing commitment and support for CHWs in Arizona. The coalition recognized the need to coordinate and amplify their efforts and work with state institutions for increased recognition of the CHW workforce.

9.2.5.2 Yanitza's Story: Involvement of the State Health Department in the Voluntary Certification Process

Yanitza Soto is the CHW Program Manager at the Arizona Department of Health Services.

> Cultivation of such a collective buy-in has promoted public health ownership of House Bill 2324-Voluntary Certification for CHWs. The Arizona CHW Workforce Coalition, the University of Arizona Prevention Resource Center, and many other community-based organizations worked to develop the language around HB 2324, which designated the Arizona Department of Health Services to serve as the certifying entity for CHW voluntary certification. Some of my roles as the ADHS CHW Program Manager include: 1) create professional development opportunities for CHWs; and 2) and strengthen the awareness of core competencies for the CHW workforce. The significance of these roles continues as the voice of the CHW workforce is brought to the forefront during the development of the infrastructure for voluntary certification for CHWs in Arizona.

9.2.6   The Legislative Process

The coalition acknowledged the need for increased workforce development and recognition and prioritized the development of a voluntary certification process in Arizona. In 2016, the coalition introduced legislation in the Arizona State Legislature to establish a CHW Certification Board (Fig. 9.1). The legislation passed out of the State House of Representatives but stalled in the Senate.

After the initial attempt at legislation failed, the coalition recognized the need for a stronger voluntary certification model led by AzCHOW as the representatives of the workforce throughout the state. The CHW Workforce Coalition took a "parallel pathway" approach to voluntary certification: legislation and systems change. The legislative pathway is fraught with uncertainty and dependent on the State Legislature, but the systems change approach allowed the Coalition to harness their collective power to create a voluntary certification process through AzCHOW. This voluntary certification process also served as a model for how ADHS might

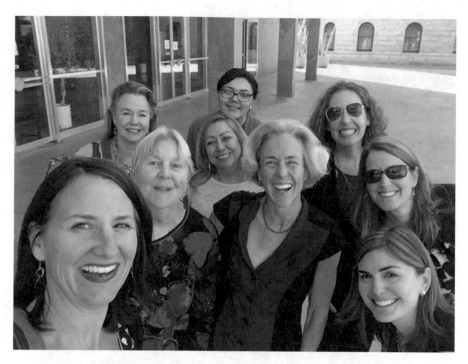

Fig. 9.1 CHWs and CHW allies at the Arizona State Legislature to support HB 2324 Voluntary Certification for Community Health Workers

structure a voluntary certification through legislation. If we were unable to pass legislation, we had a viable alternative pathway toward increased CHW recognition and sustainability in the state. Before introducing legislation, the second time, the Arizona CHW Coalition worked together to create our unified vision for voluntary certification. We worked with CHWs, clinics, public health professionals, and government officials to craft a certification process through our state association. Instead of waiting for the legislative process, we took matters into our own hands to craft the voluntary certification that we wanted. During this time, we piloted our materials and approved one CHW training program and certified four CHWs!

After we created and tested the voluntary certification process, we were more prepared for the 2018 legislative session. We had spent the year building a relationship with other legislators, finding more allies and growing our alliance. There were many people interested in CHWs, and we used this excitement to gather support from different places. We had support from lobbyists, health insurance plans, state health agencies, tribal organizations, academic institutions, and the health centers where we worked. There were so many individuals and organizations who already recognize the importance of CHWs, and we harnessed their power to help us in the process.

CHWs continued to be front and center in the process and provided the face of the legislation. CHWs testified in front of legislative committees, called their state representatives, and provided feedback and support for the legislation as it moved forward.

9.2.6.1　Floribella's Story: Describing the Legislative Process

To me, this process was very frustrating because I did not know how the legislation func-tioned. I thought we would write what we want and send our proposal in and wait to see if we were going to be called to present. Little did I know that here is where we had to bring out one of our strongest skill: outreach. I learned that to get to legislation, you have to reach out to your closest friends and see who they know that knows someone that sits around the legislative table. Yes, legislative work is time consuming, and you have to wear many hats; but at the same time, you have to make sure that your CHW hat stands above all.

What can I say about the experience of going through legislation for our CHW work-force in our state? For starters, this was an unreal feeling. We joined as a workforce and talked about what other states are doing. I spent a lot of time working with other CHWs at the state level and national levels. Even so, standing in front of the legislators for the first time was very stressful. I didn't know who supported us and who did not, and I didn't even know if they knew what CHWs do!

Knowing that I represented the voice of all of the CHWs not present was also stressful. My fellow CHWs trusted me to know what was best, and they counted on my voice to advance our workforce at the state level.

For me to testify in front of the legislatures was an opportunity to advocate for myself and my workforce and to bring the voice CHWs working in communities across our state (Fig. 9.2). I felt like this was a time to ensure our workforce was recognized and respected as integral part of the health care services. At least, that's what I say!

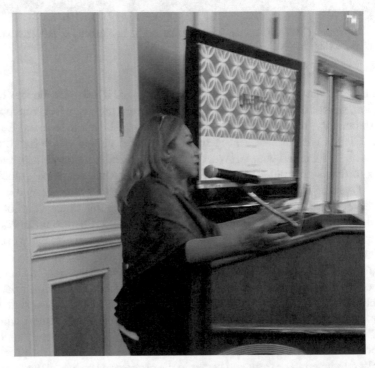

Fig. 9.2　Floribella Redondo-Martinez, President of AzCHOW, presenting on the process of advo-cating for Arizona's HB 2324 Voluntary Certification for Community Health Workers

Ok, let me tell you how it really felt to testify in front of the legislature. The first time I spoke in front of them, I felt like I was speaking to the wall. I felt as if no one cared about what I had to say. I was very overwhelmed and intimidated because I am a Hispanic/ Mexican woman whose first language is Spanish. I was speaking to a room filled with lawyers, professors, doctors and other powerful, highly educated people.

At one point in the legislative process, I had to stop, breath, and weigh whether we should continue with the legislation process or just continue with the process of having the state association certify CHWs. This was a very difficult decision since this not only meant that we had worked very hard to have our bill heard and passed through the house, but there were many stakeholders, health systems, and allies interested in moving forward with the state certification through legislation. We began reaching out to our CHW workforce coalition members to talk about the CHW voluntary certification process and to strategize how we should move forward. The CHWs overwhelmingly assured me they would support the decisions we made. Clearly, we had to continue advocating for our workforce with legislators and state healthcare plans.

We decided to continue with our legislation process because we knew this was the best way to achieve sustainability of the CHW workforce. Yet, pursing voluntary certification that was easy and accessible for all CHWs was not an easy task. However, during each meeting, we clearly saw that "our ask" was changing based on the need identified by some key persons with lots of experience in legislation. This made pursuing this path difficult. I clearly remember sending an email asking if we could stop this and maybe rethink if we (CHW workforce) wanted to continue with this process. At that point, we (CHWs) were ready to throw in the towel, but then one of our key supporters came to me and told me something that I will never forget. He said to me, "Floribella, in school I tell my advocacy students that many times we begin with a dream of what we want to see at the end, but the reality is that in every situation, once you begin a process of advocacy for legislation, at the end, you will not have what you want, but you will have what you need to advance your process."

I thought this made a lot of sense since what we wanted was specific. We were not considering all the key pieces that make the puzzle complete—the health systems, health plans, community organizations, clinics, and academic institutions. The benefits of certification would be not only for our workforce but ultimately to our communities and partners.

9.2.6.2 Difficult Decisions in the Legislative Process

The legislative process moves at an unpredictable speed. Sometimes, many things happened in the span of a few days, and we could hardly keep up with the process. However, other times we had to wait for weeks for a specific hearing or a vote, and there was a lot of uncertainty. We had to wait for a hearing, or a vote, or for news from our allies and other legislators. Usually, we would hear about an important hearing or vote just a day or 2 before its scheduled appearance. The legislative season is busy and chaotic; since we were not physically present in the room, we had to trust our allies to move things forward for us.

We also had to give up some control over the process. We worked very carefully with our allies to craft legislation based on the feedback from CHWs, coalition members, and other allies, but everything can change during the legislative process. Legislators can change the bill, add amendments, and take away language until the legislation hardly resembles the original bill created. At some point, we had to decide if we wanted to move forward or not.

9.2.6.3 Knowing Your Allies and Your Opponents

As we mentioned earlier, we had many allies in the legislative process. Some very powerful people also opposed our legislation, and we had to find the right message to gain their support. We had to take the time to sit down with both our allies and our opponents, understand their worries, and find a way to move forward together.

9.2.6.4 Floribella's Story: Knowing Your Allies

At times, we had to think and ask ourselves: who has a stake in the CHW voluntary certification of our workforce? You have to know that many sitting around the table at one point will not be there at the end but also that at the end, many more will join your efforts. What I can say is that when you are organizing a movement for your cause, in this case our CHW workforce, you will see that building relationships, trust, and commitment from your friends, allies and special interest groups takes time. But, once that trusting relationship comes to fruition, you will see how all moving parts fall into place. And yes, you can advocate at the highest level in your state for your own workforce; after all, you have to remember that you will not do it by yourself. You might remember hearing that "it takes a village" but I can tell you by experience that for us, we needed a whole state of committed CHWs, allies and supporters to advocate, design and build a path for our CHW workforce and then turn that path into a law.

9.2.6.5 Legislative Success

Every state has a different legislative process, which means that each state will have its own challenges and opportunities. In Arizona, our bill had to pass through the State House of Representatives and the State Senate and then be approved by the governor. Figure 9.3 depicts the entire process of legislation that our bill had to complete before the governor signed the bill into law. Note the complexity of the process and how long the process took, and imagine all of the work that happened between the lines. Each phase of our journey required meetings with the CHW workforce and coalition members; many phone calls and trips to Arizona's capitol to meet with our key supporters and champions; but, most of all, ensuring the Arizona Department of Health Services agreed and supported our strategies and next steps.

9.2.7 The Work of an Advocate Is Never Done

We achieved a monumental victory for CHWs in Arizona, but our work is not over. After the legislation passed, we had to immediately start to work with the Arizona Department of Health Services to ensure that the voices of the CHWs are included in the development of the rules that will oversee the voluntary certification process. Once the voluntary certification process is in place, we will

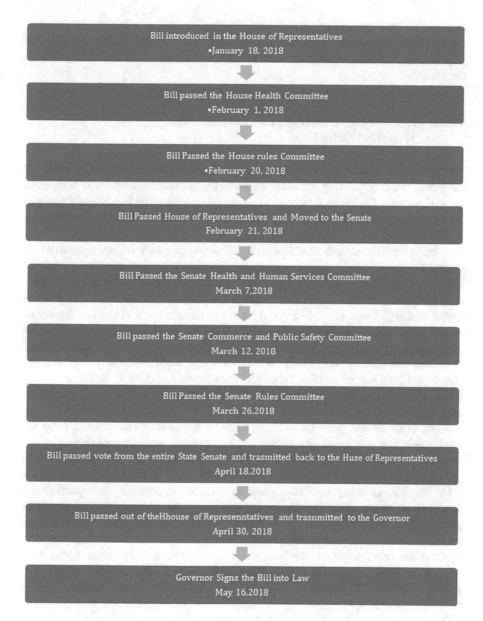

Fig. 9.3 Our legislative journey toward voluntary certification in Arizona

continue to work on other CHW workforce goals in Arizona. Passing a law is not enough; we must continue to educate organizations and agencies about the unique roles and competencies of CHWs, work toward finding more sustainable funding sources for our work with communities, and respond to new and emerging challenges to the CHW profession. In Arizona, the first step was to pass this legislation, but that was not the end goal. The legislation process brought together many CHW supporters, and we plan to continue to use this momentum to improve the respect, recognition, and sustainability of the CHW workforce into the future.

9.2.7.1 Heather Carter: Advice from the Other Side of the Legislative Dais

As the Chairwoman of the Arizona House of Representatives Health Committee, I have the honor of meeting a variety of professional associations from across the state of Arizona. Each association typically takes an active role in advocacy for both their individual professional and for the patients they serve. This was no different for the CHWs.

What *was* different was that this group of professionals were not formally recognized in the state of Arizona, yet are so critical to the functioning of numerous healthcare providers and systems in our state. Our conversation to begin the process to formally recognize the workforce via a state agency began as an informational meeting. I was invited to speak to students in a class at the University of Arizona. We did this several times, and each time we walked through the process of how a "new" profession would become licensed or certified by a state agency, including introducing legislation. While the steps are laborious, the process is clearly outlined and sequential. However, the process begins long before the legislative session and continues after the bill is signed into law. Ultimately, this was no easy task.

Only after several years of working through the exact same process were the CHWs able to realize legislative success, which entailed more than just a single passage of a bill. The bill was introduced multiple times during the interim sessions prior to the final passage, including a previous unsuccessful bill introduced the year prior. Persistence is key and having one or two elected officials committed to the issue helped ensure ultimate success. I worked with the group each year and built strong relationships within the CHW group, among other elected officials, and with stakeholders in the larger healthcare system.

Over the years, together, we built a foundation that endured when faced with opposition. For example, for 2 years, the CHW group filed a pre-session proposal for state licensing. I helped the group successfully testify during multiple interim committee meetings by requesting to hear from key witnesses and asking questions related to the proposal that would address concerns mentioned in committee and in previous hearings. During these meetings, the committee heard over 8 h of testimony on a variety of pre-session health proposals. The CHW issue was just one of several topics discussed, and in the last pre-session hearing, the CHW advocacy group waited for over 8 h to testify after traveling many hours to sit in committee. Sometimes, the testimony was limited to 2 min, which can be frustrating after waiting to speak.

However, if there is consensus to pass the proposal (or legislation), less testimony may be better than an extensive presentation. This further highlights the importance of doing the pre-work of meeting with legislators, establishing working relationships and providing information long before a hearing. Overall, committee meetings are oftentimes long and contentious and require incredible patience from all parties involved.

Another key to our success came from building a large group of stakeholders, across multiple entities who supported the legislation. Each elected official represents their own unique districts, and constituency finding support for CHWs from their specific districts proves helpful. This is a critical step in the process because things move quickly and are oftentimes unpredictable. During the session, for example, we faced opposition from individuals not affiliated with healthcare groups who were ideologically opposed to additional government regulation. While we were well organized, prepared, and engaged, we were able to enlist the help of the business community across Arizona and other entities to negotiate the final legislative proposal that would garner the votes to pass and be signed by the governor. Many times, success or failure is determined by variables not directly related to the issue. Having the greatest number of groups and organizations, including those outside of health care, supporting the work of CHWs is critical for momentum and long-lasting success.

9.2.8 Key Takeaways

In Arizona, voluntary certification was an important step for CHWs to gain recognition, adequate compensation, and financial stability from the organizations we work for and with. For you, professional advocacy may take a different path and may mean making a change in how your organization works, who supervises CHWs, or what training CHWs receive. You may also find that you can advocate with a health insurance plan or a hospital system to better recognize, support, and reward our CHW workforce. In setting on the road to advocacy, we offer some thoughts from our experience:

1. *Remember that CHWs are your community*. Make sure that you reach out to diverse communities and organizations to help you decide how to move forward.
2. *Create and grow a coalition*. Numerous people from diverse communities and organizations can help you champion the CHW workforce. Every time we ran into a roadblock, another coalition member would appear with a new idea, a new connection, or a new skill to help us maneuver through the barrier.
3. *Understand what is most important for you in the advocacy process*. For us, this was recognition and integrity of the Arizona CHW workforce. Being clear about what is most important to you will help you make important decisions along the way and will also help you communicate with others.

4. *Be prepared to be flexible.* Things will not turn out exactly the way that you hope. For this reason, professional advocacy is scary, especially when you feel you carry the welfare of your workforce on your back. But if you are surrounded by other CHWs and allies to help you make decisions, you can respond to challenges as they arrive.
5. *CHWs are our own best advocates.* We would never have succeeded without the support and wisdom of many people with years of experience in policy making and advocacy. But at the end of the day, our testimony had the greatest impact on the process by making clear to others the importance of the work we do.

In Arizona we know that the unity and collaboration make our CHW workforce strong. We hope this advocacy chapter serves as a call to action to all CHWs: we can't let others define who we are as a workforce. Let us continue advocating not only for the health and well-being of our communities but also for our own workforce. We must advocate for ourselves if we want to continue to grow, thrive, and make a difference in our own profession and the lives of those we serve.

9.2.8.1 Dedication

Some Voices Will Always Be Remembered!
We want to dedicate this section in memory of our CHR sister Preoo Johnson. Preeo was a dedicated and hardworking Community Health Representative from White Mountain Apache Tribe. Preeo's role in advocating for CHRs at the local, statewide, and national level encouraged her colleagues to also advocate for the workforce; we acknowledge Preeo's contributions and dedication to her community. Her contribution in advocating and uniting the CHW workforce will forever be remembered.

References

Ingram, M., Sabo, S., Rothers, J., Wennerstrom, A., & De Zapien, J. G. (2008). Community health workers and community advocacy: Addressing health disparities. *Journal of Community Health, 33*(6), 417–424. https://doi.org/10.1007/s10900-008-9111-y

Ingram, M., Schachter, K. A., Sabo, S. J., Reinschmidt, K. M., Gomez, S., De Zapien, J. G., & Carvajal, S. C. (2014). A community health worker intervention to address the social determinants of health through policy change. *The Journal of Primary Prevention, 35*(2), 119–123. https://doi.org/10.1007/s10935-013-0335-y

Loue, S. (2006). Community health advocacy. *Journal of Epidemiology and Community Health, 60*(6), 458–463. https://doi.org/10.1136/jech.2004.023044

Perez, L. M., & Martinez, J. (2008). Community health workers: Social justice and policy advocates for community health and well-being. *American Journal of Public Health, 98*(1), 11–14. https://doi.org/10.2105/AJPH.2006.100842

Redondo, F., Torres, E., Castro, I., Villasenor, A., & Ingram, M. (2010). *Promotora community health manual: Developing a community-based diabetes self-management program.* Retrieved from http://ces4health.info/find-products/view-product.aspx?code=NHNC44FF

Sabo, S., Flores, M., Wennerstrom, A., et al. (2017). Community health workers promote civic engagement and community capacity to impact policy. *Journal of Community Health, 42*(6), 1197–1203. https://doi.org/10.1007/s10900-017-0370-3

Sabo, S., Ingram, M., Reinschmidt, K., Schachter, K., Jacobs, L., de Zapien, J. G., & Carvajal, S. (2013). Predictors and a framework for fostering community advocacy as a community health worker core function to eliminate health disparities. *American Journal of Public Health, 103*(7), E67–E73.

Sabo, S., Wennerstrom, A., Phillips, D., Haywoord, C., Redondo, F., Bell, M. L., & Ingram, M. (2015). Community health worker professional advocacy: Voices of action from the 2014 national community health worker advocacy survey. *The Journal of Ambulatory Care Management, 38*(3), 225–235. https://doi.org/10.1097/JAC.0000000000000089

9.3 Todo Corazón: Abogacía Durante la Pandemia (All Heart: Advocacy During the Pandemic)

Ilda Hernández, Sahida Martínez, Wandy D. Hernández-Gordon, and Julie Ann St. John

9.3.1 Global Pandemic: A Repeat of History?

La historia se repite (history repeats itself) (Santayana, 2011). This certainly seems to be true with the 2020 global pandemic of the novel coronavirus, SARS-CoV-19, which causes the respiratory disease called COVID-19 (Centers for Disease Control and Prevention, 2020). Over a century ago, the world experienced the 1918 flu pandemic caused by an H1N1 virus (Centers for Disease Control and Prevention, 2019). An estimated 500 million people (one-third the world's population) became infected, and an estimated 50 million died—with about 765,000 deaths occurring in the United States. Those that suffered the most during the 1918 pandemic (and previous pandemics) included populations with social and economic inequalities—including the poor, minorities, people with limited access to medical care, and people living in severely crowded living conditions (Wade, 2020). The COVID-19 pandemic seems to be following similar trends—disproportionately affecting our communities facing social and health inequalities. This is certainly true in Chicago's Latino communities—La Villita (Little Village), Brighton Park, Gage Park, Chicago Lawn, and Belmont Cragin—which accounted for 37% of Chicago's COVID-19 cases and 25% of deaths as of May 7, 2020 (Pena, 2020). Yet, in spite of this dangerous virus, promotores de salud (CHWs) continue to serve their communities and neighbors. For them, life was business as usual in an unusual way. This section highlights the stories and experiences of two CHWs in Chicago, Illinois, who advocated for their communities and clients to meet their needs creatively in a time of uncertainty, lack of resources, and in lockdown. They tell their story of how they worked to keep history from repeating itself in their community. The CHWs are involved with two key organizations that support the work of CHWs in La Villita (Little Village), which are described in the following sections.

9.3.1.1 Enlace Chicago and PAES (CHW Networks)

Enlace Chicago

In 1990, a group of community and civic leaders in Little Village established the Little Village Community Development Corporation (LVCDC); the intent of the LVCDC was to revitalize an abandoned industrial park. Through that community engagement process, they identified the need for an organization to focus on comprehensive community development in La Villita (Enlace Chicago, n.d.-a). LVCDC opened its first office in 1998, and staff led the community in multiple organizing efforts—such as violence prevention and the development of a new high school—which eventually led to partnering with local public schools to become community schools. In 2008, LVCDC changed its name to Enlace Chicago. Enlace is constantly adapting its work to meet the priorities, needs, and interests of the La Villita community and currently has four areas of focus—education, health, immigration, and violence prevention. The organization works with more than 8000 youth and adults in La Villita and the surrounding communities. Enlace engages CHWs throughout their four focus areas (Enlace Chicago, n.d.-a).

PAES (Promoviendo, Abogando y Educando por la Salud)

PAES is a network of over 150 CHWs who represent numerous organizations in La Villita and the surrounding community areas of the southwest side of Chicago and who work together to address public health issues (Enlace Chicago, n.d.-b). Enlace facilitated a health planning process in 2015, bringing together more than three dozen stakeholders representing community-based organizations, healthcare providers, advocacy groups, faith-based institutions, and academic institutions (Enlace Chicago, n.d.-b). Participants created recommendations for strengthening the work of CHWs based on the 2013 Little Village Quality of Life Plan, with the overall goal to connect residents, community-based organizations, and healthcare providers through forming a local CHW network. PAES supports CHWs through training in health promotion and education; helps create employment opportunities; and mobilizes CHWs as community advocates (Enlace Chicago, n.d.-b).

9.3.2   Promotores with Heart

Ilda Hernández and Sahida Martínez are promotores de salud (CHWs) serving Latino communities in Southwest Chicago. Their backgrounds and experiences have enabled them, individually and collectively, to meet the needs of the community residents they serve.

9.3.2.1   Ilda Hernández

Ilda, born in Mexico, came to the United States in August of 2004 with three children (the oldest was 12 and the youngest 1–2 years old). They arrived in La Villita (Little Village) because her sister-in-law lived close to a school. Her sister-in-law encouraged her to enroll her older children in school. So she did, but she did not know anyone at the school. She was afraid because Chicago is a big city. She saw the mothers taking their children to school. In her hometown in Mexico, they walked to school by themselves because the town was safe. But in Chicago, she thought her children might be in danger or might be robbed, so she took them to school. The first day she took them, they told her that her children needed a physical and vaccinations before they could start school. She did not know what a physical was or what immunizations they needed. She took everything they gave her and waited outside; she was afraid because she did not know the way back to her house. She told herself she would not get lost, found the alley that looked familiar, and she made her way home. Thus began her daily routine.

On her route to her children's school, she saw another school that closely partnered with Enlace Chicago. Ilda asked around about the school and discovered this was a community school where they help children with homework and learning. Her children needed to learn English; her son cried when he did his homework because he did not understand the language. So, she thought to herself, "Vámonos de aquí, yo qué estamos haciendo aquí? Vámonos (Let's get out of here, what are we doing here?)." So, she took her children to the community school where they accepted him, and they told Ilda they were going to help him with his homework. They told Ilda there was an American teacher who spoke perfect Spanish, and she would help her son speak English. Her son learned to speak English quickly, and she kept going to the community school. She started volunteering in several committees and with the PTO (parent-teacher organization).

After a year and a half, one day the school asked her if she wanted to work there. She told them she was not going anywhere and started working there. She loved working and learning at the school because they spoke her language and she was with her community. After a while, they told her, "You are a leader here in the community." They saw her on the street and asked her about the school supply list or what places sold school uniforms. When she was not working at school, she volunteered at the school. She wanted to give information to everyone, and she helped those who asked—which she has done for 15 years. This is how she started with Enlace Chicago and became a CHW when Enlace began the promotora de salud (CHW) program. She worked on the project going door to door, asking parents about medical (insurance) cards for their children. She went to all the school meetings, so she knew the families, and they knew her from her volunteer work at the school. They were not afraid of her—they trusted her; they spoke the same language, were Latino or Hispanic, and had the same needs. They reached 8000 families during that project, which was a great success for this group of "pioneer" CHWs with Enlace. However, several of those 8000 families had unmet needs—such as access to medical clinics, food pantries, assistance with utility bills, etc. She and her peers told their supervisor about all the needs they saw in the community, and they worked to address their community's need.

Ilda shared that the Enlace promotora (CHW) model is not like other models. Enlace CHWs help with any needs they encounter—whether it is related to food, rent assistance, a mammogram, school help, or help getting out of a violent relationship. If they do not know of a resource, they ask their network of CHWs. This is the work they do as CHWs. She has learned a lot from her community, and she is very proud of her profession, of who she is. "Así que antes decía soy Ilda Hernández, la mamá de tres niños y ahora no. Ahora digo con orgullo que soy Ilda Hernández y soy una promotora de salud entonces y vine a este país a desarrollarme, lo que no es mi país" ("Before, I would say, I am Ilda Hernández, the mother of three children. Now, I am proud to say that I am Ilda Hernández, and I am a CHW. I came to this country to develop myself in a country, which is not my own"). She shared that in her country, she was a mother, and she helped her community. She said that was not the same as when she came to the United States and learned everything she knows now. She and other mothers who are CHWs feel proud. They encourage other mothers to grow, to learn. So, she keeps learning, improving herself, and she does not get tired of learning.

9.3.2.2 Sahida Martínez

Sahida immigrated to Chicago 20 years ago from Mexico with her husband and young children. When she first came to the United States, she did not work outside of the home because she cared for her children, and paying for childcare was too expensive. Many husbands from Mexico wanted their wives to stay home, and the husband would go to work. So, she stayed home for many years. However, she felt like she was missing something and wanted to do something for herself.

When her oldest child started school, she would take them to school, which was close to her house. The school had after-school programs, and she enrolled her children and began to get involved in the programs at the schools. Specifically, she participated in an organization that served immigrants like her—had similar characteristics, spoke Spanish—and she felt comfortable. The organization held meetings in schools and invited the parents so they could find out about activities, programs, information, etc. She started attending parent meetings and started to help with the children's programs after school hosted by an organized called Enlace Chicago. One day someone told her that she did a lot for the school and that she was a leader. She responded, "Who me? No, I do things because I like to help." She began to support other programs, and she started to get involved in more activities within the community. A lot of activities started at her children's school. She volunteered on numerous committees. Her involvement led to her interest in knowing the rights for her children; they deserved to be a part of their community. Slowly, she began to see herself as a leader.

All of these experiences—her volunteer work with the school—laid the foundation for her work that she does now. She learned how to contact and connect with the parents, to lead meetings, and to explain information. One of the people she knew told her that Enlace Chicago was creating a group of promotores de salud (CHW) for a new project. The job involved walking in the community and talking to many people, many of whom she already knew. She knocked on doors and asked parents if their children had medical (insurance) cards. Chicago Public Schools wanted to ensure all children had access to medical care. She talked with people about the public programs but also shared other programs and resources. In the same project, some CHWs helped people fill out applications and enroll them into programs. She liked helping people get access to care for their children. However, she encountered several parents who told her that their children had a medical card but that they did not. She had to explain to those parents that undocumented people could not receive public assistance program benefits. She and her fellow CHWs brought this problem to their supervisor—who taught them how to be CHWs. The supervisor asked what their communities needed. They told their supervisor that in their communities, parents needed access to health care, food, and legal assistance. The supervisor shared some resources and told them that she can help them find other resources to help them meet the needs of those they met.

When that grant ended, their paid hours reduced to only 2–4 a week—although they continued to work at least 10 h. The organization began to see how much the community needed CHWs, that CHWs needed more time to spend with the families providing services, and the CHWs needed more trainings as requested. After that projected finished, she worked on another project promoting health. About this time, Enlace helped support the creation of a CHW network called PAES: Promoviendo, Abogando y Educando por la Salud (promoting, advocating, and educating for health). PAES provided more formal training for Sahida and her peers to work as CHWs (promotores de salud). She shared that when she started receiving that training, "Algo nació en mí y yo dije 'Wow!' Acabo de descubrir lo que quiero ser en mi vida, que quiero ser una promotora de salud" ("Something was born in me and I said Wow! I just discovered what I want to be in my life, that I want to be a CHW").

Sahida loves being a CHW because she works in her community. She works with people who have the same challenges and the same barriers she has faced. She believes communication is the key; communication was what made her and her fellow CHWs build that community bridge. They created a network of CHWs in La Villita (Little Village), and they started to grow. They have started doing more and more trainings. They started looking for other mothers who want to learn. They know their community's needs—the challenges and barriers—and they approach them from thinking about what mothers may not know and what they need to know in order to address those challenges. Sharing information or phone numbers, however, is not all they do. They communicate personally with community members and help them understand that they are not alone. What they need, others need too. They help people see the need to unite and to understand that they are all in this together. Sahida and her peers gain the trust of their community members so that they feel safe, comfortable, and confident in sharing their stories. Now her community comes to her for resources—for themselves and for others. That is what she does as a CHW.

9.3.3 Advocacy During the Pandemic

9.3.3.1 Community Needs

For Ilda and Sahida, advocacy is a natural part of the work they do as CHWs. They described abogacía (advocacy) as helping others achieve some goal, to improve personally, through education, leadership development, and empowerment—giving others the confidence to meet some need or achieve some goal. While they have continuously advocated on behalf of individuals and for their communities, they shared their experiences of how they advocated for those they serve during the COVID-19 pandemic.

When asked how they decided to advocate for their community's needs during the pandemic, Ilda and Sahida said they never questioned that they would continue to advocate for their community; they just had to figure out how they would do so. They said that was a part of their values growing up in Mexico. Jumping in and helping was a way of life that carried over into their adulthoods and as a CHW. They also shared that a person starts by looking inside their own heart and needs—looking for what he/she lacks, he/she will be able to give others what they need or want because peoples' basic needs are the same. Ilda shared:

> "Aquí está, aquí está mi vecina, es mi gente. No importa que no la conozca, perdía, necesita algo de lo que yo puedo ayudarla. Yo la puedo guiar, ¿verdad? No le voy a darle, la voy a guiar. Entonces eso es bien bonito." ("Here it is, here is my neighbor, it is my people. It doesn't matter that I don't know her, she's lost, she needs something I can help her with. I can guide her, right? I'm not going to give her what she needs, I'm going to guide her. So that's very beautiful.")
>
> "Yo siempre les digo que una promotora de salud, una promotora, no se hace, se nace porque tienes que tener ese corazón para poder ayudar a los demás, ¿verdad? Tienes que tener esa, esa compasión." ("I always tell them that a CHW is not made; you are born because you have to have that heart to be able to help others, right? You have to have that, that compassion.")

Another factor leading to advocating for the community—all the time, not just during the pandemic—was their passion to overcome the injustices they see in La Villita. Sahida shared the following:

> "Y también porque conozco nuestra comunidad, las injusticias ... Por eso abogamos mucho para que haya un mejor acceso de salud, para que haya mejores tratos en clínicas, para que haya a que los padres conozcan los derechos dentro de las escuelas, para que no se dejen intimidar." ("And also because I know our community, the injustices ... That is why we advocate, so that there is better access to health, so that there is better treatment in clinics, so that parents are made aware of the rights within the schools, so that they are not intimidated.")

Their values, compassionate hearts, and desire to fight injustice motivated them to advocate for their community.

When the pandemic started to sweep across Chicago, they were surprised when the "shelter in place" or lockdown order came out. They had no idea this was coming nor how long the "shelter in place" would last. They just received news saying not to come to work for 2 weeks. On the last day in the office, they made copies of handouts with basic information from the CDC in Spanish about the coronavirus and the COVID-19 disease: how it spreads, the importance of washing your hands, etc. This was the first information they were able to distribute—about 70 flyers to local stores and public places. They needed more copies but could not get back into the office; they did not have any more physical copies of information to pass out. The first thing they did was to distribute as much information as they could before they had to stay in their homes. Then, they stayed in their homes.

The coronavirus hit La Villita hard and spread rapidly because of the large low-income population that had to go to work to be able to eat, pay rent, and other bills. As such, the CHWs there quickly began to serve their community's needs.

What did they do from home? As a CHW, the first place they started was with sharing Enlace's CHW team phone number on social networks and a resource page on the website of a local partner organization called "Únete La Villita" (Unite Little Village) that shared many community resources. One of their primary concerns was public benefits and programs for their community. They wondered how they were going to continue assisting community members in applying for medical cards (health insurance). They began to give out information from the Illinois Department of Human Services, whose offices were also closed but were accepting applications over the phone. They shared the phone number for people to call because they were told as CHWs they could not assist in the phone calls due to private information being shared on these applications. They also gave out phone numbers for commonly requested services, such as food stamps, free school meals, utility and housing assistance, health insurance, health department, legal assistance, and other public benefit programs. They then started giving out website links for families who had access to a computer and the Internet. Next, they began helping people with online applications by answering questions and clarifying requested information on the various applications. They were able to start assisting with online applications by the end of the first week. This made them happy because although phone numbers were helpful, the wait times were often long, the lines were busy, or no one answered. This led to despair and people giving up without getting what they needed. They also started sharing information about a new temporary card called P-EBT, which provides food stamps during this pandemic, and the only qualification was receiving free or reduced lunches in public schools (which most of their communities qualify for). They also continued to search for other resources shared by other CHWs.

As time passed, they received more phone calls related to housing as people began to worry about how they would pay rent and other bills. So, they found resources to share with their community. At the beginning, they gave out numbers to Catholic Charities, the Spanish Coalition for Housing, and Legal Aid Chicago. They knew there was a law to protect people from being evicted from their homes during the pandemic, and they encouraged their community that they could not be removed from their homes. Even though they shared with people they would not be evicted from their homes, their community members worried about the amount of rent owed and tried to pay a little at a time. Then they heard of efforts to help by different community organizations to raise funds for community relief efforts. For example, Enlace's Little Village Emergency Assistance Fund required only basic qualifications and provided $500 one time. They assisted with the Enlace's emergency fund program, and it involved a lot of teamwork. The funds were not nearly enough as they did not meet all the needs for the many people who had not been working and still had to pay rent.

Sahida recounted a story of how she worked to help a family during the pandemic:

> I called a family to tell them the good news about the emergency funds. The lady was very happy. She does not work. Her husband works. They reduced her husband's hours and that is why she applied for these funds … Then the lady starts to tell me that her husband has diabetes, and she is very anxious because the media is always talking about vulnerable groups and what can happen to them. She knows that diabetes is a chronic condition. So, the last thing she wants is to go outside to the bank to get the money and maybe infect her husband. I said that was fine, and we could find a solution … Then we started talking about her being a mom and having a child. She said that it was very difficult for her to care for her baby. She said she did not feel well and couldn't sleep at night. She didn't know what was happening to her and thought she was over anxious. I offered to help and started sharing many mental health resources. The lady said, 'God put you in my way' … I told her to know that you are not the only person going through something like this. This helped her a lot ….

Another key need that Ilda, Sahida, and other CHWs in La Villita helped meet during the pandemic was referring people to food pantries and other food sources, such as free meals from public schools, which were provided from day 1. They told as many parents as they could to go pick up food for their children from their schools. They also shared food resources from churches and other organizations; some organizations had food pantries, and others delivered food to people's homes.

Unemployment has been another key need and concern for their community. They received numerous calls about unemployment benefits and workers' rights. Several people in La Villita work in factories and were not being provided with personal protective equipment (PPE) such as masks. Some people were also not being paid because they were told by their employers they did not have to be paid because they were undocumented. They even received some calls from employees who had COVID-19 and were told they still had to go to work. Hence, they sought resources to share with their community to address employment and workers' rights, including programs such as Chicago Community and Worker's Rights and the Office of Business Affairs and Consumer Protection.

Another need they heard a lot was mental health and emotional health. People were anxious about not being able to pay the rent, of losing their homes, of homeschooling their children—all of which can cause uncontrollable emotions. They talked to community members who asked them for help because they could not sleep, were very afraid, and could not go outside of their homes. They shared a list of resources to send them to for mental health help, including a local mental health hospital. Further, the threat of domestic violence worried them as families had to be close together in confined spaces. They made sure to share those resources and encouraged people to use the resources as needed.

One last major request for information from their community during the crisis was where to go to get tested for the coronavirus—not only clinics and hospitals but other places as well. People were worried about going to clinics or hospitals when they were sick because they were afraid they would have to stay and not be able to pay. This, any and everything related to health, became a major focus for Ilda and Sahida during that time. Even if people were not infected with the coronavirus, they told them what to do if they had symptoms, where to go, what phone numbers to call, etc. Sahida shared that to keep track of all of the resources, she had names and numbers on Post-it Notes on her window—about 30 taped all over the frame—which gave her easy access to information and much quicker than looking up information on the computer.

In many instances, Ilda and Sahida were the only links connecting their community members to needed resources. They could share trusted resources because the information provided were organizations they had met at health fairs or collaborated with previously on various projects. They were confident in the information and assistance they provided during the pandemic. In addition to giving out the resources, they tracked this information in a data system and provided follow-up calls to make sure people were able to access services. This quote from Ilda summarized how they felt providing advocacy for their community members during the pandemic:

> "Haces tú todo lo que sea posible. Tomas los recursos de tantos entrenamientos que has tenido, tantos talleres que has tenido. De algo tienen que servirte para poder ayudar a la comunidad. ¿Y cuándo ayudas a una persona así, esa persona? Te valora, pero yo le digo no importa." ("You do everything you can. You use the resources from all the trainings and workshops you have attended. And when those resources help someone in the community? He/she thanks you, but you tell him or her it's not a big deal.")

9.3.3.2 Support for CHWs During the Pandemic

Ilda and Sahida shared about the support they received from PAES—their local CHW network in La Villita—during the pandemic. PAES provides trainings, links, and information for CHWs, even during the time they were locked down and after they returned to physical work locations. For example, PAES provided information on self-care, on assessing community and individual needs, the Census, policy advocacy to change laws to improve their communities, knowing one's rights protected by the law, and domestic violence resources.

A particular challenge they described during the pandemic was to continue to provide education classes for various programs during the shelter in place period. At first, they thought they could wait the 2 weeks and then return. However, when they discovered the time might be longer, they came up with a solution. For one particular program where they educated parents on healthier eating and chronic health conditions, they decided to continue the educational sessions via the phone and Google Meet. They shared this proved difficult at first because they had limited computer skills and training. They also had to overcome access to Internet, costs, and other technology barriers. They talked among themselves as CHW facilitators and figured out a plan. They decided that each group should work with their own individual groups of parents in a way that best met their group's needs. They listed potential barriers (which they themselves also had) and ways to address those barriers. The number of parents able to participate was less than the in-person classes, but those that attended shared the sessions greatly helped them. The parents welcomed the opportunity to share about their fears, their needs, and their struggles. Though there were challenges, the CHWs addressed them head on and adapted their plans; meeting their community's needs motivated them to continue. The CHWs shared that they learned new skills during this time; they embraced the opportunity to learn, instead of admitting defeat.

Another challenge they described in providing advocacy during the pandemic was finding a balance between helping others as much as they could while still maintaining a healthy home life. They also had children, other family members at home, and other responsibilities. Working from home meant they were tempted to work constantly—especially when people kept asking for help. For example, sometimes they found themselves cooking while watching a training webinar. They quickly learned to make time for themselves, to turn off their phones, to get some exercise, to engage in a relaxing activity, and to visit with their family members living in their homes.

They reiterated that what they liked the least about their advocacy work as CHWs during the pandemic was not being able to help everyone with every need or to help someone as much as they would like. Those limitations to what they could do affected them personally—physically, emotionally, and mentally. Sometimes they had trouble sleeping—worrying about the spread of the pandemic and the needs of their community. This is where the balance came in—setting boundaries and limits on their time, resources, and energy to appropriate levels.

Conversely, what they liked most about advocating as a CHW during the pandemic was the ability to continue to work—to help their community, their neighbors, and to make a difference, even from home. Ilda stated this point well: "Y si yo puedo abogar? Para que esas personas, las demás puedan, mi comunidad pueda tener un cuidado de salud. Lo voy a hacer mil, diez mil las veces que se pueda." ("And if I can advocate? I do so that these people, those in need, my community, can have health care. I'm going to do it a thousand, ten thousand as many times as possible.")

9.3.4 Conclusion

As exemplified in the experiences shared by Ilda and Sahida, their community, La Villita, faced numerous inequalities that led to greater challenges to address during the global pandemic—much like previous pandemics. "The idea that some lives matter less is the root of all that is wrong in the world" (Farmer, 2004). This very sentiment is what Ilda, Sahida, and their fellow CHWs sought to address through their endless, courageous advocacy. Advocacy, as described in the introduction to this chapter, refers to an act or process of supporting some cause. There are individual and community advocacy—of which CHWs often engage in both. The three sub-roles related to advocacy are advocating for community needs and perspectives; connecting people to resources and advocating for essential needs; and conducting policy advocacy. The CHWs in La Villita engaged in all three sub-roles, which they shared in detail. This was not easy in light of the lockdown, lack of resources, and a global pandemic, yet they truly embraced the adage: "Do what you can, with what you've got, where you are" (Widener, 1920). For CHWs wanting to advocate for their communities (during pandemic or not), Ilda and Sahida share the following lessons learned and recommendations:

- Advocacy often comes from and is best fueled by the desire to overcome injustices.
- Do something you enjoy in life. If you do not enjoy advocating for your community prior to a pandemic, you certainly will not enjoy advocating for them during one.
- Take care of yourself first: sleep, eat, spend time with your family, and relax. Without taking care of yourself and recharging your energy, you will not be able to do another day of advocacy on behalf of those you serve.
- Keep learning. Learning new skills, resources, and knowledge empowers you to help your communities.
- Know your limits and limitations. Create a plan to help you work, and live within them.
- Each person has his or her own gifts. Know yours and use it. If you have the gift of advocacy, then advocate.
- Be informed. That equips you with what you need to know to advocate.
- Join a nonprofit organization, and volunteer. This is one of the best ways to learn to advocate on behalf of a community and individuals.
- CHWs are leaders. Let them lead.
- CHWs fill an important role in advocacy. While CHWs often volunteer, they have homes, families, needs, and bills. Seek and find compensation to support CHWs and the great advocacy work they do.

In closing, we leave you with Sahida's words of wisdom in relation to advocating as a CHW:

> "Entonces sí, sí, tienes que tener esa empatía, ese corazón, esa compasión."
> ("So, yes, you have to have this empathy, this heart, this compassion.")

References

Centers for Disease Control and Prevention. (2019, March 20). *Influenza (Flu) 1918 pandemic (H1N1 virus)*. Retrieved from Centers for Disease Control and Prevention: https://www.cdc.gov/flu/pandemic-resources/1918-pandemic-h1n1.html
Centers for Disease Control and Prevention. (2020, May 29). *Coronavirus disease 2019 (COVID-19) frequently asked questions*. Retrieved from Centers for Disease Control and Prevention: https://www.cdc.gov/coronavirus/2019-ncov/faq.html

Enlace Chicago. (n.d.-a). *Our story*. Retrieved from Enlace Chicago: https://www.enlacechicago.org/missionandhistory

Enlace Chicago. (n.d.-b). *Promoviendo, Abogando y Educando por la Salud*. Retrieved from Enlace Chicago: https://www.enlacechicago.org/communityhealthpromoters

Farmer, P. (2004). An anthropology of structural violence. *Current Anthropology, 45*(3), 305–317.

Pena, M. (2020, May 7). *Chicago's Latino neighborhoods have most coronavirus cases in the state. Is the city doing enough to respond?* Retrieved from Block Clu Chicago: https://block-clubchicago.org/2020/05/07/chicagos-latino-neighborhoods-have-most-coronavirus-cases-in-the-state-and-city-not-doing-enough-leader-says/

Santayana, G. (2011). *The life of reason or the phases of human progress: Introduction and reason in common sense: Vol. VII: Book one*. Cambridge: The MIT Press.

Wade, L. (2020, May 14). *Science: From Black Death to fatal flu, past pandemics show why people on the margins suffer most*. Retrieved from American Association for the Advancement of Science: https://www.sciencemag.org/news/2020/05/black-death-fatal-flu-past-pandemics-show-why-people-margins-suffer-most

Widener, S. B. (1920). *Theodore Roosevelt an autobiography with illustrations*. New York, NY: Charles Scibner's Sons.

Chapter 10
Building Individual and Community Capacity

Caitlin G. Allen*, Janae Ashford, Durrell J. Fox, Rebeca Guzmán, Gail R. Hirsch, Maria Martin, Carl H. Rush, Julie Smithwick*, Katherine Sutkowi*, Claireta Thomas, Virginia Vedilago, and Mike Young

10.1 Introduction

Caitlin G. Allen, Gail R. Hirsch, Durrell J. Fox, and Carl H. Rush

The sixth core role, building individual and community capacity, has remained largely unchanged from its origins.[1] Capacity building involves the development of skills, resources, knowledge, and tools to help promote health.[2] The role includes three sub-roles: building individual capacity, building community capacity, and

---

[1] https://crh.arizona.edu/sites/default/files/pdf/publications/CAHsummaryALL.pdf

[2] Hawe P, King L, Noort M, et al. Indicators to Help with Capacity Building in Health Promotion. Australian Centre for Health Promotion and New South Wales Health Department, 2000;2. https://s3.amazonaws.com/academia.edu.documents/46735762/Community_capacity_building_A_parallel_t20160623-13669-1prxe5p.pdf?response-content-disposition=inline%3B%20filename%3DCommunity_capacity_building_a_parallel_t.pdf&X-Amz-Algorithm=AWS4-HMAC-SHA256&X-Amz-Credential=AKIAIWOWYYGZ2Y53UL3A%2F20200215%2Fus-east-1%2Fs3%2Faws4_request&X-Amz-Date=20200215T141636Z&X-Amz-Expires=3600&X-Amz-SignedHeaders=host&X-Amz-Signature=389ccf28d6bcd00e20b29867b90b1845c93588e25d5dd17a04bf559c96d25ea6

Authorship is organized alphabetically in ascending order by surname.

C. G. Allen (✉)
CGA Consulting, Charleston, SC, USA
e-mail: caitlin.gloeckner.allen@emory.edu

J. Ashford · R. Guzmán · C. Thomas
Detroit Health Department, Detroit, MI, USA

D. J. Fox
JSI Research and Training, Inc, Atlanta, GA, USA

© Springer Nature Switzerland AG 2021
J. A. St. John et al. (eds.), *Promoting the Health of the Community*,
https://doi.org/10.1007/978-3-030-56375-2_10

training and building capacity with peers and among groups of community health workers (CHWs). The final sub-role, training and building capacity within the workforce, is new.

Broadly, capacity building is focused on development and strengthening of an entity (e.g., organization, agency, community, or family) or an individual. Parallel to providing social support, this role is largely focused on building self-efficacy among clients and also includes developing resiliency, concrete skills for action, cultivating community resources, and providing social support networks. By strengthening an individual's or a community's skills and competencies, CHWs help encourage and support people's ability to overcome barriers and challenges in order to achieve their goals (health and otherwise). Individual capacity-building activities include equipping individuals and families with tools, knowledge, skills, and resources to help them take ownership of their own health and wellness.

Community capacity building is a long-term, continuous process that engages entities and community members and which requires the development and maintenance of relationships and partnerships among community members, multiple organizations, and sectors. The goal of community capacity building may include supporting an individual's and/or communities' abilities to develop new policies that encourage healthy behaviors (e.g., removing sugary drinks from schools, building parks, increasing access to healthy foods, walkable communities) and help communities take ownership of the process through equitable partnerships.

Capacity building among and within the CHW workforce is a long-term effort that is important for workforce sustainability. The new sub-role of training and building capacity with peers among groups of CHWs recognizes that CHWs are increasingly engaging in efforts to advance and support not only their clients and communities but also their peers and workforce.

The following two sections elaborate on CHWs' roles in building individual, community, and professional capacity. The first will describe CHW-led efforts undertaken in Michigan to advance the CHW workforce, and the second will discuss efforts to engage communities toward building community capacity.

G. R. Hirsch
Massachusetts Department of Public Health, Boston, MA, USA

M. Martin · M. Young
PASOs, Columbia, SC, USA

C. H. Rush
Community Resources, LLC, San Antonio, TX, USA

J. Smithwick (✉)
University of South Carolina Center for Community Health Alignment, Columbia, SC, USA
e-mail: Julie.Smithwick@sc.edu

K. Sutkowi (✉)
Queens, NY, USA
e-mail: mitchkl@umich.edu

V. Vedilago
The Fenway Institute at Fenway Health, Boston, MA, USA

10.2   CHWs and Allies: Promoting and Sustaining the CHW Profession

Katherine Sutkowi, Rebeca Guzmán, Janae Ashford, and Claireta Thomas

10.2.1   Introduction

According to the American Association of Community Health Workers (AACHW) Code of Ethics, community health workers (CHWs) have a professional obligation to advocate for the families they work with as well as the communities where they live, work, and play (American Association of Community Health Workers, 2016). While this role is unquestioned, there is a less discussed obligation to advocate for CHWs' role as a health and community professional. Building capacity of and advocating for their own profession is another level of advocacy expected of CHWs to sustain the support their work.

CHWs and allies have partnered for almost a decade to build capacity of, and advocate for, the CHW profession in Michigan. Across the state, CHWs address a range of health conditions and social determinants of health, including chronic disease, maternal-child health, housing, and food security (Michigan Community Health Worker Alliance, 2016, pp. 14–15). CHWs and allies—who include supervisors, employers, funders, researchers, community members, and other stakeholders—have the unique opportunity to develop relationships and partnerships that further the CHW role and profession while assuring authentic CHW input in leadership and decision-making roles. These partnerships can also drive development and application of ethical professional practice in the workplace and in the community; for example, CHW-ally partnerships have been integral components to the development, launch, and operations of the Michigan Community Health Worker Alliance (MiCHWA).

MiCHWA launched in August 2011 with a founding mission "to promote and sustain the integration of community health workers into Michigan's health and human service systems." MiCHWA was designed to be a voice of, and for, CHWs in Michigan. Without CHWs, MiCHWA could not have moved forward. At the same time, MiCHWA was founded as an alliance, not an association; as an alliance, there is acknowledgement of the partnership between CHWs and allies within the organization's operations and activities. CHWs serve on MiCHWA's Board of Directors, co-chair its working groups, and manage a CHW Network dedicated to peer learning and development. MiCHWA's seven guiding principles explicitly acknowledge and elevate the importance of the CHW role to the organization's functioning (Michigan Community Health Worker Alliance, 2018). Further, the first principle states that "CHWs provide active leadership at all levels of MiCHWA including its Board of Directors and its working groups" (Michigan Community Health Worker Alliance, 2018).

MiCHWA is one piece of a larger story in which CHWs have been building capacity for community and workforce change in Michigan for decades. Further, this larger story relies on various CHW-ally relationships to fuel the profession forward and elevate the CHW voice to prominence. At the center of this story is the pursuit of social justice in our communities, the undoing of decades of institutional and systematic oppression and racism. CHWs are uniquely situated to combat inequity, and allies have a responsibility and opportunity to partner ethically to facilitate change. In this section, CHWs and allies share stories of work on the ground and for the workforce. Through storytelling and discussion, we will explore three key theme areas: (1) motivation for social justice and equity, (2) ethical and professional engagement, and (3) building capacity for change through relationships. Our stories tell a small piece of a larger puzzle in which CHWs and allies together build capacity for the CHW workforce.

10.2.2 Motivation for Social Justice and Equity

CHW Story (Janae) In a world where all communities, jobs, organizations, and individuals are interdependent, there is a lack of acknowledgement around the role CHWs play in making sure everyone receives help and advocacy that is equitably deserved by the community. Community capacity building entails empowering residents, co-workers, clients, peers, and any other individual to advocate and serve for not only themselves but for others within the community and the community itself. As CHWs, we are trained to teach people how to fish. We are dedicated to knowing when a river lacks fish, or resources to thrive, and committed to knowing the strategy to dive into the river to find them.

Growing up with a parent in the public health field, I was called a "public health baby." By having a parent who worked in the public health field, I was exposed to a lot of the systems, processes, and norms of working with the community and the steps needed to help residents have their needs met and to help them thrive. I grew up watching my mom teach the community how to fish. She took me everywhere with her. I did not know it then, but she helped shape my commitment to working toward a healthy community (Fig. 10.1).

As I reached my teenage years, I began working as a public health worker. The difference between being on the outside looking in and actively working in the field is eye opening. I remember working my first job at the health department, working in a fruit market. The market, open twice a week, purchased fruit from a produce company and sold the produce at more affordable prices than the markets in town. I also worked as a summer lunch worker; I would inspect lunch sites to make sure the areas were clean and safe for children to eat. I initially looked at this opportunity as a job, not a career. Over time, as a CHW, my eyes were opened. I was able to see the social implications of community markets, knowing that most families can't afford to properly sustain their families with the (lack of) healthy food options offered

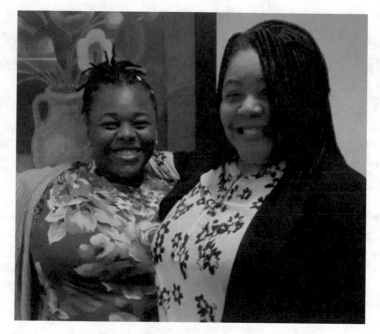

Fig. 10.1 Janae with her mom, Yolanda

throughout the city. My mother helped me grow as a community organizer by her example and by the exposure she provided me. From my experiences serving the community, I realized that you cannot properly serve them with one lens. Our eyes have to be opened, with our hearts and minds truly dedicated to the needs of the family as a part of a larger community. There are so many different levels that we need to look at when we work for and with our families. Our focus needs to be on the work in the community, with the community, and for the community (Fig. 10.2).

10.2.2.1 CHWs Motivate for Social Justice

The CHW profession is grounded in social justice. The heart of all CHW work is helping people attain the highest level of physical and mental health. CHWs recognize that the circumstances in which a person lives, works, and plays can influence their quality of life and their longevity.

Allies and CHWs have the opportunity to motivate communities and motivate each other in this work. The CHW Code of Ethics acknowledges the "promotion of equitable relationships" as a key tenet of CHW practice, emphasizing values including cultural humility, maintaining the trust of the community, respect for human rights, anti-discrimination, and client relationship (American Association of Community Health Workers, 2016).

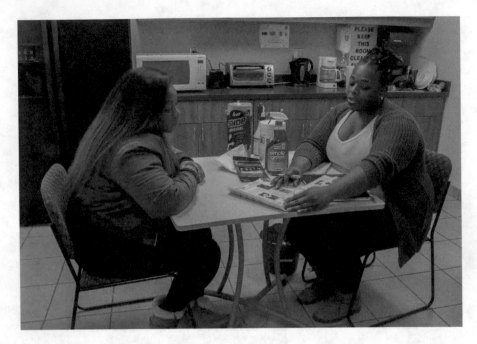

Fig. 10.2 Janae working with a client

CHWs are motivated by this pursuit of social justice. They build capacity in their communities to overcome decades of oppression and marginalization. Capacity is not only built for individual change; CHWs inspire and motivate to create change at systematic and institutional levels. Further, CHWs have been acknowledged as an essential strategy to achieving health equity in our broken, fragmented systems of care and service delivery (Wilkinson et al., 2017). As natural helpers, CHWs are true motivators for change; they support their communities through a personal connection to their friends and neighbors. Many CHWs use these personal connections to serve in non-formal roles in their communities prior to taking on a formal CHW position and are often recruited because of those experiences. This speaks to true social justice, change coming to the community, from the community. In this way, CHWs uniquely motivate change in a way that aligns with social justice ideals.

Ally Story (Katie, Ally and Advocate) We stood in hallway on the second floor of a small apartment building, a few toys scattered in the hallway. Paula[3] marched over to the red door, knocked, and entered swiftly. Within seconds, I saw a real community health worker (CHW) in action.

Standing behind Paula, a CHW serving Black and Latina pregnant and postpartum moms, I saw the beginning of real change. Paula commanded; her voice was

---

[3] The name has been changed to protect the privacy of the individual featured in this story. Story used with permission.

strong, authoritative, and direct. We were on a visit to a young couple with a 4-month-old baby. They had a pregnancy scare the week before; based on the tone of the conversation, it was not the first time. Paula did not waver to the excuses of either parent, both of whom acknowledged that they had not taken the appropriate steps to avoid another pregnancy while their daughter was so young. "Do you want to have another child right now?" she said.

I was flabbergasted. As a trained clinical social worker, I could never walk into a family's home and say something that challenging, that blunt. But Paula could.

While there was no pregnancy this time, Paula walked them through their next steps, which included getting a new ID in order to secure free contraception. The visit continued with a few questions about how the baby was doing, some tips on feeding, and a new infant carrier. Paula demonstrated how to wear the baby and had the mom try the carrier on for practice so she could take baby on the bus more easily. The visit ended all smiles—a glimmer of change on the horizon.

Paula was sparking change. That day, it was one family enrolled in a maternal infant support program, but in a week, Paula may see a dozen in similar situations. She talked about running into former clients at the grocery store and hearing about how well their children were doing in school, being thanked for her constancy during the first few years of their child's life. That's real change. Some of those former clients have moved on to be CHWs themselves, reaching their communities with the same care they had once received. That's a testament to building real capacity.

CHWs have the unique ability to build relationships that create real, socially just change in communities. They build individual and community capacity, drawing from personal experiences and drawing on ethical principles that guide an essential yet messy practice. Both the relationship and the boundaries Paula built with her client allowed her to be blunt and persuasive with the family. They trusted her as someone who could relate to them but also who was keeping the health of the baby and mother at the forefront. She was a peer but also a professional, one that kept her visit details confidential and who turned a blind eye when running into a client at the post office. She was also someone who saw and experienced the injustices in her community and fight back with compassion.

My visit with Paula that day taught me the necessity of the CHW role and opened my eyes to **the necessity of ethics-driven capacity building for creating change in pursuit of social justice**. She also helped me recognize the privilege and ethical responsibility that comes with not being a CHW—what it means to be an ally.

10.2.2.2 CHW-Ally Partnership: Bidirectional Motivation Toward Social Justice in the Community

CHW-ally partnerships can foster understanding and awareness of what actual social justice and equity look like both for communities and for professions, creating a bidirectional motivation loop wherein CHWs motivate allies and allies help equip CHWs. CHWs are experts in community, whether geographic, ethnic, health-specific, or otherwise. In most cases, allies do not have this lens. As natural helpers

(Israel, 1985), CHWs work in the community in a natural and organic way. Allies can learn from CHWs' experiences and perceptions of what's happening as insiders in these communities while also serving as professionals among their peers. The unique lens CHWs bring is invaluable to various types of other professions, including social workers (Spencer, Gunter, & Palmisano, 2010) and nurses (Roman et al., 2009), as well as researchers seeking to conduct equitable, fair research in marginalized communities (Hohl et al., 2016). The bidirectional nature of learning between CHWs and allies can further help each develop new approaches and new ways of thinking about community issues. This additional lens can help each group identify and act on opportunities to create equitable change at the community level and build capacity for community change among residents.

10.2.2.3   CHW-Ally Partnership: Bidirectional Motivation Toward Social Justice in the Workplace

Bidirectional motivation can extend to advocacy in the workplace and institutions that have historically appropriated or perpetuated injustices. Employers, for example, have the opportunity to hire CHWs from the community, provide training and supervision for them, and equip supervisors to provide support, professional development, and mentorship to those CHWs. Further, allies can partner with CHWs to advocate for job stability, fair wages, and a socially just approach to addressing community needs in program design and development. The CHW profession has historically been supported by "soft" money, relying on grant funds and other nonstable funding streams (Islam et al., 2015; Martinez, Ro, Villa, Powell, & Knickman, 2011). Allies can further partner with CHWs in pursuit of workforce standards to support professional sustainability. To pursue equity, CHWs and allies can motivate each other to work at the highest level of their respective professions as they pursue social justice in the community and in the workplace. Allies must be open to investing in the CHW workforce if equitable of service delivery and employment is valued.

10.2.3   Ethical and Professional Engagement

Ally Story (Rebeca, Ally Trainer and Supervisor) It was one of those days when I asked myself, "What am I doing with my life and my career? Am I making a difference in this world?"—then I received a note in the mail. It was a thank you card from a community health worker (CHW) who wanted to thank me for supporting her decision to move out of state. She wrote that she was married and was expecting her first child. She proudly talked about how she was walking confidently through her pregnancy, applying all she learned in the training she received from me. She said I made a difference in her life and she was thankful that our paths crossed.

The interesting bit about the note was that I did not remember who this woman was; all I knew was that she was one of several hundred CHW I had trained over the years. I must have been actively listening to her, asking the right questions, and providing her the space to make the best decision for herself. I still have the card, and I will keep it always as a reminder that supporting CHWs is a wonderful way I make a difference in this world.

I believe in social justice and equity. As a supporter of CHWs for nearly 30 years, I have come to believe that bringing out the leaders from different under-represented communities and arming them with the knowledge and confidence to go out and improve the quality of their lives and the lives of those they touch is transformative. Teaching people to become fishermen/women has taught me to be a better listener, to trust that a true CHW knows how to use their knowledge of their community to create lasting change, and to practice what I preach—trust your talent, walk with integrity, look for the strength in others and capitalize on it, and know that your every step is a teachable moment.

As a CHW ally, I make it my responsibility to bring the CHW voice to the table where ever I go. Just as they teach their clients that their voice matters, I try to do so as well in the work place. I have learned over the years that believing in social justice and equity is not always enough; many times it means putting yourself out there, being persistent, and keeping the conversation open regardless of the reception it receives.

As a founding member of MiCHWA, I have the opportunity to sit at a table with like-minded representatives from various backgrounds, disciplines, and interests. In spite of where we come from and where our personal interest lies, we share a common goal to sustain and promote the CHW workforce in Michigan.

10.2.3.1   Ethics of Being a CHW Ally

Being an ethical ally requires the ally to be familiar with their own professional code of conduct and feel confident operating within their scope of practice. The responsibility of adhering to standards of practice in the workplace goes beyond being a good role model and requires actively encouraging CHW colleagues to operate outside of their comfort zones and support them as they try new skills or explore new found interests:

> As a supervisor, I would not only encourage CHWs to attend program planning meetings, I would orient them on what to expect, what were the expectations of them, and what the formal and informal protocols were for that situation. We would discuss who would be there, what materials to take with them, and reassure them of the value of their contributions. After the meetings we would debrief the experience as well as their feelings about the experience.
>
> - Rebeca

CHWs like other professions have ethical standards that guide how they conduct themselves and how they practice their profession. The CHW Code of Ethics, adopted in 2008, reflects the core values of social justice, health equity, the value and worth of each individual, and the fidelity of service provision (American Association of Community Health Workers, 2016). The ethical responsibility to promote the CHW profession shares these core values. As CHWs promote the profession, they demonstrate the importance of human relationships beyond their interactions with the people they serve. The commitment to advancing the profession includes the support and engagement of and with their allies.

Just as CHWs engage the people they serve in self-actualization, so, too, do allies engage with CHWs in the same manner. The collaboration between the CHW and the ally is strengths-based and promotes the rights of the CHWs to make choices in their own best interest. This form of collaboration demonstrates an appreciation and respect for the human relationships that emerge through mutual respect and shared values.

Respect is a primary tenet of health and human service delivery. Just as CHWs are expected to treat the people they serve with care as they promote self-sufficiency, so too should allies rely on their own professional code of ethics to support and promote the CHW profession with respect and care. The notion of empowering CHWs to build upon their individual and collective strengths to create a workforce that reflects their unique contributions to public health and social justice is congruent with the belief that CHWs are inherently capable of expressing their needs, wants, and goals. The premise that each individual is the master of their own experience applies to CHWs as they navigate the formal and informal arenas where standards are created and formalized for their own profession.

CHW Code of Ethics: Articles

1. Responsibilities in the Delivery of Care
2. Promotion of Equitable Relationships
3. Interactions with Other Service Providers
4. Professional Rights and Responsibilities

These ethical guidelines, reflected in the CHW Code of Ethics' list of articles, align with the CHW roles and responsibilities to execute the core competencies of the profession.

CHW professional competence is defined by the code of ethics and their knowledge and understanding of CHW scope of practice. Allies, such as trainers, supervisors, mentors, and colleagues, can support the growth and development of the CHW in different ways and at different times throughout a CHW's career by creating opportunities in nonjudgmental, strengths-based, and empowering environments, building the capacity of the CHW profession ethically using their scope of practice.

Through formal and informal training and supervision, allies support the integrity of profession by presenting information and enhancing skills in a way that is recognizable and easily integrated into the CHWs' unique role. Clarifying questions through respectful discussion and relying the CHWs expertise promotes CHW confidence to explore and contribute in ways they may not have previously envisioned for themselves. The bidirectional nature of these learning exchanges creates appreciation for diversity and talents in one another.

The shift in the power dynamic of the teacher-student, supervisor-supervisee, and mentor-mentee changes to a collegial appreciation for the strengths each party brings to the relationship:

> As a CHW trainer, authenticity has been my strongest asset as an ally. CHWs, both experienced and new to the field, appreciate that I present topics for discussion rather than dominate the instruction. I embrace Paolo Freire's theoretical approach to learning where participants actively engage in the teaching and the learning by creating a space where participants share their knowledge and experiences.
>
> - Rebeca

10.2.3.2   Developing Professional Presence and Boundaries in the Workplace

Allies further have the opportunity to play a unique role in supporting the acceptance and endorsement of the CHW role among other non-CHWs in the workplace. With increased evidence showing the value of team-based care and integration of CHWs on clinical teams (Centers for Disease Control and Prevention, 2018; Klein & Hostetter, 2015), the need for supportive CHW supervision and mentoring is ever more important. There is also a need for ally team members to advocate for the CHW role. A key to CHW integration is clarifying the CHW role for all team members (Matiz et al., 2014), an activity in which allies can partner with CHWs, especially new CHWs that may be learning their role. CHWs have encountered challenges to integrating into care teams, citing the time it took to build trust between team members and an initial lack of knowledge about how to work with CHWs from other team members (Allen, Escoffery, Satsangi, & Brownstein, 2015). There are many examples of CHW programs that falter or fail all together due to lack of understanding of the CHW role or lack of a CHW champion in the workplace that can support the CHW in adapting to the culture of the workplace. In fact, accounts from the literature (Martinez et al., 2011; Rosenthal et al., 2010) and the media have elevated the role of the CHW as a key to success in the era of healthcare reform (Gorman, 2015; Luthra, 2016) and, in some cases, as the "future of health care" (Quinn, 2017); this perception can be dangerous, creating unfair expectations for the type of skillset and approach a CHW will have upon hire. Recruitment of CHWs from communities served or who have a specific connection to the community served—geographic, lived experience, of same racial or ethnic background—continues to be common (Kim et al., 2016), which means a CHW may have limited experience in the type of workplace hiring them. Allies—including supervisors, managers, and team members—can counter assumptions made about a CHW's value or effectiveness based on their ability to relate to and engage in the professional workspace and provide respectful mentoring and skill building support to CHWs. This, in turn, can affect equitable employment infrastructure and foster professional credibility of the Awareness and understanding of the CHW role continues to grow, and CHW role. CHWs and allies have the opportunity to partner to build capacity of the profession and create change through meaningful CHW-ally relationships in the community and the workplace environment.

10.2.4 Building Capacity for Change Through Relationships

CHW Story (Claireta) Building the individual capacity of CHWs enables us to go forward and become agents of change in our community. It allows us to use our skills to assist and advocate for our clients. When I first became a CHW, I was sent to a CHW training and went to other trainings through the organization that hired me. My individual capacity-building skills were further increased with trainings about type 2 diabetes, computer usage, and case management. The training I received enabled me to help my clients and their families cope with their health issues.

The organization I worked for at the time was a federally qualified health center, and my program manager was a strong supporter of the CHW profession. That support allowed us to further increase our capacity-building skills by interacting with the medical team who treated our clients. Those interactions allowed me to communicate with doctors about my clients. The doctors began to realize the bond we had with our clients and would ask us for help with problems our clients were having. One of my clients was not testing her blood sugar, and I was told that she was non-compliant because she was not following the doctor's orders. I made an appointment with her for a home visit to observe her testing her blood sugar. She started the procedure, but her hand was shaking so bad that she could not prick her finger. I asked her to put the lancing device on her leg to steady it and place her finger on top and then press the lancet. It worked, and she was able to test her blood sugar from that point on. No one had ever asked her to test in front of them before, so they did not know what the problem was.

10.2.4.1 Creating Influence

CHWs have the immense capacity to build trusting relationships with their patients. When this capacity is understood, as in Claireta's story, individuals in assumed positions of power—including physicians—can identify and appreciate the value the CHW role brings to their work. In this way, CHWs build professional capacity for the workforce by reflecting the values of the community to those around them.

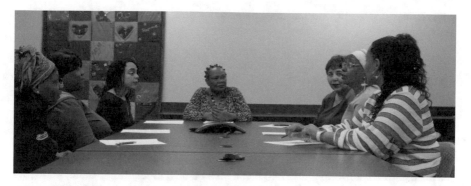

Fig. 10.3 Claireta (center) running a CHW meeting

CHW Story (Claireta)   The passage of the Affordable Care Act generated renewed interest in utilizing CHWs to reduce healthcare costs. The law named CHWs as health professionals who serve on interdisciplinary care teams while also providing new avenues for individuals—including those from low-income communities—to access insurance and preventive services like never before. Due to the renewed interested in CHWs, a new national CHW organization launched and Michigan has a statewide CHW organization, the Michigan Community Health Worker Alliance (MiCHWA).

Serving on various MiCHWA committees has given me a chance to work with CHW allies who support the CHW profession (Fig. 10.3). The allies include people from universities, health care centers, health departments, insurance companies, the State, and other health-related agencies. All the allies are committed to promoting the CHW profession so that it is sustainable. Which is important to me because I love the work that I do, but it's grant funded and when the funding ends so does my job. I have had seven jobs as a CHW in the past 16 years and they were not always consecutive. At one time I did not think that I would ever work as a CHW again.

Even when I was not working as a CHW, I continued to work on committees. My CHW Network co-leader once said to me, "once a CHW, always a CHW." She's right, so I continued to advocate for the CHW profession even though I was not working as a CHW at that time. It's important for us as CHWs to advocate for the profession. It is also in our code of ethics. In the code of ethics, it states that "CHWs are advocates for the profession. They are members, leaders, and active participants in the local, state, and national professional organizations."

Allies are committed to the CHW profession, and they bring their expertise and experience to the table. It has helped the organization to grow and become recognized as the authority of CHWs in the state. They also support CHWs by providing opportunities for professional development and supporting us to attend conferences, steering committee meetings, and participating in CHW-led activities.

10.2.4.2 Accessing Influence

CHW-ally partnerships further facilitate CHWs in accessing greater influence to further the CHW profession. Allies often have the political and financial influence to promote and sustain workforce development efforts, moving grassroots interest and organizing center stage. This can be at a local level, providing in-kind resources for a client or for a group gathering; it can also be on a much larger scale, including drafting legislation or writing policy for Medicaid payment and reimbursement for the profession. CHW-ally partnerships create opportunities for accessing influence that can further the profession while elevating the CHW voice to places of power and influence for themselves.

Allies come in all shapes and sizes. In many cases, there are unknowing allies, such as a restaurant owner that donates food to a client celebration after a CHW inquires. These relationships have an impact not only on the CHWs but also on the allies. Becoming involved with CHWs can be an opportunity to share their resources, time, and talents with communities. In the workplace, allies can also expand their own network of other like-minded people with whom they can share their expertise. Allies can learn from CHWs and expand their own understanding of community and of justice by engaging with CHWs from a place of humility and learning. As work deepens between CHWs and allies, it is essential that allies recognize the need for and practice humility in these relationships

Ally Story (Katie) I am a CHW ally. I began my journey with CHWs one summer while organizing an event focused on sustainability of CHWs in the state of Michigan. Through planning and preparation for the meeting, I learned about the roles CHWs played in Michigan's communities and how they were changing the landscape of health in Detroit, Grand Rapids, and beyond. Over 100 people attended the event, citing the need for a unified voice to support and sustain the CHW workforce statewide. Other states were further along in the work and had exciting stories to share.

The event planning committee, including CHWs and other stakeholders, held a debrief meeting the next day to figure out what to do with all the great feedback we had received through the event. There was a clear call for a new organization dedicated to building capacity of the CHW workforce while honoring and raising up the CHW profession. I remember leaving that day thinking, "wow—this might just be the beginning of something." And it was.

As MiCHWA's first full-time staff member, I provided administrative and technical support MiCHWA's efforts. Through the work, I met CHWs from urban and rural communities all over the Mitten sparking change and pursuing social justice. I also met CHW employers, supervisors, and co-workers, all of whom had varying levels of understanding and respect for the CHW profession and its unique ability to build individual and community capacity. I also met groups we wanted to be allies, ranging from state government officials to insurance company executives to health-care system leadership. I learned there are various roles allies can take, and that those roles need to be understood using an ethical framework to guide engagement with and support of CHWs, all based on relationships.

10.2.4.3   Building Capacity for the Workforce as Partners Through CHW Organizations

CHW associations, networks, or alliances can serve as vehicles through which CHWs can engage in advocacy for their profession. There are at least 40 known CHW membership organizations in the United States that go by many titles (National Association of Community Health Workers, 2018). While some of these organizations are CHW only, many include both CHWs and allies, though the make-up of boards, Steering Committees, or advisory groups is often designed to ensure CHW majority to maintain CHW leadership and power. CHW majority is a nationally recognized best practice for governance of CHW training and credential-ing (American Public Health Association, 2014), and many groups have extended that principle to groups that address CHW workforce issues. The CHW membership organization is a mechanism to funnel ally excitement toward CHW interest and connect allies and CHWs through engagement on advocacy for the CHW profes-sion. MiCHWA became a place where respect was grown between allies and CHWs in new ways: co-leading groups, facilitating meetings, planning conferences, and holding space for CHW storytelling. Alliances, associations, and other membership organizations create opportunities for that storytelling. The stories of CHWs in the field are often what drive allies to action and to partnership.

Additionally, partnerships within alliances or associations between allies and CHWs provide opportunities for policy change. While CHWs have a nationally recognized definition (American Public Health Association, 2009) and a Standard Occupational Classification through the Bureau of Labor Statistics (Bureau of Labor Statistics, 2017), formal recognition of CHW as a respected and unique pro-fession varies by state (Barbero et al., 2016).

The 2010 National Community Health Worker Advocacy Survey (NCHWAS) concluded that while the CHW profession has standardized in many ways over the past 50 years, CHWs would benefit from acknowledgement as a health profession versus a health intervention, including for increased recognition by healthcare pro-viders as a member of the healthcare team distinct from other professions and a team member positioned to address social determinants of health (Ingram et al., 2012). A second iteration of the NCHWAS in 2014 found that CHWs affiliated with a professional network or association were four times as likely to advocate on behalf of the CHW profession as compared with non-members (Sabo et al., 2015). Allies can help foster professional advocacy skills through alliances or associations; this can also help allies recognize the immense value in fostering CHW voice, including storytelling, not forcing CHW voice. Further, this partnership can support CHW and ally understanding of the value of professional advocacy. In a bidirectional way, respect for the CHW voices helps create a group of advocates unified around the CHW workforce. Through membership organizations, allies have the opportunity to connect the CHW voice and the policy voice, ensuring that policymakers—many of whom could be allies—see and hear the CHW in their communities, not just that of the ally carrying the message.

10.2.4.4   CHWs Supporting CHWs

Building spaces that create opportunities for CHW networking, which has been cited as a factor supporting CHW work, is essential (Allen et al., 2015). Allies and CHWs can partner in identifying and creating these spaces, through CHW membership organizations, workplaces, or other settings. Further, studies have indicated that CHWs request ongoing support following formal CHW training (Wennerstrom, Johnson, Gibson, Batta, & Springgate, 2014), creating an opportunity for allies to come alongside the workforce and provide infrastructure for CHW peer support internal to and external to the workplace. Allies play roles in training, hiring, and supervising CHWs; with that engagement, there is an ethical undercurrent of participation in or facilitation of ongoing professional development and peer support to sustain the workforce.

CHW membership organizations can provide this infrastructure. Many CHW membership organizations are fortunate to fund and invest in CHW leaders as paid staff members moving the workforce forward. In other cases, organizations leverage paid non-CHW staff to assist with these efforts. Allies may come with different skillsets in logistics, management, and advocacy that complement CHW organizing and capacity building. As described earlier in the section, Claireta experienced this firsthand through her work on the MiCHWA CHW Network. While the logistics were ally-facilitated, the meetings, priorities, and shared experiences were entirely CHW-led.

10.2.5   Conclusion

In Michigan, CHWs are working alongside allies of various types and in varied degrees to build the capacity of, and advocate for, their own profession. While the pursuit of equity and justice is at the heart of all CHW work, individual and community capacity building is the means by which partnerships between CHWs and allies cultivate the development and application of ethical professional practice in the workplace and in the community. Through a bidirectional motivation loop, CHW-ally partnerships create opportunities for greater understanding and awareness of what actual social justice and equity look like both for communities and for professional settings. The relationships that are developed between the CHWs and allies create influence and may allow CHWs to access power brokers they might not otherwise have. It is through many of these relationships that CHWs are mentored and provided opportunities to gain and apply leadership skills and gain additional power in new spaces in their own right.

Across the United States, CHWs are advocating for their role as health and community professionals. They are not alone: employers, health departments, health systems, universities, small business owners, and many others are walking with them, lending a hand, advice, or a word of encouragement. Partnerships between CHWs and allies are building capacity both for the community and for the CHW profession. In this way, CHWs are fulfilling professional competencies while also creating a sustainable future for their work. CHWs embody social justice, and through continued relationship building among clients and allies, CHWs are sparking and sustaining professional change.

References

Allen, C. G., Escoffery, C., Satsangi, A., & Brownstein, J. N. (2015, September). Strategies to improve the integration of community health workers into health care teams: "A little fish in a big pond". *Preventing Chronic Disease, 12*, 150199. https://doi.org/10.5888/pcd12.150199

American Association of Community Health Workers. (2016). American Association of community health workers code of ethics. In T. Berthold, E. Guillén-Núñez, & T. Berthold (Eds.), *Foundations for community health workers* (2nd ed., pp. 159–162). San Francisco, CA: Jossey-Bass.

American Public Health Association. (2009, November 10). *Support for community health workers to increase health access and to reduce health inequities.* Retrieved from American Public Health Association: https://www.apha.org/policies-and-advocacy/public-health-policy-statements/policy-database/2014/07/09/14/19/support-for-community-health-workers-to-increase-health-access-and-to-reduce-health-inequities

American Public Health Association. (2014, November 18). *Support for community health worker leadership in determining workforce standards for training and credentialing.* Retrieved from American Public Health Association: https://www.apha.org/policies-and-advocacy/public-health-policy-statements/policy-database/2015/01/28/14/15/support-for-community-health-worker-leadership

Barbero, C., Gilchrist, S., Chriqui, J. F., Martin, M. A., Wennerstrom, A., VanderVeur, J., … Brownstein, J. N. (2016). Do state community health worker laws align with best available evidence? *Journal of Community Health, 41*, 315–325.

Bureau of Labor Statistics. (2017, May). *Occupational employment and wages, May 2017: 21-1094 Community health workers.* Retrieved from Occupational Employment Statistics: https://www.bls.gov/oes/current/oes211094.htm

Centers for Disease Control and Prevention. (2018, January 18). *Integrating community health workers on clinical care teams and in the community.* Retrieved from Division of Heart Disease and Stroke Prevention: Best Practices Guide: https://www.cdc.gov/dhdsp/pubs/guides/best-practices/chw.htm

Gorman, A. (2015, October 29). *Community health workers reach some patients that doctors can't.* NPR Shots. Retrieved from https://www.npr.org/sections/health-shots/2015/10/29/452653733/community-health-workers-can-reach-some-patients-that-doctors-cant

Hohl, S. D., Thompson, B., Krok-Schoen, J. L., Weier, R. C., Martin, M., Bone, L., ... Paskett, E. D. (2016). Characterizing community health workers on research teams: Results from the centers for population health and health disparities. *American Journal of Public Health, 106*(4), 664–670.

Ingram, M., Reinschmidt, K. M., Schachter, K. A., Davidson, C. L., Sabo, S. J., De Zapien, J. G., & Carvajal, S. C. (2012). Establishing a professional profile of community health workers: Results from a national study of roles, activities and training. *Journal of Community Health, 37*, 529–537.

Islam, N., Nadkarni, S. K., Zahn, D., Skillman, M., Kwon, S. C., & Trinh-Shevrin, C. (2015). Integrating community health workers within patient protection and affordable care act implementation. *Journal of Public Health Management and Practice, 21*(1), 42–50.

Israel, B. A. (1985). Social networks and social support: Implications for natural helper and community level interventions. *Health Education Quarterly, 12*(1), 65–68.

Kim, K., Choi, J. S., Choi, E., Nieman, C. L., Joo, J. H., Lin, F. R., ... Han, H.-R. (2016, April). Effects of community-based health worker interventions to improve chronic disease management and care among vulnerable populations: A systematic review. *American Journal of Public Health, 106*(4), e3–e28.

Klein, S., & Hostetter, M. (2015, December 17). *In focus: Integrating community health workers into care teams.* Retrieved from The Commonwealth Fund: https://www.commonwealthfund.org/publications/newsletter/2015/dec/focus-integrating-community-health-workers-care-teams

Luthra, S. (2016, April 9). *Hospitals eye community health workers to cultivate patients' successes.* USA Today. Retrieved from https://www.usatoday.com/story/news/2016/04/09/kaiser-hospitals-eye-community-health-workers-cultivate-patients-successes/82802900/

Martinez, J., Ro, M., Villa, N. W., Powell, W., & Knickman, J. R. (2011, December). Transforming the delivery of care in the post–health reform era: What role will community health workers play? *American Journal of Public Health, 101*(12), e1–e5.

Matiz, L. A., Peretz, P. J., Jacotin, P. G., Cruz, C., Ramirez-Diaz, E., & Nieto, A. R. (2014). The impact of integrating community health workers into the patient-centered medical home. *Journal of Primary Care & Community Health, 5*(4), 271–274.

Michigan Community Health Worker Alliance. (2016, June 30). *Community health worker employer survey 2016: Final evaluation report for public use.* Retrieved from Michigan Community Health Worker Alliance: http://www.michwa.org/wp-content/uploads/MiCHWA-CHW-Employer-Survey-2016_Public-Report_9.30FINAL-1-1.pdf

Michigan Community Health Worker Alliance. (2018). *Our structure.* Retrieved from Michigan Community Health Worker Alliance: http://www.michwa.org/our-structure/

Quinn, M. (2017, March). *The future of health care is outside the doctor's office.* Governing. Retrieved from http://www.governing.com/topics/health-human-services/gov-community-health-workers.html

Roman, L., Gardiner, J. C., Lindsay, J. K., Moore, J. S., Luo, Z., Baer, L. J., ... Paneth, N. (2009). Alleviating perinatal depressive symptoms and stress: A nurse-community health worker randomized trial. *Archives of Women's Mental Health, 12*, 379–391.

Rosenthal, E. L., Brownstein, J. N., Rush, C. H., Hirsch, G. R., Willaert, A. M., Scott, J. R., ... Fox, D. J. (2010). Community health workers: Part of the solution. *Health Affairs, 29*(7), 1338–1342.

Sabo, S., Wennerstrom, A., Phillips, D., Haywood, C., Redondo, F., Bell, M. L., & Ingram, M. (2015, July–September). Community health worker professional advocacy: Voices of action from the 2014 National Community Health Worker Advocacy Survey. *Journal of Ambulatory Care Management, 38*(3), 225–235.

Spencer, M. S., Gunter, K. E., & Palmisano, G. (2010, April). Community Health workers and their value to social work. *Social Work, 55*(2), 169–180.

Wennerstrom, A., Johnson, L., Gibson, K., Batta, S. E., & Springgate, B. F. (2014, December). Community health workers leading the charge on workforce development: Lessons from New Orleans. *Journal of Community Health, 39*(6), 1140–1149.

Wilkinson, G. W., Sager, A., Selig, S., Antonelli, R., Morton, S., Hirsch, G., … Wachman, M. (2017). No equity, no triple aim: Strategic proposals to advance health equity in a volatile policy environment. *American Journal of Public Health, 107*, S223–S228.

10.3 Engaging Communities to Build on Strengths for Sustainable Change[4]

Julie Smithwick, Maria Martin, Virginia Vedilago, and Mike Young

10.3.1 Introduction

Between 2000 and 2014, the Latino population in South Carolina increased 172% and in 2017 accounted for 5.7% of the state's population (U.S. Census Bureau, 2017; Stepler, Lopez, & Rohal, 2016). In 2004, after noting an unprecedented increase in fertility and birth rates among this population, the Division of Perinatal Systems of the South Carolina Department of Health and Environmental Control commissioned a needs assessment of Latino maternal and child health needs (Smithwick-Leone, 2004). This research revealed significant barriers to information on and navigation of health and social service resources, as well as a lack of capacity of South Carolina's health and social service organizations to respond to the population's needs.

PASOs (meaning "steps" in Spanish) was founded in 2005 by a community health worker in response to these challenges, with initial support from Division of Women's and Neonatology Services at a local hospital and a community grant from the South Carolina March of Dimes. In August 2008, through funding provided by The Duke Endowment, PASOs initiated a partnership with the University of South Carolina Arnold School of Public Health (ASPH), which since that time has provided logistical, programmatic, and support services to the organization. In 2009, PASOs hired a second CHW and then trained its first group of volunteer CHWs, called Promotores in Spanish, after multiple community leaders expressed a desire to get more involved in the work and help the work grow. In 2010, PASOs garnered a 4-year capacity building grant from the Robert Wood Johnson Foundation, which was supported with matching funds from six local funding partners, allowing the organization to further develop its CHW model.

In 2020, the PASOs team is comprised of 21 CHWs and 7 allied professionals, most of which are also bilingual and bicultural and the majority of which are full-time and salaried. Sixteen of the CHWs provide services at community and/or clinic sites, and five CHWs provide program leadership, supervision, evaluation, and administrative support as members of the central office staff. In addition, PASOs has approximately 50 volunteer and contracted CHWs that provide outreach, support, education, and advocacy within their communities. Contracted CHWs receive funding for completion of specific deliverables related to a project or program.

---

[4]With contributions by Lorena Cervantes, Medical University of South Carolina, Charleston, South Carolina, USA; Ana Cossio, PASOs, Columbia, South Carolina, USA.

Volunteer CHWs receive incentives such as additional training, attendance at conferences, and gift cards when resources are available.

PASOs' central office continues to be supported by the ASPH, and its regional offices are partnered with local organizations in areas where significant Latino populations exist and where a host organization has committed to developing and sustaining the model. Local host agencies include a large health system, two federally qualified health centers, three pediatric clinics, a medical university, a nonprofit community service agency, an early childhood education program, and a free clinic. Partnership with these host agencies provides much of the infrastructure and networks that allow PASOs to operate sustainably within both Latino communities and formal institutional settings and to spend more of our resources on direct services. Currently, the PASOs network provides services to individuals and families from 23 of South Carolina's 46 counties.

Like most southeastern states, South Carolina has experienced rapid growth in its Latino population. In addition to the growth of the overall population, at present approximately 10% of children ages 0 to 5 are Latino, and the growth of this population over the last 20 years is over 800% (Kids Count Data Center, 2017a). In some counties, over 25% of the population of children ages 0 to 5 is Latino. An estimated 29.5% of Latinos in SC live below the poverty line, as compared to 12% of the White population of the state (Center for American Progress, 2018). Additionally, 37% of Latino children live below the poverty line—compared to 23% of all SC children— and 15% live in conditions of extreme poverty (Kids Count Data Center, 2017b, 2018). Nationally, 22% of Latinos are uninsured compared to 9% of Whites (Squires, Artiga, & Foutz, 2018). However, in South Carolina, 37% of all Latinos lack health insurance coverage (Pew Research Center, 2014). Although uninsured rates among Latinos have declined under the Affordable Care Act, Latinos are still more likely to be uninsured than non-Latino Whites (Squires et al., 2018).

The average PASOs participant is a Latina mother with young children, lives below the federal poverty level, and has resided in the United States for approximately 10 years. Up to 92% of PASOs' participants are uninsured, and most have less than a high school education. The average household income per week is $361, which is a household annual income of $18,772. Other challenges faced by Latino families in South Carolina include language access, resource navigation needs, transportation, and anti-immigrant laws and sentiments:

> Some of our Latino communities go through very difficult times. I have been through very difficult times and all of my experiences of immigrating to this country for a better life have led me to be the person I am today. This is also why, as a CHW, I am able to understand the circumstances and experiences of the community, of *my* community, of our people. They too can be in challenging situations like I used to be. They feel the same fears I had, and could be going through tough times. (A. Cossio, personal communication, June 27, 2018)

In addition to socioeconomic and political challenges faced by Latino families, service providers face a lack of capacity to serve Latino families. In the face of such rapid population growth, providers have struggled to keep up with needs and often lack the capacity to effectively serve Latino families. Examples of lack of capacity we have observed include no or insufficient bilingual staff, lack of experience serving limited English proficient clients, lack of interpreters, lack of understanding of the socio-political realities faced by immigrant populations, no connection to Latino organizations to aid in outreach or awareness of resources for this population, or no Latino representation on boards or advisory councils. All of these factors, and others, limit organizations' ability to effectively serve the target population.

Despite the barriers they face, PASOs' participants have strong individual and cultural strengths, and the PASOs team works to build on those assets, supporting their goals of self-sufficiency, leadership growth, and civic participation:

> As someone who works with the Latino population on a daily basis in the field of reproductive health, nothing touches me more than their responsiveness to this delicate yet crucial subject. Like all mothers, they want to do the best they can. The Latino families I have observed are so open to talk about a reproductive life plan and contraceptive methods despite their traditional upbringing, which would have labeled this subject as taboo. During consultations, participants often mention how important it is for them to plan their pregnancies in order to provide for their kids, focus on their education, and spend more quality time with them. Also, parents with children show enthusiasm regarding the subjects and are interested in all the resources and tools available so that they can start, maintain, or even improve the conversations [about this subject] within the family. Latino parents truly recognize how important it is to talk to their kids about reproductive health from early ages. (M. Lubov, personal communication, October 10, 2018)

10.3.2 PASOs' Work Related to Individual and Community Capacity Building

PASOs' mission is *to build a stronger South Carolina by supporting Latino communities with education, advocacy and leadership development.* PASOs' services are comprised of both community-based programs and capacity-building services. Our largest community-based program, PASOs Health Connections, uses a collective action framework through which CHWs address disparities and social determinants, while simultaneously giving voice to issues related to access to care and needed policy changes. The PASOs Connections for Child Development program enhances early childhood education opportunities for young Latino children. The PASOs for Parents program provides parenting education and support on parent-defined goals to prevent child abuse and support parents in positive parenting techniques. Other pilot programs address specific needs identified in local sites, such as early literacy and childhood obesity. With a constant goal of sustainable systemic change, PASOs also promotes equity through CHW training, advocacy, and organizational capacity building, which will be described in more detail later in this section.

All of PASOs' programs emerged and were developed in response to needs expressed by community members as well as service providers that were interested in better serving and reaching Latino families. One of our first volunteer Promotores describes the role of the CHWs/Promotores in this way:

As Promotores, we are like an umbilical cord that permanently connects the community with different services, and because of that, I think it's important that we be both present in community and institutional environments. Promotores are also like umbilical cords in that we give health and life to the community. (*N. Garcia, personal communication, January 31, 2017*)

Central to our model is an ongoing iterative dialogue based on a foundation of trust with the individuals and organizations we serve, to constantly integrate new ideas and respond to developing challenges that are identified. The programs build on each other, and incorporate PASOs' best practices of culturally and linguistically appropriate curricula; bilingual and bicultural staff; reaching the population in their natural environment; and empowering organic leadership. In this section, we introduce you to two of our Community Health Workers, Ana Cossio and Lorena Cervantes, and describe five themes related to how the PASOs team builds individual and community capacity: grounding in values; looking at empowerment in a different way; building a foundation through training and coaching; building capacity by listening; and advocacy to build sustainable capacity.

Ana Cossio is from Cuba and immigrated to the United States in 2004 with her husband and 8-year-old son, to escape what for them was an oppressive situation, and to provide a better life for their son. Dreaming of new opportunities, Ana and her family moved to the United States, but "from the beginning of our stay we realized that things were not what we envisioned and many things happened that made it very difficult for us to be able to get comfortable living here and to understand the system here" (A. Cossio, personal communication, June 27, 2018). Ana didn't know how to go to her son's school and communicate with the staff, or how to get his health insurance. The family struggled to understand a new system in a new language. Ana, trained as a teacher in Cuba, worked as a housekeeper in a hotel, which was grueling work, earning 8 dollars an hour. The family didn't have their own transportation or cell phones, making communication and integration even more challenging. Ana now says that "[this experience] has been a big part of my life because it has made me the warrior that I have become today." She explains that her experiences as a new immigrant in the U.S. make her better able to understand the circumstances and experiences of the community, *mi comunidad*, of *our people*. "They too can be in situations where they feel the same fears I had and could be going through tough times like me."

Ana was introduced to PASOs in 2009, when a nonprofit organization called South Carolina Hispanic Outreach worked with PASOs to write a grant to offer a prenatal education course in Spanish to Latina immigrants in three rural counties of SC:

I made lots of great contacts with community--key persons in my coverage area to be able to serve the community. This was work that started from zero with the community in that coverage area. I started with just one community contact, at a local clinic, and then worked my way through to meet other key people to have the most reach of the population. The program continued to grow and so did the curriculum and the education we offered the community. We also connected women to prenatal health care services. The doctors I worked with were very happy to have us in the area because they had so much support working with the pregnant women who were now coming to all of their visits. (A. Cossio, personal communication, June 27, 2018)

Ana has continued to grow professionally and personally and has recently been promoted as the statewide Training Manager for PASOs, training other CHWs on how to be effective in their work.

Lorena Cervantes is from Mexico and came to the United States with her daughter because she feared for her safety in her country. When she arrived to the United States, she quickly realized it was going to be more difficult than she thought because of the language. "Even though I had studied in the university in Mexico, I struggled a lot in the beginning. Little by little I learned what I needed to know to get by" (L. Cervantes, personal communication, June 22, 2018). She met someone she thought would be good for her and her daughter, and they had two children together, but he began to be physically and psychologically violent, which nearly destroyed her. Lorena ended up seeking services at a shelter for victims of domestic violence and spent some time there with her children. "The staff at the shelter really helped me to get back on my feet, to begin to be the strong woman I could be. They helped me find my voice and taught me that I am valuable as a person, and they gave me hope that I could move forward with my children."

As Lorena grew stronger, she started getting involved in helping people in her community. "I saw in the Latino community, people who were having the same experiences I had, the feeling of not speaking English or not having anyone to support you and tell you how to get help" (L. Cervantes, personal communication, June 22, 2018). That was when she learned about PASOs and met the local coordinator, who supported her and inspired her to do more. "She really helped me to be strong, to develop my professional skills, to reclaim my voice, to be the Lorena I was before … a woman who fights for her children. My children have seen me grow as a person and as a professional, which I am doing through the support of PASOs."

Lorena started as a volunteer CHW, going to events and health fairs and started talking more with people in her community. After gaining more knowledge and resources to help people, she was offered a part-time position as a CHW working in the PASOs Connections for Child Development program. She quickly exceeded expectations, contributed to developing the program model, and was offered a full-time CHW position. She now supervises other CHWs and has presented at statewide and regional conferences about her work.

10.3.3   Values: Our Starting Place

Many organizations have defined organizational values, and the same is true for PASOs. In addition to having and displaying our values, we are committed to regularly reflecting on and communicating our values, in order to enhance the quality and effectiveness of our work, and to hold each other accountable. Our values include *equity*, *trust*, *compromiso* (a Spanish word meaning a deep commitment and responsibility to the families we serve), *family*, *education*, and *community integration* (for a detailed description of the values, see http://www.scpasos.org/ values). We work hard to ensure that these values are woven into who we are and all we do, whether it be a workshop on positive parenting, participation in an immigrants' rights coalition, or a training to one of our organizational partners on how to effectively reach and support Latino families. Because of our commitment to equity, PASOs' team members annually choose priority partner organizations in their local sites with which they plan to partner to improve access to culturally and linguistically appropriate services. Team members work in partnership with these organizations to make sure community voices are heard and to forge systemic changes, which sometimes include policy and procedure changes.

When early childhood home visiting services were beginning to be implemented in South Carolina, PASOs' accepted the invitation to be part of the advisory board for implementation. Upon noting gaps in the capacity of home visitors to build relationships with Latino families and communities, the lead agency contracted with PASOs to provide training, technical assistance such as help hiring bilingual professionals, and ongoing participation in addressing the safety net for young Latino children in the state. Currently, all new home visitors receive training in effective outreach and engagement, and other staff receive additional training that builds on their knowledge and better equips them to reach and serve Latino families. PASOs' team members participate in various early childhood coalitions throughout the state so that collaborations are established and the Latino voice is consistently at the table.

There are multiple ways in which our organizational values influence our ability to build individual and community capacity. For example, because of our commitment to trust and community integration, we spend a lot of time focusing on relationships and the value of building and developing trusted relationships with other team members and with the communities we serve. "This is why PASOs is so important and we make our participants feel so welcome. We know what they might be going through because we have been there. Our relationships with community members are built on trust" (A. Cossio, personal communication, June 27, 2018). This focus on relationships is essential in building confidence and commitment and in our ability to overcome personal and organizational challenges. "[PASOs' leadership] models a respectful way of communication for everyone to follow. We all feel that respect and we all feel like we are part of something bigger. PASOs invests in us in the same way that we are expected to invest in our work and in our communities" (L. Cervantes, personal communication, June 22, 2018).

These trusted relationships, in turn, relate to our value of education, as they foster team members' ability to be innovative and take risks to try new things in response to experiences or requests from the communities we serve. As team members get involved in innovation and feel valued as equitable, contributing members of the team, they feel an even greater commitment to the work, the values that shape the work, and the potential to drive positive change. "Because PASOs has faith in people. They know just how to help you come out of your cocoon and become this great professional" (A. Cossio, personal communication, June 22, 2018).

As an organization, we realize that commitment to values is an active, ongoing process, and we will always have work to do in this arena. We recognize that we still have work to do to make sure we are living our values, and advancing equity, both in our individual work and the systemic changes we are promoting. For example, we spend time analyzing the words and language we use, what the true meaning and intent of these words are, and how the words we choose reflect or detract from our stated values. We have intentionally committed to eliminating particular words from our organizational language, because they do not promote dignity, equity, or strengths. There have also been instances when we've realized the need for us to step back and explore additional dimensions of our own cultures and the complexities within, so we can avoid false assumptions and more fully embrace and support the multiple diversities within cultures.

We have found that having and displaying our organizational values is essential, as well as reflecting on them regularly with the entire team involved, so that each team member has an opportunity to build our core values and determine how she will put each one of them into practice, both within the organization and in our work with community.

10.3.4 A Different Way of Looking at Empowerment

Traditionally, empowerment is thought of as the ability of one person to give power to another; however, this definition is limited in its scope. In this traditional definition, we assume that one person has the power to give, while the other person receives. Some health professionals, providers, and social service organizations purport to "empower" clients and patients with information and instructions; the organizations or professional *have* the expertise and the patients *receive* their expertise. In the organizational context of PASOs, we work from a belief that the true act of empowerment is an intentional, supported, often measurable unleashing of power from within the individual. This means eventually we can walk away, and the participants we have served will only keep getting stronger. As Lorena says, "We give support with the expectation that someone will take what they have learned and grow from it" (L. Cervantes, personal communication, June 22, 2018). Ana also comments on this: "Leadership in a person is something innate. PASOs knows and teaches its team members how to identify these natural born leaders in the community and then once they are recruited in the work, PASOs works really hard to refine their skills and to help them see their strengths to give back to community" (A. Cossio, personal communication, June 27, 2018).

The PASOs model provides the expectation that each team member will seek out opportunities for growth, far beyond the traditional trainings and conferences. In PASOs, each individual team member is held accountable for their actions, and negative perception and beliefs are challenged in a safe and supportive environment. The PASOs team provides inspiration for individual members to own their decisions as protagonists in their experiences by setting high expectations of continual growth. Additionally, the emphasis on the relationships of individuals with members of their team provides space for motivation, inspiration, debriefing of difficult situations, encouragement of self-care, and unification around a centralized set of values and goals:

> It was amazing. In the first training, I felt the humanity in PASOs. Without knowing me, everyone offered support and welcomed me, [saying] 'here I am if you need anything'. And since that moment even now I know I can always count on that support. There is a true respect and love that is really hard to find in other organizations. (L. Cervantes, personal communication, June 22, 2018)

One principal element of how PASOs engenders empowerment in our work with individuals involves the PASOs pathway model, which is designed to guide the CHW and the participant through the work of identifying goals and building on strengths. PASOs doesn't refer to those they serve with terms such as "client" or "patient." Rather, they are considered "participants" since they are stakeholders in their own success and the successes of others.

The CHW uses motivational interviewing and facilitation skills to help the participant identify what she wants to change, or achieve, and what her goals could be. The participant decides on a goal (for herself or her child), and the two discuss what steps to take, what follow-up will consist of, and how the CHW can support goal achievement. Through this method of working jointly to discuss needs and options and then determine the goal and how to work toward it, we have already begun to disrupt the traditional service model. We ask them to actively participate in every aspect of this plan, and we see the effectiveness of this model in the high success rate for goal completion throughout all of our programs. PASOs' model is predicated on trusting that others are capable of crafting their own solutions. Understanding and assisting others to reach their goals can only be accomplished through listening and believing in the capacity of others. This involves a dignified and respectful approach.

Empowerment begins with respect, understanding, and great appreciation for autonomy. In PASOs we have a great respect for each individual journey, and we know that aside from the basic interactions, referrals, and follow-up, what matters most is the mutual respect and the honoring of what each person has to offer. Decisions are made by the participant, in the best interest of his or her family. PASOs' CHWs are equipped with the ability to present options, with accurate and up-to-date information from trusted sources. As a result, PASOs' participants overcome challenges to achieve their goals and gain a new sense of control over their lives. This empowerment often encourages them to keep striving to make positive changes in their own lives and in the lives of others. "[PASOs] gives support with the expectation that someone will take what they have learned and grow from it … I want others to have the same opportunities" (Lorena). "I want to share the things that I have learned. I want to reach out and give my hand to those that do not have anybody else to help them" (A. Cossio, personal communication, June 27, 2018).

A second essential element related to empowerment in the PASOs model is the CHW's ability to connect to the participant through shared experiences. As the CHW begins to develop trust with a participant, she is also imparting (either directly or indirectly) her story of how she has faced similar struggles and overcome these barriers. Often, the participants are struggling with similar barriers in access to care or other social determinants of health, and they are able to see how another person with whom she identifies has found her way in this system. The relationship of a PASOs CHW with a participant begins with respect for one another's journey. Lorena explains:

> We are all human beings, all of us are the same and we have something to offer. I think it is so important because it really makes a difference to people. I have been where the participants sometimes are. I had the experience of meeting a woman who was suffering domestic violence and she was so … broken. She was saying 'I can't do anything, I just can't go on'. And I told her 'Do you see where I am and what I am doing? I was where you were, I want you to look at me and see yourself reflected because I was in your place, alone with my three children and I survived, I am making my dreams come true and so will you'. (L. Cervantes, personal communication, June 22, 2018)

Thirdly, the PASOs model presents a paradigm shift for the more traditional method of leadership in health, which often involves meetings, coalitions, and workgroups attended by public health specialists and clinical providers making decisions on large-scale efforts to improve health. Although these professionals often note the need to involve the communities of target, community members are often under-represented or absent from these gatherings, due to various logistical and philosophical factors. PASOs has been working to change this paradigm over the past 13 years in South Carolina. Community engagement in these efforts has been essential to elevate the voice of the Latino population in South Carolina and empower individuals to recognize the invaluable contribution they can make to improve health outcomes.

PASOs works to ensure that CHWs and PASOs participants are invited to conferences, workgroups, and task force initiatives and that they take part in the training of other health professionals such as medical and nursing students and staff from community partner organizations and state or local government. In these settings, community members are able to feel celebrated for the wealth of knowledge they bring to the table, and PASOs sets the expectation that organizations must truly hear and learn from the Latino community. When the CEO of a large hospital system approached PASOs to ask what their leadership could do to improve services for the surrounding Latino communities, PASOs' CHWs invited the entire hospital leadership team to a panel presentation, where the CHWs expressed what they appreciated about the services offered, along with the challenges they had faced throughout the years, sharing compelling stories related to barriers and ending with an offering to work with their team to make structural changes. Their voices were heard, and changes were implemented related to additional interpreter services, changing of acceptable forms of identification, more training for staff, and a stronger partnership with PASOs.

10.3.4.1 Training and Coaching: The Foundation for Success

An essential component of building individual capacity relates to the types and characteristics of the training and mentoring that the CHWs are provided.

Training

Initial training as a PASOs CHW begins with an orientation to the organization, its programs, protocols, team members, and structure. While these are important elements of introduction to PASOs, one of the most essential training components for new team members is the PASOs CHW training. The PASOs CHW training is designed to help team members learn what a CHW is and how to become a CHW, to provide direct services such as resource navigation, motivational interviewing, health education, and connection to needed services in a culturally appropriate way (Fig. 10.4). As part of the CHW training, newly trained CHWs shadow more experienced CHWs and are observed to ensure the work is carried out with quality and as it is intended to—with dignity to the people served. Lorena says that PASOs and its leadership "models a respectful way of communication for everyone to follow" (L. Cervantes, personal communication, June 22, 2018). Upon recalling when she was trained, Ana says that when the executive director used to observe her as she facilitated workshops, she would tell her to "'encourage the participants to share more than you talk' so that it could enrich discussions and create a space of trust for sharing and learning from each other" (A. Cossio, personal communication, June 27, 2018).

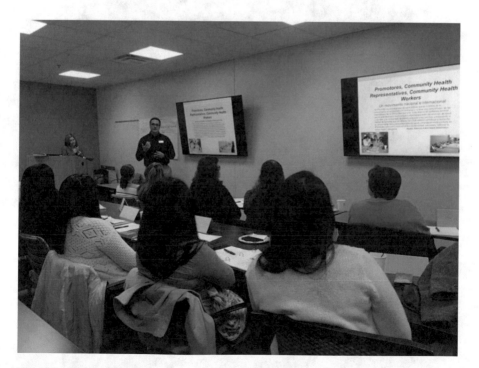

Fig. 10.4 Community Health Worker Training in Greenville, South Carolina, PASOsTM

To continue developing the capacity of our CHWs, PASOs also provides semi-annual trainings, which affect the way in which team members work from year to year. The 3-day, in-person trainings are designed to help team members strengthen their skill sets and knowledge to conduct their daily work while also including team building activities and spaces for information and resource sharing among team members (Fig. 10.5). This time together is not just important for skill building and learning from experts on given topics but also for networking and building closer working relationships between peers that can create a safe and trusting environment for sharing experiences from which all team members can grow. Lorena best explains what this means when she says that "I see how we work together as a team, how we are learning from each other. I have really learned from PASOs how to do things I had never expected to do" (L. Cervantes, personal communication, June 22, 2018). Team members leave these trainings renewed and recharged not just from professional growth and learning but also from personally connecting with other

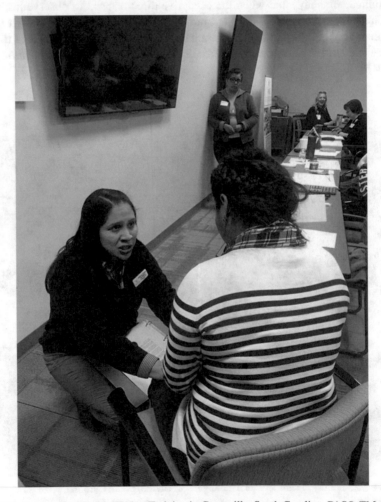

Fig. 10.5 Community Health Worker Training in Greenville, South Carolina, PASOsTM

team members which helps build up morale and support needed among each other. PASOs' CHW training team has optimistically discussed the positive impact these trainings have produced. "It is very exciting to see and have more qualified individuals who can now support individuals and families in different areas and now even in another state!" (A. Cossio, personal communication October 10, 2018).

Furthermore, PASOs holds statewide monthly team meetings, which include updates from the central office hub team, additional, training on specific topics by team members and/or invited guests. For example, if there is a team member that is working on improving their skill set in a given area that others can benefit from learning, that team member may be asked to research and put together a presentation about that topic and then present it during a monthly meeting. This helps that team member learn more about the topic, helps them sharpen their presenting skills, and teaches others as well. PASOs works conscientiously on making these monthly meetings interactive and engaging; everyone is encouraged to share information and to participate, thereby modeling the community education we provide to families and individuals.

Individual Professional Development

PASOs also supports and encourages individual professional development to continue enhancing and diversifying skill sets among team members. Professional development plans are created at the beginning of each year with the help of the team member's supervisor or mentor, based on individual goals and needs, and are updated throughout the year as needed. The activities include measurable goals to be completed in a specific amount of time. Team members' supervisors and mentors have continual check-ins with the progress of goals and provide team members support and guidance for the completion of their goals.

Peer-to-Peer Learning

PASOs also values learning and information sharing for professional development among peers. Many of PASOs' programs are innovative projects that reach the Latino population in unique ways, which require creativity and critical thinking. PASOs finds that through team peer-to-peer learning, working relationships are strengthened, trust is built, and program processes are refined to become best practices. Through shadowing, mentoring, peer-led sessions at semi-annual trainings or monthly team meetings, CHWs get to see and practice their responsibilities through action and grow to feel more confident in their skills and abilities. One of our CHWs has shared that she enjoys peer-to-peer learning because no one experience is the same for everyone. She says, "Being able to share how I dealt with a situation, and listening to the input of others facing similar situations, expands my options and provides insight, as well as, helps me think of different paths I may not have considered otherwise" (Y. Benet Uzcategui, personal communication, October 5, 2018).

Coaching

While we recognize that initial training and formal professional development is essential in building individual capacity, PASOs has also realized the importance of creating an environment of continuous support and guidance through ongoing coaching and mentorship. Participating in regular supervision and mentorship is an expectation for all team members. PASOs wants to ensure all team members feel supported in their work, have the tools needed to do their job, and are held accountable to PASOs' standards. Each team member meets with his or her PASOs supervisor or mentor at least once a month, for 1–2 h, with more frequent meetings for new team members. These monthly meetings are unique in that they are not just meetings to provide updates on program progress. While program progress is an essential part of the agenda, other topics are important to discuss for the overall health and well-being of our team and all its members during these meetings. Other items discussed during these meetings besides program progress include:

- Relationships—relevant relationships including progress, needs, and/or conflicts with either partners, team members, or collaborators.
- Data entry—data entry to ensure data is up-to-date and make sure team members correlate the progress on their outcomes and goals with their data entry and reports.
- Guidance and mentorship—including opportunities for personal growth for the CHW related to any aspects of their work and role.
- Supervision—as applicable, this is a discussion about the supervision of other team members and volunteers. PASOs has a Supervisor Competency Manual whose purpose is to serve as an aid for supervisors and mentors at PASOs to continue growing in excellence through supervision. As applicable, PASOs' supervisors/mentors review these competencies and measure growth with team members.
- Skill building and professional development—this portion of the meeting is to discuss skills that are being developed and to record any trainings completed by team members.

In PASOs every aspect of our training and ongoing coaching carries the expectation that success is imminent and the understanding that success will look different for each CHW, as well as each individual with which we work.

10.3.5 Providing Spaces for Communities to Shape Organizational Vision and Priorities

10.3.5.1 Gathering Input; Listening to Voices

Inspired by the teachings of Paulo Freire, the Brazilian educator and philosopher, who said "a change-maker is marked by their ability to trust others, to believe in the capacity of others to think, dream, create, build, to know, and to act," (Freire & Ramos, 1970), PASOs recognizes the necessity of involving and listening to a multitude of individual voices in order to achieve success and build collective capacity.

PASOs' approach to supporting the well-being of individuals and community is focused on the strengths that each individual brings to the table, which is why we say we work *with*, and not *for*, the communities we serve. In the words of CHW Lorena reflecting on how PASOs is a collaborative movement built from the work of many, "we see how we can accomplish more together" (L. Cervantes, personal communication, June 22, 2018).

The ability to build on individual capacity in PASOs' model comes from its focus on recognizing and valuing what others have to offer. By intentionally listening to CHWs and other community members, PASOs incorporates their voices and perspectives in the crafting process of innovative strategies that lead to enhanced collective capacity. Similar to the ways we uplift the voices and experiences of individual CHWs, PASOs employs a variety of methods that have proven successful in providing platforms and venues for individuals and communities we work with to speak freely, candidly, and confidently about our work, programs, direction, and projects.

PASOs conducts community assessments through several means, one of which is through surveys, providing opportunities for individuals to respond to questions anonymously. Surveys may be focused on experiences with accessing a specific resource, on current community needs, or reactions to a new PASOs' program. To conduct surveys, PASOs team members find ways to make them accessible to the population we serve, going to the community, as opposed to waiting for the community to come to us. Limitations to this method involve potentially excluding individuals that are not able to respond. A benefit to this method is the ability to acquire a larger number of voices that can then demonstrate trends where attention needs to be placed regarding services, access, and barriers.

Another method for acquiring community perspectives is focus groups. Small groups of Latino community members or organizational partners are invited to participate in a guided discussion that prompts them to share experiences based on a particular topic or theme. Lasting between 1 and 2 h, this method has been utilized to get individual narratives that provide a personal and detailed account for how a certain issue has affected their livelihood. PASOs uses a trained facilitator that speaks the language of participants fluently and has a deep cultural understanding of group participants. We also provide monetary incentives for participants' time and partner with other organizations to facilitate logistics and collaboration. The information gained can then be taken to agencies and organizations with power to change policies or procedures or can be used to adjust or change an internal program. In this way, community voices directly inform the systemic changes that would most benefit them. Benefits to this method include highly detailed and personal accounts, yet this method also requires more time and can only include a small number of perspectives.

10.3.5.2 Using Input and Perspectives to Drive Systemic Change

PASOs seeks to elevate the voices and perspectives of the Latino communities in South Carolina in order not only to improve the health of individual participants but also to make changes in systems and policies so that these systems can better meet the needs of the community. The PASOs model is based on the recognition that for change to be sustained, you must support an individual while simultaneously promoting and facilitating systemic change to organizations and systems. PASOs' CHWs engage in system change through work we call "organizational capacity building" and through advocacy, which is focused on bringing the Latino community perspective to the table, so it is heard alongside other perspectives and considered when decisions are being made and resources are being allocated.

PASOs helps build the capacity of other organizations to effectively serve Latino families and communities, which also improves the organizations' ability to address population health needs of other disadvantaged groups, through policy and procedure changes that help improve service delivery. The PASOs Organizational Capacity Building program works with organizations across the state of South Carolina, and recently outside of the state, to provide training and technical assistance, so that the communities served are better able to access what they need. As noted in the Journal of Community Practice (Matthew et al., 2017):

> The organization not only trains Promotores using nationally recommended core competencies—to include empowerment and advocacy skills—and provides ongoing training and professional development but also fosters embedded opportunities for Promotores to engage as community—(e.g., involvement with Comite Popular) and system-level advocates by working collaboratively with over 175 local, regional, and statewide partners to ensure their voice (and that of the community) is represented in decision making to enhance culturally attuned service access and quality for Latinos throughout South Carolina. (p. 15)

Just in the past year, PASOs has worked with 50 organizations to provide cultural competence training to 1004 professionals. These trainings include social, historical, and economic factors related to immigration, cultural norms and differences, and the firsthand lived experiences of Latino communities in SC and the United States. Focusing on the diversity and strengths of these vibrant communities, cultural competency trainings help organizations better understand the Latino individuals they serve and give a stronger sense of humanity for Latino communities, in the midst of turbulent political debates over immigration and immigrants. A Nurse Manager at a pediatric clinic where a PASOs' CHW works stated that "having a Latino CHW has really bridged the gap that we had, and increased the trust we have with our Latino patient population" (A. Baez, 2017).

Governmental and nongovernmental organizations have collaborated with PASOs to increase their capacity to reach and better serve Latino families. The Home Visiting Manager at a statewide child advocacy organization said that PASOs' organizational support has allowed for their partners to be more "understanding and more cognizant of how we are working with these families … working with our partners through organizational assessments to figure out where they are and where they need to be" (Baez, 2017). PASOs facilitates in-depth organizational assessments in order to identify areas where improvements can be made within an agency or organization.

Concrete changes from these partnerships that benefit Latino families have included hiring more bilingual and bicultural staff, developing targeted outreach initiatives for Latino communities, and the inclusion and elevation of community voices, concerns, challenges, and strengths so that decision-makers within organizations are able to include their perspectives when planning programs or making policy decisions. For example, one statewide agency contracted with PASOs to conduct language testing of their bilingual employees,[5] which resulted in salary raises for staff. PASOs effectively raised the value of bilingual staff by providing support and structure for how this skill level can be applied to benefit Latino families. There is currently a team of bilingual employees within this agency that now receive extra trainings and are coordinated for outreach event, all of which were recommendations provided by PASOs.

The PASOs team of staff and volunteers regularly receives requests to be members of advisory councils, boards of directors, and other influential bodies. Team members participate in local, regional, and statewide coalitions and decision-making bodies, bringing forward their community perspective and the voices of the thousands of families served by the organization. A health-focused organizational partner commented that "[Prior to partnering with PASOs] the bills we sent were not in Spanish; now they are. Also, city transportation information was not in Spanish, so the city is now working on that" (Matthew et al., 2017).

PASOs' also believes in and encourages staff involvement in strengthening the Community Health Worker profession. In 2015, PASOs helped form the South Carolina Community Health Workers Association in order to gain more visibility and strengthen the role and value provided by Community Health Workers.

10.3.6 Building Capacity Through Advocacy

PASOs' CHWs and allies develop a yearly advocacy plan, the purpose of which is to affect policies that benefit the population we serve, and build the capacity of CHWs and community members to elevate their own voices and ideas. Advocacy goals center on health, issues affecting social determinants of health, early childhood education, and community leadership development. The PASOs team has achieved multiple advocacy successes, including making sure Latino families are represented in the state's health action plans, garnering increased funding allocations for Latino population needs, and changing policy that inhibits access to care due to documentation status.

One example of our advocacy plan in practice is when in 2017, PASOs initiated *Voces Comunitarias* (Community Voices), South Carolina's first all-Spanish Latino community leadership summit, which facilitated peer-to-peer learning, awareness, and action planning. The planning committee for the event is made up of several Latino and allied organizations that understand the needs and benefits for self-representation and building capacity within the Latino communities of South

---

[5] As of this publication, 15 employees have been tested and certified.

Carolina. The success of and positive feedback from *Voces Comunitarias* has inspired the organizational partners to make it an annual event. Each year there have been almost 100 attendees, and a common expression is how much everyone appreciates connecting with and learning about other active individuals working with the Latino community throughout the state and in the region. Even though this summit is for a much larger audience than PASOs' CHWs, because of our *compromiso* to community and our commitment to community integration, we make grassroots leadership development a priority in our work.

In 2016, as immigrants faced increased uncertainty and fear related to national politics, PASOs collaborated with partner organizations to establish a coalition called "South Carolina United with Immigrants" which collectively provides resources, education, and support to immigrant communities throughout the state. In this way PASOs facilitates and builds community capacity by elevating and connecting.

10.3.7 PASOs' Impact

10.3.7.1 Individual Impact

One of the ways we are able to measure the impact of our work is through the successful individual connection to services and achievement of personal goals, which may include getting a needed health service, establishing primary care, addressing a developmental concern with their child, and choosing and learning to use a family planning method, among many others, which we track via a cloud-based data collection system. Participants across the state who received interventions from our team of CHWs have high rates of connection (80–95%), meaning they completed their goal. With PASOs, participants experience a meaningful connection to their health and feel empowered to improve their health. Lorena tells the story of one participant who had been referred several times to the Women, Infants, and Children (WIC) program through the pediatrician:

> She had stopped going to the WIC office and to the pediatrician because they kept telling her that her children were suffering from obesity and she didn't know what to do about it. She knew about these services but didn't really know how to access them. When I took the time to really sit down with her and help her see that her children were getting tired easily and not able to run around with their friends, she got inspired to do something about it. We talked for a long time, and she called me several times after that to tell me about an article she read or something she saw about health. Before PASOs, she wasn't taking them to the pediatrician and now I see her in the clinic. She has lost weight too and I also see her husband sometimes. She says he now spends more time with the children after he gets home from work. I see how that whole family was influenced by the mom who decided to make changes. I see this a lot with our families, because we are not just helping them with one aspect of health but rather helping families to see how they can be stronger and more unified, and this helps them to be happier and have more confidence too. (L. Cervantes, personal communication, June 22, 2018)

In 2017, through our community-based programs, PASOs connected 4542 Latino individuals, most of them recent immigrants, to needed resources and services;

reached 867 participants with educational information on health, social determinants of health, and child development in their language; and provided information in their language to 3768 people at community-based outreach events.

10.3.7.2   Systems Change Impact

The capacity of communities improves greatly when they feel confident to access services, but it is also important that community members have continual support to communicate concerns and contribute to health policy when it has a direct impact on their neighborhoods and families. PASOs works to empower Latino community members in South Carolina to participate in leadership roles on policy workgroups and in panels to train future clinical professionals. The impact of this work affects communities by giving them a seat at the table but also has a tremendous impact on the partner organizations who can better connect with community members:

> For me, it was an exciting opportunity to participate in the Family Engagement workgroup and get to know other professionals in my area. I was so surprised because everyone wanted to hear what I had to say, they wanted to know how to better serve the Latino community and that made me feel like they really do care. And I had the chance to tell them about all the obstacles that Latino people face when they are trying to get healthy. (L. Cervantes, personal communication, June 22, 2018)

In our work to address systemic barriers over the past year, PASOs worked with 216 partners statewide to bring forward the voices of the Latino community to inform the decisions being made that affect the health of their families and helped 23 organizations make documented policy or procedure changes to improve access for Latino families. One major achievement involved a state agency working with PASOs to conduct a community survey to better understand the Latino community's needs, then making changes to address needs at various levels throughout the agency. In addition, a hospital system changed its financial aid policy to improve access to care for thousands of immigrants that had previously been denied services, based on feedback and advocacy of our CHW team. Lastly, our Capacity Building team provided training and technical assistance to 1029 health, social service, and education providers to help them effectively meet the unique needs of South Carolina's Latino population while advocating for effective, culturally appropriate policies and services.

10.3.8   Challenges/Barriers

As in all things, PASOs has seen its share of challenges and barriers in the work. A few challenges related to building individual and community capacity are finding the right people for the job; inability to respond to all the needs identified by CHWs and other community members; lack of understanding or support from organizations and funders; and stigmatizing political environments and policies.

Finding the right people for CHW positions is crucial, and not all people have the lived experience, connections with, and interpersonal skills to build trusting relationships with community members. Finding individuals able to meet all of the demands of the job is also challenging. The job of a CHW requires flexibility to meet the needs of community members who might need to schedule a home visit on a Saturday morning instead of during a typical daytime shift. CHWs also need to be flexible in the work they do and be able to manage a wide range of needs for a single participant and their family. Successful CHWs are open to self-examination and continuously seek out professional development opportunities. Having a shared experience is essential to the ability to establish trust, but CHWs must also be able to understand how to work with diverse cultures without assuming that their background will help them to be culturally competent in every situation. This is also true of the distinct cultures and political climates that can be found in the Federally Qualified Health Centers and free clinics, which require an ability to adapt to the environment in which they find themselves on any given day. Bilingualism is often put to the test as CHWs navigate relationships with community members and the clinics and health systems partners where they work. Additionally, CHWs are members of teams working on projects with complicated evaluations databases, and this requires great attention to detail as well as a familiarity with computer and software systems.

In order to build community capacity, as we mentioned above, you must ask CHWs and communities what they want and need. However, sometimes we find that the needs are so great and that due to capacity and resources, we cannot meet all the needs identified, which can lead to frustration for the team and for the communities we serve. This inability to respond to all needs identified and, in the speed and capacity families would like, can create doubt among communities about why we are not able to help them.

Some health systems, social support organizations, state institutions, and funders do not recognize the potential of CHWs or fully understand the model. Oftentimes these systems doubt the potential of CHWs to affect change and drive outcomes, which can lead to insufficient resource allocation, slow policy change, and stagnated goal achievement. Sometimes state agencies or funding organizations prefer to drive programming because they do not trust in their ability to do so themselves.

Lastly, periods of stigmatizing political discourse and action affect our ability to support and reach the population we serve. A stigmatized or negative national landscape or policy implications can create fears among our participants making it difficult for us to reach them and for them to trust in service providers in general. This also affects team morale, and concerns for our own families and loved ones make daily work more challenging. Building individual and community capacity is more difficult when the population served is experiencing enhanced trauma and has valid concerns related to everyday activities and needs. However, when there are periods of heightened stigma, we must continue to build and support the community's capacity to respond to the stigma—to feel comfortable bringing forward their voices, ideas, and concerns. By consistently showing up to be part of the conversation, and by building power of combining each person's individual voice with the voices of others in their communities, individuals being oppressed by stigma and national discourse can effectively begin to turn the tide and change the conversation.

10.3.9   Successes and Lessons Learned

PASOs' exponential growth since its inception in 2005 is one testament to our success. What started as a small program serving two counties is now a statewide community-based organization reaching over 8000 individuals a year, bringing voices forward to create systems change, and investing in grassroots leadership development. Every time a pregnant mother who faced challenges getting insurance is able to receive coverage due to our advocacy, or a police department sits down with one of our CHWs to listen to the concerns we bring, PASOs is creating change and helping make the Latino community more visible, more understood, stronger, and healthier.

Another success is having built a reputation that is consistently synonymous with excellence, and being a trusted organization that other organizations want to partner with and invest in is a success that cannot be quantified. Each year PASOs' programmatic numbers increase, local sites gain the ability to hire more staff, partnerships get stronger, and the recognition of the work becomes more known.

As we have built this organization together, we have learned many valuable lessons related to capacity building—what works, what doesn't, how to overcome challenges, and when to go back to the drawing board. One important lesson learned is the importance of spending vital time and resources building each other up, connecting to one another, and supporting each other's successes and failures. Focusing on relationships, on individual strengths, as well as on the assets and needs of the team should not just through occasional "team building activities" but as an essential component of the organizational model. Organizational leaders must dedicate time to listening, encouraging, and sharing power, so that each team member feels valued and committed to the vision.

Another lesson learned is the importance of both community work with individuals and families, as well as the promotion of sustainable, systemic change, and how both components feed and nourish the other. By working with individuals and families, we increase our capacity to inform policy and to advocate. By being connected to policymakers and health system leaders, we can better inform and support community members. As a bridge between the two, we can make sure organizations and institutions are listening to communities, and communities have more power to influence the decisions being made related to the health and well-being of their families.

Lizbet Herranz, PASOs' Community Health Worker/Promotora, reflecting on our multi-year partnership with a statewide public health program, says:

> The change in [the statewide program] is immensely felt. The staff ask us for suggestions to improve their services, and we get to be voices for Latino families across the state. As a result, there's now an online site in Spanish for nutrition classes, more openness on the part of the community to connect to the resources for their children's health, and families are beginning to make nutrition choices that make sense in their cultural norms, and that will help improve their family's overall health. The families are better off and the statewide program has improved its services! (L. Herranz, personal communication, October 12, 2018)

Dr. Richard Foster, former Executive Director of the Alliance for a Healthier South Carolina, a multi-stakeholder coalition of state agency leaders, funders, health systems directors, and community organizations, views PASOs' team of

CHWs as bridge builders: "This organization serves as a shining example of the value of the community health worker model in building trust and social support with individuals and communities most vulnerable to social inequities and health disparities. As a key member of the Alliance, PASOs is helping to shape our collective commitment to improving health for all in our state through an equity lens" (R. Foster, personal communication, October 16, 2018).

References

Baez, A. (2017, June 20). *PASOs' capacity building services* [video file]. Retrieved from https://www.youtube.com/watch?v=fIpaJazEQ1Y

Center for American Progress. (2018). *Talk poverty: Poverty by state, South Carolina, 2016*. Retrieved July 15, 2018, from https://talkpoverty.org/state-year-report/south-carolina-2018-report/, https://www.youtube.com/watch?v=fIpaJazEQ1Yrg/state-year-report/south-carolina-2016-report/

Freire, P., & Ramos, M. B. (1970). *Pedagogy of the oppressed*. New York, NY: Continuum.

Kids Count Data Center. (2017a). *Child population by race and age group*. Retrieved July 16, 2018, from https://datacenter.kidscount.org/data/tables/8446-child-population-by-race-and-age-group?loc=42&loct=2#detailed/2/42/false/870,573,869,36,868,867,133/68,69,67,12,70,66,71,13%7C/17077,17078

Kids Count Data Center. (2017b). *Children in poverty by race and ethnicity*. Retrieved July 16, 2018, from https://datacenter.kidscount.org/data/tables/44-children-in-poverty-by-race-and-ethnicity?loc=42&loct=2#detailed/2/42/false/870,573,869,36,868,867,133,38,35,18/10,11,9,12,1,185,13/324,323

Kids Count Data Center. (2018). *Children in extreme poverty (50 percent poverty) by race and ethnicity*. Retrieved July 16, 2018, from https://datacenter.kidscount.org/data/tables/8783-children-in-extreme-poverty-50-percent-poverty-by-race-and-ethnicity?loc=42&loct=2#detailed/2/42/false/870,573,869,36,133,35,16/4038,4040,4039,2638,2597,4758,1353/17619,17620

Matthew, R., Willms, L., Voravudhi, A., Smithwick, J., Jennings, P., & Machado-Escudero, Y. (2017). Advocates for community health and social justice: A case example of a multisystemic promotores organization in South Carolina. *Journal of Community Practice, 25*(3–4), 344–364. https://doi.org/10.1080/10705422.2017.1359720

Pew Research Center. (2014). *Demographic and economic profiles of Hispanics by state and county*. Retrieved July 16, 2018, from http://www.pewhispanic.org/states/state/sc/

Smithwick-Leone, J. (2004). *Looking at the present and towards the future: The perinatal outlook for Latina women and children in the midlands region of South Carolina*. Columbia, SC: University of South Carolina Press. Retrieved from http://www.asph.sc.edu/cli/documents/PerinatalCare.pdf

Squires, E., Artiga, S., & Foutz, J. (2018). *Health and health care for Hispanics in the United States*. Retrieved from http://kk.org/infographic/health-and-health-care-for-hispanics-in-the-united-states

Stepler, R., Lopez, M. H., & Rohal, M. (2016). *U.S. Latino population growth and dispersion has slowed since onset of the great recession* (Vol. 8). Retrieved from http://www.pewhispanic.org/files/2016/09/PH_2016.09.08_Geography.pdf

U.S. Census Bureau. (2017). *U.S. Census Bureau QuickFacts: South Carolina*. Retrieved July 2, 2018, from https://www.census.gov/quickfacts/fact/table/sc/PST045217#qf-headnote-b

Chapter 11
Providing Direct Services

Caitlin G. Allen*, Mae-Gilene Begay, Tom Bornstein, J. Nell Brownstein, Ramona Dillard*, Durrell J. Fox, Dana Hughes, Dane Lenaker, Elizabeth Mallott, Susan L. Mayfield-Johnson, Kimberly Moler, Nadereh Pourat, E. Lee Rosenthal, and Joanne Spetz*

11.1 Introduction

Caitlin G. Allen, J. Nell Brownstein, Durrell J. Fox, and Susan L. Mayfield-Johnson

The role of providing direct services focuses on health-related services that are delivered in person or face-to-face and involves three sub-roles: providing basic screening tests; providing basic services; and meeting basic needs. This role and corresponding sub-roles have shifted from the originally identified roles and sub-roles from the National Community Health Advisor Study in 1998. Originally, this role specified that community health workers (CHWs) provide clinical services and meet basic needs. The recent version removed language regarding clinical services and shifted the "meeting basic needs" to part of the sub-roles. Removal of "clinical services" from this role was due, in part, to the need to clarify boundary-spanning

---

Authorship is organized alphabetically in ascending order by surname.

C. G. Allen (✉)
CGA Consulting, Charleston, SC, USA
e-mail: caitlin.gloeckner.allen@emory.edu

M. G. Begay
Navajo Nation Community Health Representative (CHR)/Outreach Program, Window Rock, AZ, USA

T. Bornstein · D. Lenaker · E. Mallott
SEARHC Dental, Juneau, AK, USA

J. N. Brownstein · E. L. Rosenthal
Texas Tech Health Sciences Center El Paso, El Paso, TX, USA

R. Dillard (✉)
Pueblo of Laguna Community Health, Albuquerque, NM, USA
e-mail: rdillard@pol-nsn.gov

© Springer Nature Switzerland AG 2021
J. A. St. John et al. (eds.), *Promoting the Health of the Community*,
https://doi.org/10.1007/978-3-030-56375-2_11

issues. That is, CHWs are generally not licensed individuals and do not have the proper credentials to perform clinical services. Primarily, CHWs provide social services and education but can attain additional knowledge and skills to support clients in ways that are more direct.

The sub-roles identified provide examples of specific ways that CHWs may provide direct services, which may be especially relevant in rural areas where clinical services are limited. For example, providing training to a CHW who conducts home visits in providing basic screening tests such as height and weight, checking blood pressure, or performing diabetic foot checks may be a viable option to address the needs of rural and underserved areas. This could ease some of the barriers clients face in accessing services and encourage opportunities for health education. In addition, the role includes providing direct services using service networks and resources. This is a newly added sub-role, which reflects the important link CHWs play for vulnerable populations. Being able to provide access to food and other resources may be especially important for CHWs who work with clients that are experiencing homelessness.

The two stories included in this chapter describe ways CHWs, Community Health Representatives (CHRs), and Community Health Aides (CHAs), and specifically Primary Dental Health Aides (PDHAs), are engaged in providing direct services.

D. J. Fox
JSI Research and Training, Inc, Atlanta, GA, USA

D. Hughes · J. Spetz (✉)
Philip R. Lee Institute for Health Policy Studies, University of California, San Francisco, San Francisco, CA, USA
e-mail: joanne.spetz@ucsf.edu

S. L. Mayfield-Johnson
Department of Public Health, School of Health Professions, The University of Southern Mississippi, Hattiesburg, MS, USA

K. Moler
SEARHC Dental, Kake, AK, USA

N. Pourat
Fielding School of Public Health, UCLA Center for Health Policy Research, Los Angeles, CA, USA

11.2 Alaska's Primary Dental Health Aides: Adapting a Community Health Worker Program to Preventive Dental Care

Joanne Spetz, Nadereh Pourat, Kimberly Moler, Elizabeth Mallott, Tom Bornstein, Dane Lenaker, and Dana Hughes

11.2.1 Introduction

American Indians and Alaskan Natives experience more serious oral health problems than any population in the United States while also facing severe problems of access to dental care (Center for Native American Youth, 2014). The lack of access to oral health care is of particular concern in Alaska, where approximately 15% of the population is Alaska Native and more than 83% of Alaska Native third graders are reported to have caries experience (Whistler, 2012). In 1999 the Southeast Alaska Regional Health Consortium (SEARHC) documented the extent and severity of oral disease and described the difficulties Alaskan Natives faced in obtaining care, especially among the 70% of Alaskan Natives who live in the state's 200 remote villages that are reachable only by boat, snowmobile, or bush plane (Southeast Alaska Regional Health Consortium, 1999). Many villagers receive only sporadic care provided by traveling dentists and hygienists since they do not have consistent on-site dental services. The US Health Resources and Services Administration (HRSA) estimates that about 144,115 Alaskans live in dental shortage areas, and the shortage of dentists is expected to worsen due to impending retirements (Section of Health Planning and Systems Development, 2016).

To address these severe oral health access problems, Alaskan Native communities and Tribal Health dentists have developed and refined an innovative workforce program over the past 15 years. In 2001, in response to the SEARHC report, the Alaska Dental Health Aide Program (DHA program) was launched as a specialty area under the Community Health Aide Program (CHAP), which has provided medical services in Alaska's remote communities since the 1960s. There are approximately 550 Community Health Aides/Practitioners (CHA/Ps) who are selected by and work in over 170 rural Alaska villages as frontline healthcare providers who provide culturally appropriate care including assessing patients, providing treatment according to standardized procedures, and developing and executing health education programs (Alaska Native Tribal Health Consortium, n.d.).

The DHA program is operated by Alaska tribal health programs and was initially authorized by federal law only for operation in Alaska. There are four categories of professionals in the program: (1) *Dental Health Aide Therapists (DHATs)*, who provide oral exams, preventive dental services, simple restorations, stainless steel crowns, and extractions and take X-rays; (2) *Expanded Function Dental Health*

Aides (EFDHA) I and II, who serve as expanded-duty dental assistants in regional dental clinics, depending on training; (3) *Dental Health Aide Hygienists*, who serve as expanded-duty dental hygienists in regional dental clinics and villages; and (4) *Primary Dental Health Aides (PDHAs) I and II*, who provide dental education and preventive dentistry services, including the application of topical fluoride. PDHAs focus on prevention of dental disease, providing oral health education, screening, fluoride varnish application, anti-microbial (anti-bacterial) application, and, in some cases, taking dental X-rays, applying sealants, and performing simple dental prophylaxis and atraumatic restorative technique (ART). Most were born and raised in the communities they serve. This section describes the training, work, and impact of PDHAs on the prevention of oral disease through the role of providing direct services and assesses the prospects for adopting this model outside of Alaska in areas with similarly severe access problems.

11.2.2 Program Context

Established in 1975, SEARHC is a nonprofit tribal health consortium of 18 Native communities, mandated to serve the health interests of the Tlingit, Haida, Tsimshian, and other Native people within the 30,000 square miles of Southeast Alaska. SEARHC was created under the provisions of the Indian Self-Determination Act, which was designed to turn Indian Health Service programs and facilities over to tribal management. In 1976, SEARHC assumed management responsibility for implementing the Community Health Aide Program (CHAP) in their region. Over the years, SEARHC has taken over management of various IHS facilities and programs in Southeast Alaska. Services include inpatient care, primary care, specialty clinics, behavioral health, health promotion, and a variety of other clinics, along with dental services. Clinical oral health services are provided in 45 operatories throughout the region, as well as hospital-based services for surgery and services requiring anesthesia.

The SEARHC Dental Program has two pillars: risk assessment for determining caries risk and making dental treatment and restoration recommendations and prevention through health education and fluoride application. SEARHC providers actively use Caries Management by Risk Assessment (CAMBRA) protocols, categorize patients by their risk levels, and prioritize preventive and restorative care accordingly. Both approaches are employed in seven full clinic sites, ten direct care villages, and two "contract care" villages. In fiscal year 2014, SEARHC provided 29,685 dental visits.

As described above, the DHA program dates from the early 2000s. Recruitment for all types of DHA positions is conducted by the individual Alaskan tribes; the jobs are generally held by tribal members who live, work, and serve in their community. This both maximizes the chances that they will remain in the community and ensures that care is delivered by individuals who share the customs and traditions of the patient population.

11.2.3 Education of Primary Dental Health Aides

SEARHC PDHAs receive training at the Sitka and Juneau clinics with a curriculum developed by the Alaskan Native Tribal Health Consortium (ANTHC). This curriculum drew from the education program designed for Community Health Aides/Practitioners (CHA/P), which is overseen by the federally recognized Community Health Aide Program Certification Board (CHAP CB). ANTHC provides support for the CHAP and CHAP CB, and SEARHC is one of many tribal health organizations that implements the CHAP and utilizes CHA/Ps. PDHA training is in accordance with CHAP CB Standards and Procedures.

PHDA I training includes a Core Module, consisting of an introduction to health/disease processes, anatomy and dental anatomy, medical history taking, interviewing skills, medical ethics, and other topics (see Table 11.1). Additional training at the PDHA I level includes topics such as primary oral health promotion and disease prevention and basic dental procedures. PDHAs also have a preceptorship covering the delivery of fluoride treatments, delivery of oral health information, diet education, and 40 h of work experience before certification. PDHA II training includes an additional 14 to 32 h on more advanced diagnostic techniques, such as using intraoral cameras. PDHA IIs also must complete specialized training in at least one area of certification: sealants, dental prophylaxis, radiology, or ART. After completing their training program and preceptorship, PDHAs apply to the CHAP CB for a federally authorized certificate that permits PDHAs to provide services in the areas in which they have demonstrated competency. They must be employees of the IHS, a tribe, or a tribal health organization and work under the general supervision of a licensed dentist. The certificate allows the PDHA to work under standing orders of a supervising dentist, and the orders can be tailored to align with the skills of the PDHA. Certification is for 2 years, and PDHAs must meet recertification requirements established by the CHAP CB every 2 years.

DHATs, who specialize in diagnosis and restorative treatment, are educated in a 2-year program. The first year involves didactic classroom education in Anchorage, and the second year is clinical training in Bethel, Alaska. Upon completion of their clinical training in Bethel, the students return to their sponsoring Tribal Health Organization and complete a minimum of 400 h of preceptorship under direct supervision. Upon successful completion of the preceptorship, the DHATs can receive a federal certification allowing them to work under the general supervision of their collaborative dentist. As is the case with PDHAs, the DHATs are required to be recertified every 2 years. Some PDHAs have pursued DHAT education after having worked as a PDHA for several years. Pursuing the DHAT credential requires exceptional dedication due to the length of time that learners are away from their villages and families. After returning to their villages, DHATs usually provide the preventive services of a PDHA as well as diagnostic and treatment services.

Table 11.1 PDHA training

PDHA core training	PDHA level 1	PDHA level II
Role of DHA in village and general scope of work	*PDHA core training*	*PDHA core training*
Medical ethics and legal issues	Introduction to caries and periodontal processes	*PDHA level 1 training*
State of Alaska reporting requirements and consent for treatment	Theory of oral health promotion and disease prevention	More comprehensive dental anatomy, caries and periodontal disease process, dental charting, handling/sterilization of dental instruments
Interviewing skills	Fluoride as a drug and related issues including toxicity	Disinfection of operatory
Health/disease process, infection and communicable disease	Topical fluoride treatments, including gel, foam, varnish, and rinse	Patient record documentation
Introductory anatomy, dental anatomy, and medical history taking	Patient education: diet counseling, oral hygiene instructions, prevention strategies including sealants, fluoride, and caries risk protocol	Use of telemedicine technology, including intra- and extraoral cameras
Vocabulary, abbreviations, and documentation (including HEAP and SOAP documentation)	Toothbrush prophylaxis	Problem-specific medical and dental history taking
Introduction to pharmacology and clinical management	Introduction to dental anatomy	Recognition of medical and dental conditions and the relations between medical conditions and oral health
Healthcare system access, including Medicaid and third-party insurance	Introductory identification of dental problems, including oral cancer and referral	Must obtain one of the following skill sets[a] through completion of training module and preceptorship: sealants, dental prophylaxis, radiology, dental assisting, ART
Scheduling	General medical history taking	

Sources: Community Health Aide Program Certification Board, Standards and Procedures, Amended January 25, 2018
[a]SEARHC requires 2 skill sets

11.2.3.1 Role of PDHAs in Prevention

SEARHC provides dental services with a multidisciplinary team approach, though village services are anchored by PDHAs and/or DHATs, with periodic, usually scheduled, visits by dentists and hygienists to provide more extensive cleanings and restorations. Altogether, SEARHC employs 12 dentists and 2 pediatric dentists (all of whom are residency-trained), 1 prosthodontist, 3 dental residents, 4 DHATs, 6 hygienists, 2 Certified Dental Assistants, 24 dental assistants (DA), and 7 PDHA IIs (providing 6.5 PDHA full-time equivalents).

PDHAs supplement the SEARHC Dental Program and are particularly critical in remote villages where they are the only consistently present oral health provider. PDHAs also practice in more urban areas as well; two PDHA IIs are employed at each of the Juneau and Sitka clinics. But, more commonly, they live and work in small villages, such as Kake and Angoon. In these two communities, the PDHAs are the sole dental provider continuously on-site; in the other villages, they work along-side a dental team.

I work with all ages – kids 0 to 3 through the Parents As Teachers Program, preschoolers through Head Start, K-12 students and staff at Kake Schools, and older adults through the Elders Program. I help to educate the students about the importance of good oral hygiene. I talk with the patient about eating healthy food, and educate them about the high amounts of sugar in different foods and drinks. PDHAs try to educate as much as we can and also talk about the other health risks you can develop if you do not make lifestyle changes to improve your health.

The biggest challenge is when I have a patient come in with a dental emergency and I am unable to help because it is out of my scope of practice. This is when I will take an X-ray and contact a provider to read it, and set up a treatment plan for the patient. If they should need anything for pain or infection, I am able to contact the on-site nurse practitioner to fill the prescription. I also schedule the patient for an exam and follow up with the dental team.

—Kimberly Moler, PDHA II, Kake, Alaska

The scope of work for SEARHC PDHAs is variable, depending on level of training (PDHA I vs. PDHA II) and the site of service. Because urban clinics typically have a broad range of staff working on-site, including dentists and dental hygienists, the PDHA's role tends to be focused on caries prevention, provision of education and oral health coaching, application of fluoride varnish and silver diamine fluoride, application of sealants, prophylaxis (above the gum line only), and dental assisting. In villages, the utilization within the clinic setting is broader, especially when PDHAs are the sole provider, because they are responsible for all aspects of the dental clinic. In the villages, their work often includes the same services as in larger clinics, as well as scheduling and receptionist duties and inventory and management of dental equipment. Village-based PDHAs are the vital link between the hub dental clinics and their community by knowing their community's dental needs and advocating for higher-level dental services that a visiting dental team can provide. They inform residents of visiting dental trips and provide follow-up care when the team leaves.

In remote communities, PDHAs' long-standing relationships are invaluable to promoting oral health. They know the families in the community, and having intimate knowledge such as who has recently given birth and how to best find family members is a key component of their success in supporting oral health education and services for their fellow village residents. They know how to best communicate with individuals and groups within the community and provide an important bridge between the traveling dental team and residents. Another contributor to the success of village-based PDHAs is that they provide community members with the opportunity for positive dental experiences. The PDHA provides education, applies fluoride, and performs noninvasive procedures, developing a culture that some dental visits are for maintenance and prevention. Prior to SEARHC establishing their current model of care, as well as utilization of the DHAs (DHATs and PDHAs), dental teams did not visit villages frequently enough to meet the needs of the community; thus, residents would only see the dentist when there was something significantly wrong due to the financial and logistical challenges of seeking dental care.

In both urban and rural areas, PDHAs plan and execute outreach programs, such as fluoride application and oral health education in Head Start programs, schools, and nursing homes. PDHAs are expected to take leadership in community outreach, in both the larger clinics and small villages. All of the PDHAs we interviewed visited schools two or three times per year, providing oral health education and applying fluoride varnish. In one village, the PDHA also provides education to teachers and encouraged teachers to offer students 5 min after lunch to brush their teeth. PDHAs provide students with toothbrushes, which in remote village settings are expensive to purchase due to high transportation costs for grocery items. An elementary school principal in a small village reported, "The teachers have them brush their teeth after lunch. The teachers weren't doing this until [the DHA] started bringing in the toothbrushes. Now the teachers and the kids brush every day." PDHAs in the larger clinics reported a broader range of outreach activities, including managing dedicated programs within nursing homes and visiting a boarding high school for Alaska Native students for dental evaluation and education.

11.2.4 Impact of PDHAs on Their Communities

PDHAs are the "the prevention specialists" for oral health in their communities. They provide oral health and hygiene education at schools, Head Start sites, and nursing homes on subjects such as the importance of tooth brushing, reducing consumption of sugar-sweetened beverages, and prevention of early childhood caries. In these settings PDHAs also apply fluoride varnish to children, screen them to detect potential problems, and help guide patients to treatment with visiting dentists. Residents of villages in which PDHAs work, as well as community leaders, educators, and medical providers, attribute improvements in oral health to increased access to dental services and the work of PDHAs, especially among children. Education from PDHAs about the health effects of sugar and encouragement to reduce its consumption are provided at health fairs and in schools, as well as with patients individually.

> I can honestly say that our dental clinic has had the support of the community and schools, which has made our dental program successful. Over the years I have seen so many positive changes – preventive programs for all ages are making a difference. I am thankful that I am allowed to go into the schools and help educate about oral hygiene and do the fluoride program, provide dental supplies for each student so they can brush and floss after breakfast and lunch at school. Changes like this are making a difference.
>
> —Kimberly Moler, PDHA II, Kake, Alaska

School leaders believe that having a PDHA in their community has resulted in the majority of students now not having pain issues from dental health problems, unlike in the past. School principals and childhood education program leaders point to differences in behavior such as consumption of soda as well as greater engagement by parents in ensuring children get regular checkups. Principals of schools in remote villages have seen in attendance records that kids go to larger clinics in Juneau and Sitka less frequently for serious dental care, which they attribute to the preventive services provided by PDHAs as well as increased frequency of visits by general and pediatric dentists.

> Baby bottle mouth was epidemic prior to the PDHA, but has been turned around. PDHAs teach parents about the importance of baby teeth and how to protect them.
> It's rare now to see little kids lose teeth. Young kids no longer have bombed-out mouths.
> Our PDHA brings toothbrushes for the kids, which are expensive to buy. That means the teachers can have the kids brush their teeth after lunch, which they were not doing before.

> —School Principals in rural Alaskan villages

Dentists and program leaders believe PDHAs are a key component of preventive oral health care and also are essential in triaging emergency cases and scheduling patients for visiting dentist, dental hygienist, and dental therapist teams. They also point to the increased comfort of community members in receiving preventive care due to the "normalization" of having somebody routinely inspect the mouth.

> In the 1980s and 1990s it was unusual to see a caries-free child from a village, and at least one child presented with an eye swollen shut due to a dental infection on nearly every field trip. By 2015, that kind of severe caries was very unusual.
> It used to be that all kids had swollen mouths...bombed-out mouths. Now people want routine care. There has been a shift from a common belief that losing teeth, even among the young, was normal, to a growing acceptance that caries are avoidable, which is largely the result of the PDHAs.

> —Leaders of oral health programs at SEARHC

11.2.4.1 Data Demonstrating Success

The perceptions of PDHAs, community members, and community leaders that PDHAs have had a positive impact on oral health are substantiated by positive oral health trends among SEARHC patients from 2012 through 2015. During this period, the number of patients found to be at High Risk with Caries declined modestly from 2439 to 2138. However, during the same period, the number of patients deemed to be High Risk with No Caries rose from 163 to 621, and the percentage of High Risk with Caries Control Completed rose from 18% to 39%. While these marked improvements cannot be attributed to PDHAs alone, but rather likely reflect the constellation of innovations that SEARHC has employed, PDHAs are a critical component of the overall approach (Sekiguchi, Guay, Brown, & Spanger, 2005).

11.2.5   Financing and Sustainability

Services provided by Primary Dental Health Aides are reimbursable through private insurance and Medicaid. Medicaid and private insurance reimbursement rates generate sufficient funds to support the program, and the program is highly important to SEARHC due to the high incidence of caries in the population and the evidence that expanding preventive health services and offering fluoride varnish to all children improve oral health. PDHAs are skilled at implementing fluoride varnish programs and educational programs, allowing other professionals to focus on restorative services.

A very high proportion of eligible children are enrolled in Medicaid, but their eligibility has to be recertified every 6 months. SEARHC staff, particularly DHATs and PDHAs, work closely with families to complete the recertification process. As one PDHA has said, "I have to work hard to keep my families' [Medicaid coverage] current." Staying current with Medicaid increases families' access to dental care by reducing the financial barrier to it. In addition, if the family has to travel out of the community to receive higher-level dental services, Medicaid will pay to cover the cost.

PDHA IIs can bill additionally for radiographs, dental prophylaxis, sealants, and other minor procedures, depending on their training and certification. While these covered services do not encompass the full range of services provided by PDHAs—such as the programs they develop to educate community members about the causes of caries, the importance of oral health care and reduced sugar consumption, and proper tooth brushing technique—reimbursement rates are sufficient to support this additional and highly complementary work. As long as reimbursement rates do not decline substantially, the PDHA program is sustainable.

11.2.6   Lessons Learned

All evidence points to major health benefits of PDHAs in Southeast Alaska. There are also community development benefits as the availability of PDHA positions produces critical jobs in low-employment, low-resource communities. Moreover, the sequential training structure of the Dental Health Aide Program in Alaska creates ladders for advancement for individuals who are interested in building their skills and training to assume increasing levels of responsibility.

> I am happy when I look back on all the positive changes that our dental clinics have made over the years – and with these changes, we are able to provide better services. We can provide and schedule more clinics here in the community. My main goal as a dental health aide is to continue to bring in more services, so we can continue to see more positive change. The program has been very effective in educating me as a PDHA so I can provide better services.
>
> —Kimberly Moler, PDHA II, Kake, Alaska

The personal attributes of PDHAs—their personality, organization, and motivation—are key to their success as oral healthcare providers. Since usually there is only one PDHA in a community and they primarily work independently, they need to be motivated and well-liked in the community. Their eagerness to serve their community and understanding of oral health disease prevention are reflected in the ongoing efforts of PDHAs to expand their services to all demographic groups, including new mothers, nursing home residents, and other populations often overlooked in oral health programs. A motivated, personable, talented PDHA can make a large difference, and one without those skills will have much less impact.

But could this program work elsewhere? Some suggest that SEARHC may be a special case even in Alaska, because other regions have not had SEARHC's level of success. In the Yukon-Kuskokwim region, for example, budget cuts led to the elimination of PDHAs in their dental program, despite the fact that the region has among the highest rates of dental disease in Alaska. Other Alaska regions have experienced significant turnover of PDHAs, making it difficult for the model to take hold. Some argue that SEARHC's oral health successes may be more about the effects of their overall model—which involves multidisciplinary teams, designating resources to manage the PDHA program, use of CAMBRA, use of pediatric dentists, regular application of fluoride varnish, and support for other innovations like offering Xylitol products—than a single component such as PDHAs.

With leadership to promote and prioritize PDHAs, along with reimbursement mechanisms to finance them, PDHAs can be a successful approach elsewhere in Alaska and other regions with severe oral health workforce shortage. A DHAT in Sitka has said, "People say it works here just because we're in Alaska, but this model could work anywhere there is need, inner-cities, other rural areas." In June 2016, the IHS announced a new draft policy statement that called for a process of expanding the use of Community Health Aides at IHS facilities around the country in order to improve access among Native Americans (Indian Health Service, 2016). With federal IHS leadership encouraging use of Community Health Aides, including Dental Health Aides, opportunities to replicate this model in other dental-underserved communities in Indian Country are likely. At a minimum, the experience of the SEARHC PDHA model, particularly in demonstrating the role of providing direct oral health services, is an excellent guide for others interested in exploring adopting this innovative workforce approach. This also provides an exemplar of the adaptation of the CHW role into a specialized clinical area, demonstrating that the fundamental competencies of CHWs can be leveraged to address a plethora of healthcare needs.

References

Alaska Native Tribal Health Consortium. (n.d.). *Alaska Community Health Aide Program*. Retrieved February 17, 2020, from http://www.akchap.org/html/home-page.html.

Center for Native American Youth. (2014). *Oral health and Native American youth*. Denver, CO: Aspen Institute. Retrieved February 17, 2020, http://www.aspeninstitute.org/sites/default/files/content/docs/cnay/Oral-Health-and-Native-American-Youth.pdf.

Indian Health Service. (2016). *IHS initiates Tribal consultation on draft policy to expand Community Health Aide Program* [Press release]. Retrieved February 17, 2020, http://www.ihs.gov/newsroom/pressreleases/2016pressreleases/ihs-initiates-tribal-consultation-on-draft-policy-to-expand-community-health-aide-program/.

Section of Health Planning and Systems Development. (2016). *Alaska 2015–2016 primary care needs assessment*. Juneau, AK: Alaska Department of Health and Social Services. Retrieved February 17, 2020, from http://dhss.alaska.gov/dph/HealthPlanning/Documents/Primary%20Care%20Needs%20Assessment/AlaskaPrimaryCareNeedsAssessment_2015-2016.pdf.

Sekiguchi, E., Guay, A. H., Brown, L. J., & Spanger, T. J. (2005). Improving the oral health of Alaska Natives. *American Journal of Public Health, 95*(5), 769–773. https://doi.org/10.2105/AJPH.2004.053546.

Southeast Alaska Regional Health Consortium. (1999). *Crisis in access to dental care: A white paper*. Juneau, AK: Southeast Alaska Regional Health Consortium.

Whistler, B. J. (2012). *Alaska oral health plan: 2012–2016*. Juneau, AK: Alaska Department of Health and Social Services. Retrieved February 17, 2020, from http://dhss.alaska.gov/dph/wcfh/Documents/oralhealth/docs/OralHealthPlan2012.pdf.

11.3 Community Health Representatives (CHRs) as Direct Service Providers in Native American Communities: When the Pavement Ends, the Dirt Road to Patient Health Care Begins[1]

Ramona Dillard, Mae-Gilene Begay, E. Lee Rosenthal, and Susan L. Mayfield-Johnson

11.3.1 Introduction

Native American tribal communities' introductions to public health services began under Indian Health Services (IHS, n.d.-a) in 1954. They were united through the Public Health Services (PHS) staff to address chronic disease and communicable outbreaks. IHS was established to take over health care of American Indian and Alaska Natives from the Bureau of Indian Affairs (U.S. Department of the Interior, n.d.) so that the PHS could take the lead in hopes of improving the health care of Native Americans living on reservations. During this evolution of PHS and IHS, many tribal communities continued to live, adapt, and rely on their cultural practices for health, wellness, and healing. Tribes also relied on highly trusted and innately skilled individuals in the community to interpret and bridge an understanding of the Western way of care with health promotion and traditional healing. Tribes fostered public health and direct health services to their people in their own ways through traditional native practices and worked towards bridging understanding of health through knowledgeable, trustworthy, and action-oriented individuals in the community. Many of these individuals later became Community Health Representatives (CHRs).

11.3.2 Community Health Representatives (CHRs): A Historical Overview

The IHS is divided into 12 physical areas of the United States: Alaska, Albuquerque, Bemidji, Billings, California, Great Plains, Nashville, Navajo, Oklahoma, Phoenix, Portland, and Tucson. The map (IHS, n.d.-c) identifies the 12 areas of IHS in which hospitals, clinics, and other facilities are operated by the IHS and tribal governments, even today. There are 573 federally recognized Tribes in 37 states across the country, as illustrated in Fig. 11.1.

---

[1] With contributions by Hondo Lewis, Iris V. Reano, Laurene Sarracino, Jean Pino, Sabrina Baca, and Jicarilla CHR Program.

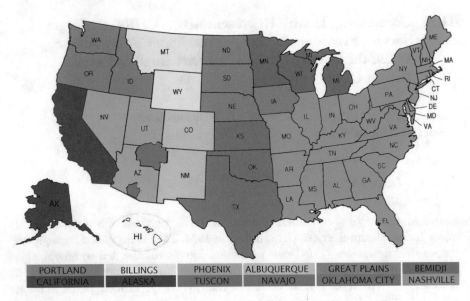

Fig. 11.1 US tribal map

The CHR Program (USDHHS, 2015) was established by Congress in 1968 in response to the voiced needs of American Indian and Alaska Native governments, organizations, and the IHS for a healthcare program that would provide outreach to meet specific Tribal Healthcare needs. It was based on the concept that community members, trained in the basic skills of healthcare provision and disease control and prevention, would be able to achieve the most success in effecting change in community acceptance and utilization of limited healthcare resources. CHRs are frontline public health workers who are trusted members of the community with a close understanding of the community, language, and traditions. They serve as a link between clinical settings and the community to facilitate access to services and improve the quality of cultural service delivery. CHRs meet the needs of Tribal Communities through transportation to clinic appointments, conducting outreach, providing community education, facilitating informal counseling, offering social support, and promoting advocacy (Division of Behavioral Health, Indian Health Services, n.d.). The National IHS CHR Program (n.d.) provides funding, training, and technical assistance to tribal CHR programs to address the healthcare needs through the provision of community-oriented health services.

CHRs, themselves, were key in providing historical knowledge and information on tribal members and services within the community. CHRs facilitate access to the history of the evolution of health care that involved CHRs in the community. Laurene Sarracino, CHR at Laguna, Pueblo, who began with the program in December 1996, recalls the history and role of the CHR program:

> The program has evolved over the years with many changes to keep abreast with the changing times and services needed. The CHR Program provides health/health related services in

areas identified under the SOW of the Indian Health Service, which also aligns with identified community health needs, and priorities for health set by our Pueblo government, as
well as established policies and procedures, the program's Standard Operating Procedures
and national health practice guidelines, state/federal guidelines for staff, and approved best
practices.

From the 1960s to around the early 1980s, the Community Health Representative provided services to the "then" times of what the community was in need of – this included
home visiting of community members in their homes; to check on their health or illness –
both short term and long term; assisting with historical needs from long ago, such as helping a household patch/repair their adobe home; white washing the inside to keep the home
in best repair; helping the elders of the community by way of chopping wood; or fixing a
meal if a member was ailing.

A former, retired CHR recalls a story of assisting the local EMS 'back when' riding in
the ambulance to take a mother in labor to the hospital some 50 miles away. Another former,
retired CHR also remembers dressing up as a tooth fairy to provide dental health education
to elementary aged students so they would be comfortable and lessen some of the fear when
going to the dentist for care. Another CHR recollects being stationed at the local IHS
Optometry department to assist patients, especially if there was a need for speaking Keres
so the patient would be able to understand what would take place at the appointment.
(Fig. 11.2)

The Indian Health Transfer Act included language that recognized tribal sover-
eignty and afforded a degree of tribal self-determination in health policy decision-
making (Warne & Frizzell, 2014). The importance of tribal decision-making in tribal
affairs and the primacy of the nation-to-nation relationship between the United States

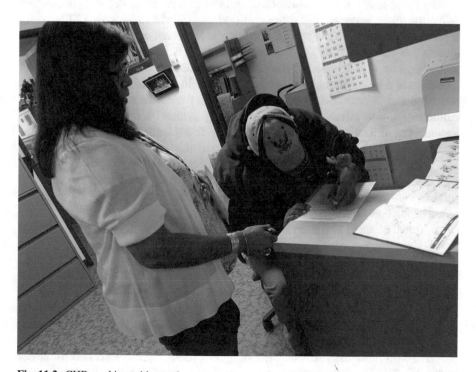

Fig. 11.2 CHR working with a patient

and Tribes led to the passage of the Indian Self-Determination and Education Assistance Act (ISDEAA), Public Law 93-638 in 1975 (IHS, n.d.-b). Under the ISDEAA, Tribes and Tribal Organizations have the option to "(1) administer programs and services the IHS would otherwise provide (referred to as Title I Self-Determination Contracting) or (2) assume control over health care programs and services that the IHS would otherwise provide (referred to as Title V Self-Governance Compacting or the TSGP)" (IHS, n.d.-d, para 4) through avenues called 638 contracts. While there are two options, they are not exclusive and can be combined based on Tribal needs and circumstances. Both options are grounded by local tribal leadership to set priorities and develop assets and meet the identified needs within the Tribal Organization by the Tribe. Please note that each Tribal nation is different, and this section presents Tribes and Pueblos within the greater IHS Albuquerque Area that have selected Title I under the P.L. 93-638 contract.

Within IHS areas, there are 638 funded and tribally funded CHR programs that implement the scope of work of the P.L. 93-638 Title I contract (Sabo, O'Meara, & Camplain, 2019). CHR programs under IHS implement a scope of work (SOW) that is in line with the core functions identified in the regulation, but scopes vary based on the needs, assets, and resources of the community and approval by the Tribal government. While CHR program's SOW vary based on community needs, core services for most CHR programs are set and include translation for non-native providers and clients, transportation, referrals, home visiting, health education, and care coordination.

The IHS-funded, tribally contracted, and directed program began to implement SOW for direct services. Individuals who were selected to become CHRs under contracts to work as CHRs received training in the areas of health promotion and disease prevention (HP/DP), to work as community-based health paraprofessionals providing care and services in their tribal communities (USDHHS, 2015). Most CHRs were native community members, trained in the basic skills of healthcare provision and disease control and prevention. They used their innate knowledge of cultural norms to effectively aid in translating medical terms and practices and encouraging utilization of healthcare resources. Tribal leaders, Indian Tribal healthcare organizations, IHS, and DHHS recognized that the CHR Programs had an important role and contribution to make in improving Indian health. CHRs, both then and now, addressed a myriad of areas, ranging from basic health care, social service, care coordination, emergency incident command responses, community-based health care, and HP/DP services.

A critical element to the services provided by CHRs is data collection through the IHS records payment management system (RPMS) under their P.L. 638 contracts. Data collection, including documentation of services performed and encounter data for core services provided by CHRs, is critical to the sustainability of funding and CHR program validation, especially in rationale for continued federal support. Some programs have additional private or external grant funding to support their work. RPMS access is not available to all CHR programs due to various issues.

Today, the CHR program serves as the largest tribally contracted and compacted program with more than 90% of CHR programs being directly operated by Tribes under P.L. 93-638 of the Indian Self-Determination and Education Assistance Act, as amended. There are more than 1600 CHRs representing over 250 tribes in all 12 IHS areas.

11.3.3   CHR Direct Service Impacts

CHR programs provide a myriad of services to meet the needs of Tribal members, Native American individuals, and their families within the reservation boundaries and near reservation communities. Providing direct services by well-trained, certified, and competent CHRs is lifesaving in rural and remote tribal communities where CHRs are often the only culturally appropriate linkage to the individual and the care needed. The overarching goal of the CHR Program (Fig. 11.3) is to address healthcare needs through the provision of community-oriented, public health, primary care services, including traditional native concepts in multiple settings, utilizing community-based, well-trained, medically guided workers. The majority of the work of CHRs occurs in the community—in homes of tribal and community members on or near reservations. Some CHRs are stationed in clinics and provide services from those locations.

CHR programs largely provide services within the Tribal SOW that identifies the areas of concentration for the program. These include:

- Health Education/Counseling
- Monitor Client/Community
- Case Management/Coordination
- Case Finding/Screening
- Non-emergency Care

Fig. 11.3 CHR seal

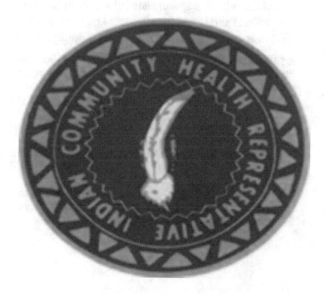

- Health Promotion/Disease Prevention
- Translation/Interpretation
- Transportation/Delivery

These direct services are part of the framework for care provided by CHRs. While the above listed service areas of concentration are common to most Tribal nations in their SOW, other areas of concentration specific to Tribal nation may also be included. Programs are able to develop standard operating procedures that guide how the direct services will be provided. Programs can adopt regulations and standards of practice to ensure overall quality in performing these direct services. Tribal CHR programs utilize the knowledge and skills of well-trained staff, who work with cultural relevance to meet the needs of individuals and families within the community.

CHRs provide direct services to meet the myriad of health, chronic disease, mental health, care coordination, and natural disaster needs of their patients as they utilize their knowledge, skills, and abilities in health promotion/disease prevention, public health, motivational interviewing, mental health, and clinical screening knowledge. Highlighted in this chapter are vignettes that CHRs in various Southwest Tribes, Navajo nation, and Pueblos in the greater Albuquerque area have selected to emphasize CHRs' direct services and the level of expertise demonstrated to address patients' needs. These are true stories linked to real CHR scenarios of actual services provided.

11.3.4 Health Education/Counseling

The Health Education practice is designed to provide individuals, families, and communities with the appropriate information to practice a healthy lifestyle. Each CHR is trained and tested for adequate knowledge in the health area to be practiced. Education is provided on topics from community resources to disease etiology.

A CHR received a referral to approach a client about her interest in receiving diabetes self-management education. The person was suspicious when approached and asked in a loud voice "Who told you this?" Once I explained how I received the referral, the client changed her tone. I explained how I was there to support her and provide information about her health condition.

We continued our one-to-one health education sessions, and I encouraged her to make it to our local gym to work out and use our treadmills. This went on for some time. At the start of the New Year, I was busy helping a college intern. I was walking to my office and noticed a familiar figure at the front desk. I didn't investigate at that time, but I kind of wondered "Is that her?"

A couple of weeks later, I was looking around the gym and to my amazement I ran into my client. She said she had been coming in for several weeks. She expressed to me that she had taken my advice and was very happy she did!

This example demonstrates how CHRs must utilize cultural sensitivity in relaying referral sources and how one-on-one health education sessions and encouragement make a difference in quality of life.

11.3.5 Monitor Client/Community

Patient monitoring involves making periodic personal contact with a patient with a known health problem or a client that is at high risk for illness or disablement. Contact is often made by telephone or in person at a patient's home. Activities may include asking questions to see if the patient is feeling well or has enough food and/or medicine, conducting an environmental scan to see if the community member has any unmet home healthcare needs (like adequate heating, water, etc.), and taking immediate action to provide care for patient needs detected through monitoring.

Sabrina Baca, CHR, relates a story of how monitoring the health of a 73-year-old female client in a northern New Mexico tribal community left an impact and imprint on her heart:

Most recently my work as a CHR was truly tested. I had a 73-year-old client whom I had done home visit with two to three times a month for over the last two years. At these visits, I would check her vitals and talk to her about her eating habits and daily activities. We often discussed her hypertension and medications she was taking. At my last home visit with her she had told me that she had not been feeling well for a couple of weeks. She noticed that she had gained some weight for an unknown reason and did not have much energy or appetite. Her vitals were normal for her, and she had stated that she had a doctor's appointment at the end of the week and that her daughter was taking her. I told her I would return on Monday to check on her and find out what the doctors had to say.

On that Monday I returned to visit her, but she was not home. Her daughter notified me that she was in the hospital and was expected to be released by the end of the week. The following week I contacted the family and was told that she was home and doing better. They informed me that that the insurance was sending out a nurse three times a week to visit with her. I called her and she said she was feeling better and asked that I stop by in a week. So, that following week I called her to schedule a home visit, I was to go see her on a Friday. On that Friday I went to visit, and no one was home, so I figured she had an appointment. Then on Tuesday, I received a call from the family letting me know that she had been in the hospital again, and at this time they were sending her home as there was nothing left they could do. The Hospice nurse would be returning home with her and the family was requesting that I be there as they wanted me to administer her morphine and other medications to help keep her comfortable, as the family was not confident in doing so.

I met with the Hospice nurse and family and got the instructions on what I needed to do. So, for the next 36 hours I stayed with the family and kept my client comfortable. This is not in our scope of work. However, I know the family needed my assistance and I was happy to help my client. Sometimes in this line of work you are called to do things that you never thought you were capable of doing or that are not part of the job. I am glad that when needed I was able to step up to the challenge and be of help to my client. She has left an imprint on my heart and truly challenged my abilities as a CHR. She will forever remain in my heart.

Jean Pino, CHR Coordinator, Five Sandoval Indian Pueblos in New Mexico, shares why monitoring clients in the community makes CHR work "personal":

On an early Monday morning, I was on my way to work. I noticed a 63-year-old female sitting on the clinic porch, holding a tissue to her face. I asked her why she was sitting outside the clinic so early in the morning; it was before 8:00 am. She mentioned she wanted to get in to see the Dentist as soon as possible. She informed them she had a root canal abscess the week before and felt some pain that Friday evening but could tolerate it. Then on Saturday morning, she woke up swollen and was having severe pain. I checked her face and noticed the swelling was close to her eye. She explained that the swelling and pain had existed for two days. I talked with her about the pros and cons of a root canal and asked if she had gone to Urgent Care over the weekend. She said she could tolerate the pain and didn't want to go due to having a workshop for childcare; she was having pain off and on and was using Anbesol.

Once the dentist came to the clinic front door, I stopped him and had him take a look at her face. He mentioned that he would have her be seen as soon as possible and had her start antibiotics. Once she finished with her visit with the dentist, she was to make a follow up appointment. I asked when she was scheduled for her follow up, and she said a week out. I mentioned to her that usually a person on antibiotics should be seen in 2-3 days after, to check the swelling. I went up to the front desk and asked the receptionist if there were any available appointments other than a week away. I then spoke to the receptionist and asked her to cancel my appointment for dental and to place the patient in that appointment instead. I put the patient in my place for follow up. Without proper care and follow up, I thought about what could happen due to knowing her health issues and the impact of her swollen face. My concern was severe infection and further loss of teeth.

She kept her appointment that Wednesday and for the next two days. I followed up on Monday with her, and she was so happy and grateful that I helped to advocate for her. I informed the patient that this comes with being a CHR and advocating for our people. I gained her trust from being honest in letting her know the pros and/cons of a root canal procedure. She said this information was not given to her by the staff. I mentioned there are times others don't feel comfortable giving information, due to their lack of knowledge on the subject.

Both of these snapshots demonstrate how close CHRs are to community members and the importance of their care to the community.

11.3.5.1 Case Management/Coordination

Case management and coordination include helping individuals with complex health conditions navigate the healthcare system. They advocate for and liaise between the community member and a variety of health, human, and social services organizations. CHRs also support individuals by providing information on health and community resources; coordinating transportation; making appointments; or developing a care management plan and using tools to track their progress over time (e.g., food and exercise logs).

CHR programs are involved in the provision of information and/or education to individuals, families, and communities that encourage family unity, community commitment, and traditional spirituality that make positive contributions to their health status, such as cessation of tobacco smoking, reduction in the misuse of alcohol and drugs, improvement in nutrition, improvement in physical fitness, family planning, control of stress, pregnancy, and infant care (including prevention of fetal alcohol syndrome).

CHRs also focus on health literacy for families in tribal communities to ensure they understand health benefits available to them through IHS and other third-party resources. Oftentimes, the CHR serves as the interpreter and navigates information with the patient. Such was the work of Iris Reano, Health Director/CHR/Benefits Coordinator, as she provides services to a client regarding medical bills.

On a raining Friday afternoon, a 69-year-old female community resident came to our CHR office to get assistance and help understanding a letter regarding her visit to the doctor's office. In this small, north central New Mexico Pueblo community, we only have specific days for IHS clinic providers. There is no business office on site, and the nearest IHS business office is 35 miles away. As a certified CHR/Benefits Coordinator, I listen to her concerns, issues, and questions. Knowing her, her level of understanding, and insurance language and demands cited in the letter, I wanted to make sure she understood. I proceeded to read the letter out loud to the patient and explained the purpose of the letter, translated in our native language KERES. KERES is our spoken language, which most of our Elders understand either by showing visuals or hand gestures. The letter was, in fact, an actual bill from a private doctors' office visit.

As a CHR/Benefits Coordinator, I formerly enrolled this person for QMB benefits, and I had her records on file in my office. I had previously explained the benefits of both New Mexico Medicaid and Medicare Part A, B, and D at time of enrollment (I explain to all patients the benefits of New Mexico Managed Care Organization and Medicare Part A, B, C, D, E, & F benefit examples). We had discussed the coverage, and she used the 20/80 coverage of benefits. She had a one-day surgery done with an outside provider, but because it was referred by an IHS Provider, we made a call to Indian Health Service's Referred Purchase Care or contract health. She was afraid to call on her own to the PRC office because she does not know medical terminology or understand the jargon. After explaining to her in KERES language, she understood the bill letter. She felt comfortable after reviewing the case, and she proceeded to discuss her current family situation.

She was disappointed that one of her sons started drinking again and was worried about her finances. Apparently, she had a joint account with her son. She stated, "if he finds out I have money, he may take it from me." Based on her response I asked if she might be in fear of her finances, or perhaps her life. I suggested a referral to the social service department so they could alert law enforcement, if needed. She denied social services assistance; she didn't want all the Tribal officials and social service personnel at her home. We sat and talked a little more, and she thanked me for always keeping our health department doors open to our community. She stated, "it feels good to vent out my problems and get recommendations." She requested a CHR to continue with home visits to her to check vital signs and continue home talking sessions.

I see a lot of our community members getting more frustrated with medical bills. They have difficulty understanding all of the various options and patient responsibilities. Patients don't understand about FFS (Fee for Service) and MCO (Managed Care Organization) is. Patients usually ask, "who do we pick?" and "what services do they offer?" Most of my explanations are done in my native tongue, and usage of visual aids are helpful in communication.

As a CHR in our communities, we are the focal point of bringing in providers, insurers, MCOs, health partners, and contractors together to inform patients, provide health literacy, and explain health conditions, medications, prevention and interventions services. ACCESS to third-party benefits is critical. This third-party information is presented via transportation rides, home visits, community health prevention, and education presentations but simply giving the time to sit and hear their concerns is perhaps one of the most vital services I can provide.

11.3.5.2 Non-emergency Care and Emergency Care

Providing non-emergency care includes taking vital signs; providing other clinical services, such as foot care, to persons with a diagnosed illness; or counseling for social, emotional, mental, or other related problems. When appropriate, CHRs provide for traditional tribal services for the sick and other services requiring individual assessment, therapeutic care, and follow-up care. Home health care and maintenance of patient equipment (e.g., crutches, wheelchairs, eyeglasses, and hearing aids) are included. Non-emergency care services are provided to patients with diagnosed illnesses.

In contrast, some CHRs that provide emergency care services are licensed and certified Emergency Medical Technicians (EMTs). Some CHRs, more often in the Oklahoma area, work as EMTs in their SOW. Oftentimes, these CHRs work long hours. Providing emergency patient care includes giving care to a sick or injured person while arranging or waiting for transportation to a hospital or clinic, contracting an ambulance or hospital driver, transporting a seriously ill patient to medical care, or performing a crisis intervention with an emotionally upset or suicidal patient.

A Navajo Nation CHR used her skills to assess the client and then accessed the critical care needed for her patient. She shares this story:

> When there is no one else, CHWs are there for emergency transport to the emergency room (ER). When an elder was experiencing chest pains, a CHW answered the call, took the drive into the mountains and transported the gentlemen to the hospital. She saved his life. When an elder has missed consecutive medical appointments, the CHW drives to the local Senior Citizen center to locate the patient and to check on him. During her visit, she conducted a patient assessment and noticed that her patient became disoriented and shaking; he was unable to keep eye contact, which lead the CHW to check his vitals and his blood glucose level. She also ran a quick Face, Arm, Speech, and Time (FAST) stroke assessment. Her continued assessments, vitals, and blood glucose readings indicted "HI" as it was clear his condition could be related to hyperglycemia. She called the ER, but they couldn't get to him in time. She transported the patient to the ER and saved his life.

Saving community members' lives through training, skills, and assessments are vital for CHRs in providing non-emergency and emergency care.

11.3.5.3 Health Promotion/Disease Prevention

Disease prevention and health promotion are operationally defined within the SOW to address both individual and population-based interventions. This service area is primarily focused on primary and secondary (including early detection) levels of prevention, aiming to minimize the burden of diseases and associated risk factors. *Primary prevention* includes those measures aimed at avoiding the onset of a disease or condition and may include actions to improve health through changing the impact of social and economic determinants on health. It can also involve information on behavioral and medical health risks, alongside consultation and measures to decrease them at the personal and community level. Examples can include nutritional and food supplementation, oral and dental hygiene education, and clinical preventive services such as immunization and vaccination of children, adults, and the elderly, as well as vaccination or post-exposure prophylaxis for people exposed to a communicable disease. Secondary prevention deals with early detection when this improves the chances for positive health outcomes (McKenzie, Neiger, & Thackeray, 2013).

Health promotion is the process of working with individuals and communities to increase their control over their health and its determinants and usually addresses behavioral risk factors such as tobacco use, obesity, diet, and physical inactivity, as well as the areas of mental health, injury prevention, drug abuse control, alcohol control, health behavior related to HIV, and sexual health. Disease prevention and health promotion share many goals, and there is considerable overlap between functions.

A Jicarilla Apache Nation CHR recounts this experience to emphasize the importance of disease prevention and health promotion from the early 1980s:

> "Thank you for caring." These four words always bring back a memory of my tour of duty during the HIV outbreak in the early 1990s. I served as health educator for our community and had attended several area trainings by the Albuquerque Area Task force.
>
> As part of my community outreach activity, I would go to the "Zoo", the name of a local bar. The frequent customers referred to this gathering as "roll call", a gathering and lining up for the purchase of alcohol beverages upon the opening of the facility.
>
> I took HIV pamphlets and condoms to this gathering. At first, this crowd seemed a little suspicious. It took several days but eventually I gained acceptance as part of their morning gatherings. Soon I had a captive audience. We would sit in the nearby arroyos, out of sight of law enforcement.
>
> This was my classroom. I shared the HIV education and distributed condoms. I even had a nickname amongst them. "Rubber Man" was not exactly a superhero name, but it worked for me. I took this time to educate and give positive outlooks to this group that most had given up on. As I was leaving one day, a lady expressed her appreciation with the comment, "Thank you for caring." That was over 25 years ago, and I still remember like it was yesterday.

While this event happened in the past, the lasting impression it left to the CHR demonstrates that every act of direct service, even providing education and helping share information on an epidemic, leaves a lasting impression on CHRs for the impact they make in the community.

11.3.5.4   Translation/Interpretation

Interpreting or translation is the taking of a statement from one language and expressing the meaning, either orally or in writing, in another language; this enables people who do not speak the same language to communicate with one another. Having fluent speakers of native languages is a major benefit in providing and navigating patient care in Tribal communities. Translation of medical and health terms into native language concepts is a key for many CHRs as they work with elderly tribal members. Many CHRs are fluent in native languages and have been able to develop phrases and terms to explain procedures, conditions, and medications. There are many Western words that are foreign concepts for elder tribal members.

For example, the Laguna CHR program recounted a time when they were required to translate to an elder male the colonoscopy procedure he was to have. The concept of a colonoscopy is foreign in native cultures as tribal members did not routinely have colonoscopies as a part of daily living. The CHR consulted with key persons in the community, who were able to advise on words that should be used to explain the testing procedure. In addition, there was an added layer of sensitivity and respect that needed to be addressed, especially for an older respected elder male, considering the physical anatomical location of the procedure. In supporting the elder male, the CHR escorted the male to the appointment on the day of the test and supported him through the procedure.

These types of translation and interpretation services differ than merely converting words or phrases from one language to another. They require intelligence of the culture (including physical environment, history, traditions, beliefs, and customs) to interpreting to others this philosophy of ethos, layered in the understanding, sensitivity, and respect of the culture.

11.3.5.5   Transportation/Delivery

A key function of the CHR is transportation of a patient. On reservations and in many Tribal community areas, it is difficult to get from one place to another. Many community members are low-income and have no dependable vehicle to make it from one place to another of significant distance. Without other means of transport, getting to/from an IHS or tribal hospital/clinic when necessary for routine, non-emergency procedures, transportation can become a barrier to access of care if not provided. This Jicarilla Apache CHR offers an account of the importance of her role for providing both transportation and support to her client on her day of surgery:

> This client did not have a relative or friend that could go with her that day. The CHR stepped in as the support person comforting and reassuring the patient that everything would be okay. She accompanied the client to the exam room and stayed with her until the nurse came to take her to surgery. She reassured the client that she would be there when she came out of surgery. In the recovery room the patient woke up to the CHR sitting beside her. The look on the client's face was priceless as she woke up from anesthesia, she was relieved that she had a support person close by.
>
> The CHR received post-op instructions from the nurse on wound care and what to expect after surgery (Fig. 11.4). She in turn provided that information to the client's significant other when they arrived home. Throughout the day, the CHR checked in with the client's babysitter to make sure the kids were okay at home. They also stopped to pick up prescribed medication from a pharmacy, and food that the physician recommended for the

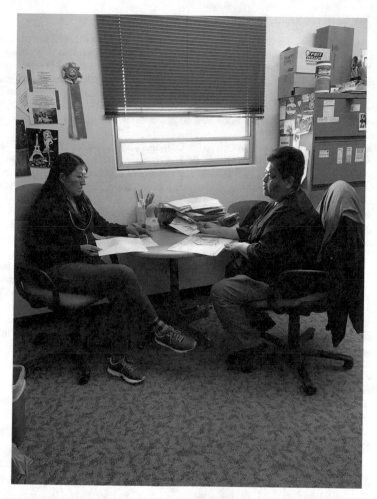

Fig. 11.4 CHR and Public Health Nurse (PHN) working together

post-op diet. On the way home, the client was nauseated, and about every 15 minutes throughout the drive home the patient had to stop due to emesis. The CHR reassured the client that she would stop even every 5 minutes if she had to. The CHR explains, "She was in my care, so I was going to make sure and do a damn good job! It was a long day, but it was worth it. I love my job!"

Transportation is a critical service for many CHR programs and provides a critical linkage to patients to medical and dental services provided on and off reservations. Many CHRs travel extremely long distances, over 100 miles in one direction, to connect patients to specialty services. Many patients and families have no means of transportation, so CHRs are their only link to health care and other services to support patient needs. Often the CHR is the only resource for transportation and support for patients.

Another CHR recounted:

The CHR received the call and was asked if the CHR could assist with the situation. The CHR was able to contact the Indian Health Service and was able to pick up the grandma's medications. The CHR then started the trip to the grandma's house. During this time of the year, the area had just received a ton of snow, and there was on-going snow fall in the area. The CHR was aware that getting to the grandma's house would be a chore, as CHRs were informed to be mindful of treacherous areas. However, this CHR knew that the grandma needed her medications, and she wanted to conduct a welfare check.

The CHR then arrived at the turn off to the Grandma's house and realized that the snow was at least above knee high deep. The CHR had requested for the Grader to go out and make an attempt to grade the roads prior to her arrival to the grandma's area. To no avail, there were no tire tracks and the road was not visible; the falling snow was impairing visibility.

The CHR then walked on foot for about a mile up to the Grandma's home, and she found the Grandma at home, alone. The CHR was able to bring wood into the home and start a fire for the grandma. The Grandma was so thankful; she stated that she would not have known what to do if she spent another night without wood and her medications. The Grandma stated she felt better and was able to warm up, and the CHR assisted the Grandma to warm some food. The CHR also fed the grandma's dogs and cats. Finally, the CHR heard the grader at the road and told the grandma that they might be able to clear her road. The CHR walked back out to the main road and found that the grader was there; the grader was ready to grade the road to the grandma's home. Also, the CHR was met by the grandma's daughter and grandson, who thanked the CHR for going above and beyond for their mother to get medications and ensure her safety. The Grandma's daughter knew the roads were treacherous and was thankful that the CHR was able to request for the Grandma's roads to be cleared.

The CHR did get stuck while attempting to leave the area (turning around), but there was enough help there to help the CHR get out of the highly snowy area of the Chilchiltah community. This CHR presented bravery, determination, and compassion for the Grandma's needs and knew she had to reach the Grandma at all cost to ensure the safety of the Grandma and to get medications to her.

CHRs use their knowledge and understanding of the patient's environment to successfully assist the patient. Knowing the patient's history is important to care delivery, as was the case with this 70-year-old Navajo elder living in a remote chapter house needing assistance with medications.

11.3.6   CHR Direct Service Impacts

Why is CHR direct service delivery so important? Service delivery has previously been distinguished in terms of a medical paradigm of providing clinical services to meet basic needs. While some CHRs do have specified clinical training to provide specialized services, CHRs have been meeting basic needs across Tribes and Pueblos since the beginning of time. Considering the distances where many of our

Tribal brothers and sisters reside, providing these types of direct services are particularly relevant, especially in rural areas where medical and social services are limited.

Meeting basic needs is fundamentally a characteristic of our humanization. According to Maslow (1943) and his hierarchy of needs, he outlines a pyramid with the largest, most fundamental needs at the bottom and the need for self-actualization and transcendence at the top. In other words, the theory is that individuals' most basic needs must be met before they become motivated to achieve higher-level needs. CHRs meet these needs through their SOW and provisions provided under the role of direct service.

However, CHR direct service delivery is vital in that CHRs serve as a link between the clinical setting and the community to facilitate access to services and improve the quality and cultural competence of service delivery (Division of Behavioral Health, Indian Health Services, n.d.). In the words of a CHR from Jicarilla Apache CHR Program:

> The CHR title comes with many roles. A greeter, an aid, an ear to listen, an encourager, a person to boost them up to go to their appointments and even a shoulder to cry on when news is too much. There is so much joy you see in a patient's face when you tell them you are not in a rush and you are there for them.
>
> By taking patients to their appointment, you gain friendship, trust, and bonds that are comforting to them, and you, yourself, know you did your job right. By being the support person, you establish comfort so that the client is able to see things in a more positive way and realize it is worth the try to fight and keep going to their appointments. I like to leave them with a clean home, full belly, and a good feeling that they had a productive day. By helping patients want to stay alive and live a longer healthier life, it creates a positive feeling for the CHR, and is what makes me love my job. Being a CHR is important to the community and it's important for the future.
>
> When we look at the statistics for the CHR programs, we see just that -- statistics...data...numbers. These numbers for direct services do not capture the true extent of CHR worth in the tribal communities. When I simply state, "We did a home visit and checked her blood pressure," how did that capture the quality of education, the kindness, the empathy, the enthusiasm, and passion that the CHR provided?
>
> We establish trust with clients and their families. We speak the language and practice the same culture and customs as they do. We understand how Jicarilla's are taught to view the world and treat one another. We knowingly establish a relationship with that client and are impacted when we lose a client. Our ability to remain resilient after such loss merits recognition.
>
> What helps us to continue on after the loss is that all of us know that in the end, we did exactly what was needed to be done, we did it with quality, enthusiasm, and kindness. It is valuable to us as CHRs to help our clients to feel better, to comfort, and provide needed support. This is the rewarding experience that makes us able to continue our work. This is why if you ask any CHR to describe how they view their work, more than likely you will hear the sentiment, "I love my job!"

As you can distinguish, CHRs make a difference. They make a difference one person, one story, and one community at a time.

11.3.6.1 Dedication

This section is dedicated to Community Health Representatives who work with great respect, sensitivity, and honor in their Pueblo villages, communities, plains lands, Hogans, and Teepees providing quality care and services to ensure good health and wellness of their native people.

Special thanks to the Laguna CHR program and the Albuquerque area CHR programs representing the Pueblos and tribes and to the Navajo Nation CHR programs in Arizona and New Mexico.

> *Da wa ee (Thank you~ Keresan)*
> *Ahéhee' (Thank you~ Navajo)*

References

Division of Behavioral Health, Indian Health Services. (n.d.). *Community Health Representatives fact sheet*. Retrieved from https://www.ihs.gov/sites/chr/themes/responsive2017/display_objects/documents/chrfactsheet2018.pdf.

Indian Health Services [IHS]. (n.d.-a). *About us*. Retrieved from https://www.ihs.gov/chr/aboutus/.

Indian Health Services [IHS]. (n.d.-b). *Legislation*. Retrieved from https://www.ihs.gov/aboutihs/legislation/.

Indian Health Services [IHS]. (n.d.-c). *Locations*. Retrieved from https://www.ihs.gov/locations/.

Indian Health Services [IHS]. (n.d.-d). *Title 1*. Retrieved from https://www.ihs.gov/odsct/title1/.

Maslow, A. H. (1943). A theory of human motivation. *Psychological Review, 50*(4), 370–396. https://doi.org/10.1037/h0054346.

McKenzie, J. F., Neiger, B. L., & Thackeray, R. (2013). *Planning, implementing, & evaluating health promotion programs: A primer* (6th ed.). Boston, MA: Pearson.

Sabo, S., O'Meara, L., & Camplain, R. (2019). *Community health representative workforce assessment: A report to the Arizona advisory council on Indian health care in collaboration with the Arizona community health representative coalition*. Flagstaff, AZ: Center for Health Equity Research, Northern Arizona University.

U.S. Department of Health and Human Services [USDHHS]. (2015, January). *Basis for health services. Fact sheet*. Indian Health Services. Retrieved from https://www.ihs.gov/newsroom/factsheets/basisforhealthservices/.

U.S. Department of the Interior, Indian Affairs. (n.d.). *About us*. Retrieved from https://www.bia.gov/bia.

Warne, D., & Frizzell, L. B. (2014). American Indian health policy: Historical trends and contemporary issues. *American Journal of Public Health, 104*(S3), S263–S267. https://doi.org/10.2105/AJPH.2013.301682.

Chapter 12
Implementing Individual and Community Assessments

Jeffrey Tangonan Acido, Jermaine Agustin, Caitlin G. Allen*,
Rebecca Anderson*, Melanie Apodaca, Rachel Arasato, Roshni Biswa,
Gretchen Bondoc, J. Nell Brownstein, Chasity Nohealani Cadaoas,
Kristy Canionero, Ashley Corpuz, Dennis Dunmyer, Selena Gaui,
Leina'ala Kanana, Shawna Koahou, Dominique Lucas, Sara S. Masoud,
June Munoz, Susan Oshiro-Taogoshi, Kelly Pilialoha-Cypriano,
E. Lee Rosenthal, Desiree Santana, Dalia Solia, R. Napualani Spock,
Julie Ann St. John*, Malia Talbert, Nathan Tarvers, Lani Untalan,
Wes Warner, Shannon Watson, and Deborah White

12.1 Introduction

Caitlin G. Allen, E. Lee Rosenthal, Sara S. Masoud, and J. Nell Brownstein

As the C3 Project continued to explore community health worker (CHW) roles, the importance of the implementation of individual- and community-level assessments became increasingly apparent. By assessment, we mean the process of identifying the strengths, assets, needs, and challenges of a specified individual and/or community.[1] While the common CHW practice of structured health assessment was not originally included as a "lead role," in initial phases of the C3 Project, this role came to prominence as the project unfolded. This role includes two sub-roles, which demonstrated the multilevel nature of the assessment role: participating in design,

Authorship is organized alphabetically in ascending order by surname.

[1] https://ohioline.osu.edu/factsheet/CDFS-7

J. T. Acido
Kokua Kalihi Valley Community Health Center, Kalilhi, HI, USA

J. Agustin · R. Arasato · G. Bondoc · K. Canionero · A. Corpuz · S. Gaui · L. Kanana ·
S. Koahou · K. Pilialoha-Cypriano · D. Santana · D. Solia · M. Talbert · N. Tarvers ·
L. Untalan · S. Watson
Wai'anae Coast Comprehensive Community Health Center, Wai'anae, HI, USA

C. G. Allen (✉)
CGA Consulting, Charleston, SC, USA
e-mail: caitlin.gloeckner.allen@emory.edu

© Springer Nature Switzerland AG 2021
J. A. St. John et al. (eds.), *Promoting the Health of the Community*,
https://doi.org/10.1007/978-3-030-56375-2_12

implementation, and interpretation of individual-level assessments and participating in design, implementation, and interpretation of community-level assessments. While there were antecedents of this role in the original 1998 National Community Health Advisory Study, this role became prominent and distinct from the other nine roles included in the study. The assessment role, similar to the role of participating in research and evaluation, demonstrates that CHWs are part of a wide variety of teams and provide services at both the individual and community level.

Individual assessments, or health assessment, are a way for a CHW to determine and address an individual's goals and needs. A CHW can perform an individual assessment focused on health or social issues to develop an action plan. Individual assessment could include the delivery of a home environmental scan to help identify and reduce falls among older adults. Increasingly, CHWs are using tools which "flip the script" by identifying strengths and resources in individuals' and families' lives and creating action plans building on those strengths.

There are also a number of specific assessment instruments designed to focus attention on issues such as substance use, health literacy, food insecurity, and housing status. CHWs can determine which of these assessment tools is most appropriate in a given situation, as often multiple assessments are needed. In all such work, the CHW must be able to suggest changes to assessment tools that reflect local cultural preferences and understanding.

At the community level, assessments may include identification of the strengths, assets, and challenges within a specific community. A CHW is well-equipped to conduct community assessments and/or help establish efforts (e.g., coalitions) to address the concerns raised through a community-level assessment. Community-level assessments could include the implementation of a windshield survey or community asset mapping, which are two well-established techniques to help consider opportunities for growth within a community.

The following two sections expand on this new role with examples of how findings from individual and community assessments were implemented in different settings.

R. Anderson (✉) · M. Apodaca · R. Biswa · D. Dunmyer · D. Lucas · W. Warner · D. White
KC CARE Health Center, Kansas City, MO, USA
e-mail: rebeccab@kccare.org

J. N. Brownstein · E. L. Rosenthal
Texas Tech University Health Sciences Center El Paso, El Paso, TX, USA

C. N. Cadaoas
Maui Aids Foundation, Wailuku, HI, USA

S. S. Masoud
UT Health San Antonio, San Antonio, TX, USA

J. Munoz · S. Oshiro-Taogoshi
Ho'ola Lahui Hawai'i Kauai Community Health Center, Lihue, HI, USA

R. N. Spock
Hawaiian Community Capacity Building Resources, Makawao, HI, USA

J. A. St. John (✉)
Department of Public Health, Texas Tech University Health Sciences Center,
Abilene, TX, USA
e-mail: julie.st-john@ttuhsc.edu

12.2 CHWs Implementing Individual and Community Assessments: Examples from Hawai'i

R. Napualani Spock, Julie Ann St. John, Leina'ala Kanana,
Jeffrey Tangonan Acido, Jermaine Agustin, Kristy Canionero, Malia Talbert,
Dalia Solia, Rachel Arasato, Kelly Pilialoha-Cypriano, Shawna Koahou,
Shannon Watson, Gretchen Bondoc, Selena Gaui, Nathan Tarvers,
Lani Untalan, Desiree Santana, Ashley Corpuz, Chasity Nohealani Cadaoas,
June Munoz, and Susan Oshiro-Taogoshi

12.2.1 Introduction

In traditional Hawai'i, values such as *pono* (balance, justice), *alu like* (working together), *malama* (to nurture, lovingly care for)*, kako'o* (support), *kuleana* (responsibility, role), and *aloha* (love of community, environment, all of creation) provided the foundation for our worldview, human relationships, and community. These traditional values of the host culture of Hawai'i continue to thrive and influence our diverse community of modern-day Native Hawaiians, kama'aina (longtime residents), and immigrants from all over the world.

In Hawai'i today, similar values are held by community health workers (CHWs) from the diverse cultures that comprise our population: Native Hawaiians, kama'aina, and immigrants from Asia, the Pacific Islands, the American continents, Europe, and many other parts of the world. A commitment to social justice and community engagement, compassion, advocacy, servant leadership, support, collaboration, deep caring, and love of community are qualities that are found in CHWs serving in nonprofit organizations, community health settings, clinics, and volunteer agencies across the pae 'aina (archipelago) of Hawai'i, from Hawai'i to Maui, Moloka'i, O'ahu, and Kaua'i.

12.2.2 Community Health Workers in Hawai'i

Hawai'i's CHWs work in a wide range of health and human service organizations such as community health centers, Native Hawaiian Health Care Systems, hospitals, the State Department of Health, Offices on Aging, Head Start, and many others. They are hired into a wide range of job titles: outreach worker, patient service representative, health educator, bilingual health aide, enabling services worker, care coordinator, service coordinator, case manager, health aide, eligibility worker, and, of course, community health worker.

Coming from the communities they serve, they are dedicated in service to the neighbors and 'ohana (*family*) surrounding them. They are mission-centered, community-centered, inherently aware of culturally appropriate engagement and communication, and privy to culturally relevant approaches and strategies. Hawai'i's CHWs contribute these irreplaceable strengths to the organizations they work with and serve as strong bridges that allow those organizations to implement their missions in service of community. As one CHW coined: "We bring the community to community health."

Contrary to Hawai'i's image as a vacation paradise, the reality for the majority of the roughly 1.5 million people living in Hawai'i includes a skyrocketing cost of living and low wages (United States Census Bureau, 2019). Hawai'i has a growing population of people experiencing homelessness, poverty, and no health insurance. In fact, Hawai'i has the lowest wages in the United States after adjusting for cost of living, which is also the highest in the nation. The current minimum wage is $10.10 per hour or an annual wage of $21,000; average rent, however, is comparable to San Francisco and New York City—cities with significantly higher wages.

Disparities between the "haves" and "have nots" have grown exponentially in recent years as new multi-million-dollar high-rise condominiums pop up, attracting millionaires and billionaires from around the world. The booming, unregulated vacation rental industry has dominated the availability of smaller studios and one-bedroom apartments, leaving a significantly reduced inventory of long-term affordable rentals for kama'āina (longtime residents). This has resulted in increased houselessness for many and a mass exodus of Native Hawaiians and other kama'āina moving out of Hawai'i, relocating to Las Vegas, Southern California, Arizona, Washington, and Oregon for a better ratio of income to expenses. We call this "houselessness," because for Native Hawaiians, Hawai'i is our homeland, and we are born of this land with an unbreakable deep spiritual, emotional, and physical bond which cannot be broken by the lack of a house. Although the temporary condition of houselessness may exist for months or years, the 'aina itself is Papahanaumoku, our ancestor, from whom we cannot be disenfranchised.

Besides affordable housing shortages, and in contrast to Hawai'i's reputation as a very healthy state, certain populations experience considerable disparities in health and the social determinants of health, primarily Native Hawaiians, other Pacific Islanders, Filipinos, and other immigrant populations. Native Hawaiians and other Pacific Islanders bear a disproportionate burden of chronic physical (diabetes and heart disease) and mental health conditions (depression and suicide) compared with other ethnic groups in Hawai'i.

Researchers further describe health disparities affecting Native Hawaiians:

> The Native Hawaiian population experiences numerous social and health disparities. In Hawai'i, Native Hawaiians have the shortest life expectancy and exhibit higher mortality rates than the total population due to heart disease, cancer, stroke, and diabetes. Poor health is inextricably linked to socioeconomic factors, and Native Hawaiians are more likely to live below the poverty level, experience higher rates of unemployment, live in crowded and impoverished conditions, and experience imprisonment. Noteworthy and disturbing are the high percentage of Native Hawaiians who are homeless in their own island homeland.

The Native Hawaiian community has suffered numerous historical traumas, including severe depopulation due to introduced diseases in the nineteenth century, the overthrow of the Hawaiian Kingdom in 1893, the outlawing of '*olelo Hawai'i* (Hawaiian language) from 1898–1978, ongoing systemic racism, and all of its accompanying discrimination. These historical traumatic events are considered factors in the disparities mentioned above.

In addition to lower wages and housing challenges, Native Hawaiians, other Pacific Islanders, Filipinos, and other immigrants face significant disparities in the social determinants of health. For example, 10% of the population are Veterans, and 18% of the population was born in other countries. Twenty-six percent of the population speaks a language other than English at home (United States Census Bureau, 2019). Eleven percent of the population has a disability (Hawai'i Health Matters, 2014–2018).

Rural communities on neighbor islands and parts of O'ahu face higher health disparities when compared to urban centers, in part due to a lack of primary care providers and other health promotion resources. For example, the islands of Maui, Moloka'i, Lana'i, and Kaua'i each have only one hospital for their populations. On the biggest island of Hawai'i, significant geographic barriers frequently affect timely access to care.

In all of these cases, community-based CHWs serve to bridge their communities to services, promoting access to care, addressing social determinants of health, and ultimately reducing health disparities. The first step in their service is to assess the needs of individual members and communities as a whole. In the next section, we describe the importance of CHWs' assessment roles. Next, CHWs will share personal accounts of conducting both individual client assessments and community-wide assessments. These personal accounts include their impressions of how the service that began with the assessment resulted in improved health and lives of community members. In the final section, CHWs share how they used assessment results to address identified needs. Highlighted communities include Kalihi Valley and Wai'anae on O'ahu island, Maui island, and Kaua'i island. The section concludes with a discussion of key factors in conducting assessments and lessons learned and recommendations for the CHW field regarding assessment.

12.2.3 The Importance of CHW Assessment

In Kalihi Valley, the Kokua Kalihi Valley Comprehensive Family Services (KKV) actively recruits CHWs from the community and engages CHWs in strategizing the best ways to reach community members. The Kalihi community is extremely diverse, bringing together Native Hawaiians, Pacific Islander immigrants from the Federated States of Micronesia and the Republic of the Marshall Islands, and Asian immigrants from the Philippines, Korea, China, and Vietnam. Jeffrey Acido shares his perspective on the importance of CHWs for the community and the value of their assessment role:

Looking at the history of Kokua Kalihi Valley, I realize that CHWs and a community-oriented pastor together founded our organization and rooted in us the values of the people we serve. Today we depend on CHWs to carrying our mission of healing and reconciliation and alleviation of suffering in Kalihi Valley. We cannot do this without CHWs! I have observed that the participation of CHWs in the planning and implementation of programs we have had at KKV have been essential to its success. Because CHWs are the frontline staff, or "frontline healers", in our community, they are able to assess the heartbeat of our community—listening to its aches and pains, joys and suffering, resilience and liberation of the people who we serve.

CHWs are unique because they are neither provider nor stranger; they are the community, breathing and living in the heart of Kalihi. A common practice for KKV is to hire within Kalihi, which allows us to have CHWs really invested in the healing of Kalihi. As a coordinator of various programs, I do not think we can work effectively with our community without the diverse gifts that CHWs bring. Because they are from the community, they speak the language, eat the same food, and live in the same houses as our patients. CHWs are extensions of our clinic into the homes of our patients or that the home of our patients become extended into our clinics. As CHCs face the challenges of envisioning and implementing a patient-centered/community-centered health care home, we recognize that the perspectives of CHWs who live in the community we serve are essential. What would it look like for a patient to see the clinic as the extension of their home? CHWs are critical component of our efforts to embody patient-centeredness.

We strive, from the organization's standpoint--to place a higher value in the lived experiences, as a reflection of our community, embodied by the CHWs as a way to inform the practices and policies that affect our community. In valuing their relationships to our larger community of focus, we are able to articulate better what kinds of programs we need or what type of healing opportunities we can provide for our community. CHWs serve as both the ear and the heart of the larger community. CHWs have a gift of realizing the context of the community's life and are able to, when empowered and given the agency to effect change, transform the social context of our community health centers (CHCs).

When we realize that CHWs belong in the spectrum of healing and are healers, in the same way providers and front-line medical staff are, then we can achieve an equitable way of seeing CHWs' contributions to the vocation of health and the goal of healing. When we can switch the framework of CHWs as not simply handing over healing to the providers but see them as the first responder to the needs of our community, then we can begin to undermine the arrogance of the hierarchy of medicine and health/care.

In the final analysis, CHWs become the very people that can strengthen the bridges that medicine and health care has neglected—primarily the ability to listen with an open heart, so that in the end, when the patient comes into the exam room, we are able to tell each other's story—the story that can ultimately heal both the provider and the patient.
> —Jeffrey Tangonan Acido, PhD, Education and Training Specialist,
> Kokua Kalihi Valley

From this perspective, CHWs can more readily assess individual and community needs because they understand the context of living in a particular community and social content. They have direct access to the community and the ability to listen—both critical elements in assessments, which we explore next, individual followed by community assessments.

12.2.4   Individual Assessment

A key role of CHW work is conducting individual assessments. Individual assessment refers to the identification of the specific needs of an individual, including physical, mental (social, psychological, and social well-being), and spiritual, and setting up interventions to meet these identified needs. This involves one-on-one interviewing skills, putting the client at ease, and speaking their language or using recognizable terms in a way that helps them feel comfortable sharing personal information with the CHW. The Wai'anae Coast of O'ahu is home to the largest community of Native Hawaiians in the world. CHWs from the Wai'anae Coast Comprehensive Health Center (WCCHC) share their experiences in conducting individual assessments with community-based clients. Below, Leina'ala Kanana introduces the CHW team who, one by one, will share their own stories of assessment and impact in subsequent paragraphs:

> My department has staff with varying levels of education, from high school graduates with no experience, to master's degrees. No matter the education or pay grade, the most important aspect of our work is to assure everyone feels valued. Each member, each team, brings to the department their own strengths, skillset, and perspective that make the department unique. The CHW team in particular holds great value. What makes this team just as unique is their various backgrounds, knowledge of community resources and their community connections. No degree in the world can amount to the value of their community connections. On numerous occasions, our social workers or nurses find themselves reaching out to our CHWs for a community resource to assist a patient.

> The team conducts assessments with every client they meet, looking for socio-economic barriers to achieving their health goals. Barriers include transportation, financial, housing, access to healthy food, access to exercise opportunities, mental health concerns, substance use disorders, and other comorbidities. The following stories from our CHW team illustrate the specific encounters our staff has experienced and how they addressed the needs identified in the assessment.
>
> —Leina'ala Kanana, Director of Community Health Services

12.2.4.1   Assessing Barriers

Barriers often limit or prevent people from receiving adequate health care and/or social service. Some of the most common access barriers—several discussed in the following stories—include finances; lack of insurance; geographic location; health needs; transportation; literacy; and language (Office of Disease Prevention and Health Promotion, HRSA, 2020b). Assessing and then addressing barriers are critical because barriers can lead to unmet health needs; delayed care; inability to receive preventive services; financial burdens; preventable hospitalizations; and poorer health outcomes. Further barriers to accessing care often vary by race, ethnicity, socioeconomic status, age, sex, disability status, sexual orientation, gender identity, and residential location (Office of Disease Prevention and Health Promotion, HRSA, 2020a). This first set of stories describes CHWs' assessment of individual client barriers:

A thorough assessment can really lead to a more thorough solution to problems affecting a patient. One example of this was a 40-year-old male with multiple Emergency Room (ER) visits for abdominal pain. He frequented at least 3 times a week and his Primary Care Physician (PCP) could not figure out the cause of his pain. Every PCP visit resulted in a medical cocktail to treat his abdominal pain.

After receiving a referral from the patient's PCP, I met the patient in a comfortable setting, his home. The conversation began with a discussion of his perceived barriers and health problems. During the assessment, the patient revealed a history of abdominal pain when experiencing nervousness.

After learning of this, I inquired if he was willing to talk to a Behavioral Health specialist. He accepted my referral, and after the first session, his ER visits drastically reduced from three per week to two more visits, then no more at all! After reviewing his clinical visits over the past 6 months, he has had 6 behavioral health appointments and no ER visits. In our six-month follow-up assessment, his health has improved, and his demeanor is positive.

—Jermaine Agustin, Care Coordinator

A 61-year-old male with recurrent hospitalizations due to congestive heart failure (CHF). The patient's chart said he smoked cigarettes, ate whatever pleased him, and did not understand what was causing his shortness of breath and generalized swelling. I met with this patient face to face to do my assessment for barriers to care and opportunities to educate him on his chronic condition. During this assessment meeting, he mentioned he did not have transportation, he lives alone, he can't exercise due to shortness of breath and poor footwear, and only eats canned goods because he's on a fixed income.

As a result of this assessment, I assisted him in getting connected with the Handi-van (a public transit service for persons with disabilities). He was able to go to his cardiologist appointments. I also educated him on a proper CHF diet, risks of CHF, connected him with a program for monitoring of patient's weight electronically, and referred him to a registered dietitian and smoking cessation program. I scheduled him with his primary care provider (PCP) and ensured his appointments were in the morning, as he preferred in an effort to help him increase compliance (or likelihood to attend). I also worked with his PCP to get him diabetic shoes for exercising. I worked with his community case case manager to order a medical ID necklace. The patient kept all of his appointments with the specialist and PCP, complied with health monitoring program, made dietary changes, and quit smoking cigarettes.

This patient has not been readmitted to the hospital for CHF since 2014. He is still seeing all specialists and his PCP and remains tobacco-free. He still has his medical ID necklace, which he wears daily. He is thriving and is now able to walk to the bus stop and rides his bike with his diabetic shoes (gets a new pair annually) and swims.

—Kristy Canionero, Care Coordinator

Being a CHW has been one of the most rewarding experiences for me. I remember one particular home visit I did for a patient who had multiple no-shows to our health center, outstanding wellness goals, and was very difficult to reach. During a home visit, this patient expressed that their family only had one car, and her husband took the car to work. After identifying transportation as a barrier to care, I informed her that our health center's transportation services to and from medical appointments. She was almost shocked to hear that those services were available for her and her children. We scheduled her an appointment and transportation services during this home visit. This family is now aware and able to utilize transportation for their appointments.

—Malia Talbert, Service Coordinator

In my experience, home visits can be scheduled or unannounced. Home visits are conducted in an attempt to locate clients for case management services, notify clients of immediate treatment/appointment that is needed, complete Advance Healthcare Directives, and visit face-to-face to address progress with case management goals. Home visits help with breaking down barriers for those without transportation and/or has mobility issues. Home visits are crucial to help clients meet their needs. A majority of my home visits have been successful. If the client is not home, then a family member is usually cooperative with relaying the message. As a result of the assessments I do during home visits, I have identified a critical need: housing. With the rising cost of living in Hawaii, housing has been difficult to obtain for many clients given most have fixed income from Supplemental Security Income (SSI, $760) or General Assistance (GA, $360) per month. Shelters have a wait list, which makes finding immediate housing for clients challenging. This causes families to double up or become homeless. Hawaii needs more affordable housing to help clients help themselves.

—Dalia Solia, Service Coordinator

I was assigned to a 70-year-old part-Hawaiian male who was seen at our facility for a hospital follow-up. Previously, he was admitted for dyspnea and shortness of breath due to Afib (Atrial fibrillation) and CHF (congestive heart failure). The patient lived alone, was homeless with no cell phone, had difficult access to food or clean facilities (bathroom/shower), no insurance and received $300/month from social security. At the time of my first encounter with him, the patient was doubling up with a friend but stated his main residence was in a remote location that barely had access to cars and was a mile's walk from the main road/nearest bus stop. The patient declined shelter and preferred to remain on his family's land. Due to all these barriers, I could see that this was a complex situation that required me to think creatively to get patient access to health care/basic needs.

By collaborating with our Patient Assistance team and utilizing the resources at our campus, I signed the patient up for Medquest (Medicaid) and got him SNAP (food stamps) benefits. I scheduled appointments in advance and made referrals for the patient so that he was aware of the plan of care prior to leaving the clinic. Unfortunately, the patient no showed to the first appointment and still had not means of contact. I searched for him and was fortunate to find his residence. He missed his first appointment because he sprained his ankle tripping over one of his dogs, which made him unable to walk to the bus stop. I found him transportation that day to the ER to address his foot wound. After his ankle swelling decreased, I set up transportation to pick him up near his living location, and he was able to keep all his appointments. The patient connected with a cardiologist for his heart issues and other providers. The patient also got a car from a friend to live in and utilized the car to get groceries and go to his appointments.

As a Care Coordinator, I have faced many instances such as these in which I often need to dig a little deeper to find the root cause to a problem that my patient maybe facing. I have to assess the situation from the patient's viewpoint in order to understand their driving factors. If not, I may overlook crucial information that could have been addressed. As CHWs in the West Oʻahu Community, we have to think outside of the box and collaborate with resources in order to address the challenges that our population faces.

—Rachel Arasato, Care Coordinator

These CHWs clearly demonstrated the need for assessing their clients' barriers and engaged specific strategies for eliciting these barriers. Some of these included motivational interviewing, guided discussions, and assessment tools (such as surveys, forms, and checklists). An important principle here is to gain trust through empathy, which facilitates a more accurate list of barriers, which can then be addressed to improve health status.

12.2.4.2 Assessing Eligibility

The next couple of stories share CHWs' experiences in assessing eligibility of clients for various programs and services, which is often a critical first step in helping a client overcome a major barrier to accessing services and improving health: finances:

> Assessing patients' qualification for sliding fee scales and insurance through our Patient Assistant Services has given me a broader perspective that the problems we face individually are common to most people in Waianae. I think it's fair to say we are all struggling to get by and get coverage somehow, someway. We would like to believe that we are organized people, and all we need to do is bring in our documents. However, obtaining these records takes time and effort; scrambling to complete our applications can be discouraging due to time and circumstances.
>
> Patients come to Patient Assistant Services every day with an ordinary need. They need to see a doctor. Often, they don't have insurance, or their insurance was terminated, and they don't know why. Now because of MEC (minimum essential coverage), we must ensure every patient is accounted for and that they understand the steps we need to take to get that coverage.
>
> Income is something we talk about every day. Do they have income and are they twenty dollars above or below the Federal Poverty guidelines that will determine no pay eligibility? The process can be especially discouraging for immigrants who have some money but not enough to get coverage through the Federal Marketplace. However, my job is to find a way for everyone.
>
> People walk into the pod with clouds over their heads sometimes. When I start asking them about their situation and answers are vague or foggy (of course their minds are everywhere but medical insurance, which is probably why his coverage got terminated in the first place), I try to be as specific as possible. The application process shouldn't be an ambiguous and sketchy process that I am making them do. Specific directions and specific goals get better results for me. I print out the Pending Document worksheet we have and make a checklist for them. I offer my phone number and email address because if mom is working part time with three children, she can take a picture of her documents, pay stubs or whatever she needs to complete her application and email them to me because she has go pick the kids up from soccer.
>
> We are blind if we do not address the homelessness in Wai'anae. Typical human reasons like laziness, apathy, despair, hopelessness, financial crisis and mental illness are everywhere around me. I talk to them in the Center, I see them at Tamura's Grocery. I live on the same street. Problems become overwhelming for all of us. I try my best to use this crucial twenty minutes of their time to convey an earnestness about what we need to do by when or else Med Quest/SFS (sliding fee schedule) is going to deny coverage because we didn't get this information to them in time.
>
> Med Quest Office is a sterling example of assessing the population on a community level. Department of Human Services sets a great example of stating what they need and expectations for patient compliance. Being accessible facilitators provides great opportunity to reach out and assist our patients, which hopefully helps patients acquire and maintain coverage. Having integrity with our expectations obtains results, which is what we do and works.

—Kelly Pilialoha-Cypriano, Eligibility Coordinator

> Meeting with families not of my culture or same language is pretty common in what I do. I help many different ethnicities, U.S. citizens, and non-citizens. Over the years, I have learned to first be patient. Whenever there is a language barrier, assisting patients can be difficult. I use the Center's Interpretive Services when needed, but I've learned that you

need to slow down in all that you do and take your time, especially when speaking to the patient. When I first helped these patients, I found that unknowingly, I would speak louder to them. I've since learned that the patients are not deaf; they just can't understand me. At times, I would get frustrated because I want to help these families, but it's not always easy. I have my own beliefs and values, and I've learned that regardless of what they are, I cannot judge anyone for their beliefs. When I first started in this position, I struggled. I had to learn to watch not only what I say but how I spoke and also had to watch my body language. Doing that is now natural, and I understand that I'm here to help families, not judge them. I'm still true to my beliefs, but I've learned that the priority is to help these families. Personally, I have a heart for our non-citizens, especially our COFA (Compact of Free Association) Migrants (migrants from the Federated States of Micronesia, The Republic of the Marshall Islands and the Republic of Palau). They are discriminated in Hawai'i, but I've found that they are great people. I've gotten to know a few of them well and have become friends with them. I currently have the same families coming to me for assistance and bringing their families and friends as well. Overall, I have learned that we all come from different backgrounds, race, and cultures but we need to have respect for one another and cannot be judgmental—have cultural humility.

There is one patient I will always remember. He is an older gentleman that lives on his own, has no transportation besides his bicycle, no phone, and is over the federal poverty income limit by $100, so he doesn't qualify for Med Quest (Medicaid). He came into my office where I first assisted him with a sliding fee scale application. He qualified but at a very low percentage because of his income. His only source of income was workmen's compensation due to a chemical injury he experienced years ago at his job. He is not considered disabled although the condition makes returning to work impossible. He is constantly requested to do exams by his company to ensure he still qualifies for workmen's compensation. He returned every six months for two years to reapply for the sliding fee scale until one day I got a call from a hospital stating that he was admitted there and needed to apply for medical insurance; he gave them my name. I already knew that he didn't qualify due to his income, but I teamed up with a care coordinator and due to his condition and the length of his stay in the hospital, he qualified for Long-Term Care insurance. We knew that he was in the hospital but could not get in touch with him or contact his sister that he listed as a contact in his chart due to HIPAA laws. A waiting game began where we waited for him to call us. Eventually he did, and I was able to assist him with a Med Quest (Medicare) application and had the care coordinator assist with Long-term care services. I recently saw him at our main clinic and talked with him. He looks great and was so thankful for our services. He now has his own phone and car, which makes getting to and from his appointment easier. I think of this man often and worry about him. I couldn't figure out how a man of his age had no family support. Through all his trouble and struggles, he is remains a sweet man, always smiling. Knowing we helped him and that he was doing well produced a great sense of accomplishment. And to help him, I had to assess his personal needs through listening to him.

—Shawna Koahou, CHW, Eligibility Outreach Worker/CHW

My experience with meeting a family that is not of my culture was with a COFA family that came into our pod at the main clinic that needed to apply for Medical Coverage, primarily for her children. This mother of four came in with little knowledge of speaking English and struggled to operate the phone we placed in front of her. Luckily for her and I, her 12-year-old child helped her mom out with questions that she didn't understand in English as well as helping her mom with the phone headset. I assisted the mom and family in applying for the SFS program, Med Quest for her children, and the Federal Marketplace Insurance—all done in a timely manner.

Upon completion of the Med Quest Assistance and SFS Program, mom was in tears— thanking me for being so patient with her as everything here in Hawai'i is so new to her. I then thanked her and her daughter as well for their awesomeness in having patience with me. As of today, all her kids are still covered with medical insurance and keep up with their doctor visits with the WCCHC. Cultural barriers can be worked out through assessing needs and a little Aloha that we as Hawaiians can share with others and hopefully be of great help to those in need of our assistance.

—Shannon Watson, Eligibility Worker

These CHWs highlighted how assessing eligibility for various programs—frequently based on financial need, disabilities, or other requirements—and then assisting clients in enrolling into these programs often serves as a first step to better health and quality of life. To conduct CHW assessments, CHWs should have a deep knowledge base of program requirements, utilize multiple eligibility tools and forms, and have the ability to communicate clearly and plainly to clients in a way that is helpful and eases anxiety and overwhelming feelings that clients often experience when faced with multiple needs and barriers.

12.2.4.3 Assessing Social Determinants

Three main types of factors include our health: biological or physical; environmental; and social. Specifically, more and more research has emphasized the social determinants of health. Social determinants of health are the conditions in which people are born, live, learn, work, play, worship, and age that affect health and quality-of-life outcomes (Office of Disease Prevention and Health Promotion, HRSA, 2020a). Distribution of wealth, power, and resources often influences these conditions, and social determinants often lead to health inequities. CHWs expertly help address social determinants of health, which means they first know how to assess social determinants. The next three stories depict different ways to assess social determinants in order to help their clients improve their health and well-being:

I received a list of patients to assist. I recall a specific instance where I had difficulty contacting the patient, and the patient met the criteria for intensive level of care for Care Coordinator (CHW) services. The patient had uncontrollable Diabetes Mellitus (A1C >10), and wellness goals were not up to date. I attempted to meet patient on scheduled appointments, but the patient either cancelled or did not show up. So, I consulted with the providers regarding the patient's current status. The provider's feedback was the patient was noncompliant with the scheduled appointments and hard to reach.

One day, while at the satellite clinics, I received a warm hand off from a provider, who requested assistance in coordinating the patient's care at the center. I finally had a face-to-face encounter with the patient. The patient completed the social determinants health assessment, and I identified the patient's barriers in meeting his/her healthcare needs, which was transportation. I provided the patient with education on transportation and assisted the patient in arranging transportation through the health plan. I also activated the patient for intensive level of care monitoring. I then helped the patient create goals, such as to decrease the A1C level by 10% and to complete/update wellness goals for the next 3 months. In less than 3 months, the patient's A1C decreased more than 10%, and all wellness goals were up to date! As days passed, we received feedback from the providers that the patient had been compliant with scheduled appointments, and the patient's A1C was nearly within the normal range.

—Gretchen Bondoc, Care Coordinator

One day a man walked in to our facility wanting to see a doctor. Our eligibility office referred him to us because he did not have any medical insurance. I sat down with him for an initial assessment interview, which consists of me asking him about his financial situation so that I can complete the Medicaid application and identify any other potential public benefits that he may be eligible to enroll. During the interview, he revealed he lost his job due to the company restructuring. His wife didn't work, and they had three children. Though receiving unemployment, the amount didn't pay all the bills and help them stay above water. They eventually fell so deep into debt that they lost everything.

His wife's parents offered to take in their daughter and grandchildren, but he was not welcomed. In their culture, the husband is supposed to take care and provide for his family, and because he failed, he was considered a disgrace in his in-laws' eyes and not welcomed.

He convinced his wife to move in with her parents; that way, he knew that they were safe. He decided he would live in his car. He cashed his unemployment check and kept $100 for himself and gave the rest to his wife and kids for their living expenses. He kept applying for jobs—hoping someone would hire him. After 6 months, he still had no calls for work. His in-laws refused to let him spend time with his wife and children.

So, he found himself in our facility—sick, depressed, frustrated, unemployed, and broken, with only $100 a month to live on. A middle-aged man who had worked his entire life, now down on his luck, no higher education other than high school, no trade schooling, no family here in the islands and all his friends that he once thought was friends now looked down on him, finally broke down and cried. I sat there with him in silence and let him have his time. He finally pulled himself together, apologized, felt embarrassed, and started to gather his belongings to leave. I assured him this was nothing to be embarrassed about and should he choose to sit back down, together, we would figure out a plan to start his climb back out of this darkness.

Based on the information I gathered from the initial assessment above, with his input, I came up with a plan. His health was the first concern, so I assisted him with our health center's Sliding Fee Scale discount program; due to his unemployment income, he qualified only for a small discount. We then completed the State MedQuest (Medicare) application, which again because of his unemployment income, he qualified for limited coverage. This was a start. We also submitted an application for food stamps, which was denied again due to his unemployment income.

He was relieved that at least he was able to go to the doctor and to start to take care of his health again. He was, however, worried about all the balances that were building, so luckily we helped him work out a payment plan. He picked up his prescriptions with help from an additional discount program we found. We gave him information on our facilities' assistances, farmer's markets, food banks, churches and homeless shelters.

We also set up future doctor appointments and got him to our gym to get his health back on track. He also agreed to see our behavioral health provider so that he had someone to talk to. He had a car parked on the side of a road but could not afford the gas, registration, insurance and safety check, so we set him up with our transportation department to pick him up and return him after his appointments and exercising were done.

Eventually, he found himself at one of the churches that had a food pantry and ended up volunteering to do odds and ends, fixer-upper jobs in exchange for room and board and hot meals. He also started to maintain the church grounds. A fellow parishioner saw his work ethics and offered him a job.

I'm so glad to say that he now has a full-time job with medical coverage and his health has improved. He is sad that his marriage ended, but at least he is allowed to see his children. He found a room to rent from a church parishioner and continues to volunteer as the church's handy man, groundskeeper, cook, and anything else they need him to do. He is now very happy with his new life.

Not all cases end up with a happy ending, but this is the one case that has definitely touched my heart and soul, and I can truly say that I was a part of a team that made a dif-

ference in this man's life. This shows if you can be that one listening ear, helping hand or guidance to someone down on their luck—truly take the time to assess one's needs—this can make all the difference in the world to that individual. Community health work is not work but is how we, as human beings, should always be, compassionate to others. You don't have to be a professional to make a difference someone's life, you just need to be human.
                                    —Selena Gaui, WCCHC, Care Enabling Manager, Non-Clinical

Working as a Care Coordinator with the Waianae Coast Comprehensive Health Center (WCCHC) is a rewarding job because we get to do help our patients to understand their health needs, identify patient goals related to their physical and psychosocial health, provide education and assistance, and link patients to community resources to assist them in achieving their goals and meeting their needs. We are empowered to meet our patients in the clinic and to conduct home visits or meet with patients in the community. Our first step is to conduct an assessment of their needs while building a relationship. I have found establishing rapport with patients and fostering trust is a key first step in effectively collaborating with patients to help them to identify and achieve their health management goals. Once a relationship is developed through listening to patients' stories, concerns and understanding about their health, we identify potential barriers to enhance their understanding and management of their health. Often there are psychosocial factors or physical barriers preventing them from improving their disease management or health maintenance. This is our psychosocial assessment. These potential barriers must be addressed first so that focus can be ultimately shifted to health management.

I recall one patient with multiple chronic conditions, including end-stage renal disease, diabetes, and hypertension. Clearly, the patient had difficulty managing his health, with a history of missed appointments including with dialysis. Also evident, the patient was not consistent with taking his medications, adhering to diet, or monitoring his blood sugar. I connected with the patient via a telephone call initially, and we made plans to meet at his upcoming appointment. Through my assessment, I determined immediately that lack of transportation and financial constraints were barriers for him in meeting his health care needs. I connected him with his health plan and effectively collaborated with his insurance service coordinator to provide vouchers for him to use a community transportation service. I set up this service immediately by submitting a medical necessity form to the service. He was approved, and after education on how to effectively use this resource to get to his appointments, he used the service to greatly improve his compliance with keeping follow-up appointments.

We again met at his next appointment and continued to build rapport. Trust was already being fostered with him seeing that I was able to assist him with his transportation. From here, we collaborated to identify needs and create a service plan to establish goals for him to start making behavioral changes to increase health maintenance and management. We started bubble-packing his medications to make medication compliance easier. He stopped missing dialysis appointments and kept appointments with his primary care provider and specialist. The patient has continued to demonstrate improved health management with improved labs and overall health. He agreed to see a nutritionist and is managing his diet better. He enrolled in a hypertension management program and his blood pressure is improved and stable. He has established treatment with a behavioral health provider and continues to follow up frequently. All of these changes have led to him having a more positive outlook and proactive approach to managing his health. I have continued to work with him but on a less intensive basis as he is able to effectively manage his appointments, transportation, and medications independently. He has improved to the point where he is now a candidate for a kidney transplant.

This is just one story. Not all stories are as positive as this one, though we continue to reach out to our patients to try to engage them in an active approach to their health. Establishing a connection, collaborating with patients to assess needs, providing educa-

tion, linking to resources, and providing encouragement and assistance to our patients in achieving empowerment to improve their health is how we try to make a positive change in the health of our patients and our community.

—Nathan Tarvers, Care Coordinator

Commonalities across these examples involved the utilization of specific assessments tools (such as surveys, forms, checklists) and the development of trust and rapport with their clients. A key point addressed in these stories is consistent, clear communication and the ability to connect their client's stories to specific determinants in order to develop an action plan to address these determinants and, subsequently, overall health.

12.2.4.4   Assessing Communication, Culture, and Language Needs

This last section of individual assessment covers communication, cultural competency, and language needs assessment. In these shared experiences, CHWs stress the importance of cultural humility and putting oneself in another's shoes:

As a CHW, our services we provide must be respectful of and responsive to the needs, health practices and beliefs of diverse patients. This provision of care can help close the gap in health outcomes. Culturally and linguistically appropriate services (CLAS) are respectful and responsive to the patient's culture and their communication needs: "Respect the whole individual and Respond to the individual's health needs and preferences" (U.S. Department of Health & Human Services, n.d.).

I received a case management referral for a patient from the island of Chuuk. Prior to meeting with the patient to introduce case management services, I reviewed the patient's chart to obtain information to help me provide CLAS, such as gender, age, languages spoken. Upon making the first contact via telephone, I assessed the patient's verbal communication needs. A critical component of care is the patient's ability to communicate effectively with the CHW. If the patient needed an interpreter, I had to keep in mind that arranging for an interpreter for this population may not be as easy. A recent study done on Guam showed Chuukese women did not trust Chuukese interpreters to know about their health problems and that they preferred to have a family member interpret for them (Smith, 2008). In this case, although the patient's primary language was Chuukese, she spoke and understood English. When reviewing a patient's chart for health information in preparation for providing any type of health services, I must also review the patient's social history for information that will ensure that I provide culturally and linguistically appropriate services, which is part of individual assessment.

—Lani Untalan, Service Coordinator/CHW

Working at WCCHC has been such a robust experience for me because this is the one place that I have had the opportunity to work with individuals/families with diverse cultures, ethnicity, race, and beliefs. At the Waipahu clinic, the majority of the ethnicities are Filipino, Micronesian, Marshallese, and Chuukese.

I have learned to be more mindful about how their culture and beliefs may be different from my own. Most of my patients at this clinic were born and raised in the Marshall Islands, Chuuk, or the Philippines and were not raised to believe in Western medicine. The information that I discuss with my patients and their family, such as general health care, continued obstetric care, well child visits, medications, birth control, domestic violence, depression, etc., are not something that most are used to hearing or talking about in their daily lives. When I do a patient encounter, I like to take some time (if possible, considering the fast pace of our clinic) and ask questions about where they are from and who is in their support system. I don't just ask them these questions because I have to but to really hear and understand where they are coming from. This can help me understand more about who will be helping them at home during their pregnancy or even encouraging them to come in for their appointments and what sort of barriers this individual may experience.

Sometimes I find that some of my patients who are Marshallese, Chuuk, or Filipino may have been born in a country different from me, but they have been raised in the U.S. for several years and have a good understanding about the medical system and the same or similar belief system as me. I have learned to not make assumptions just because an individual or family is in a certain ethnic/culture or race different from my own, and I continue to keep a mindful perspective in my daily work.

—Desiree Santana, Women's Health Case Manager

When doing assessments, CHWs must be culturally competent when working with families of another ethnicity as they may have different traditions, values, and social norms. With such a diverse population, CHWs should demonstrate self-awareness of racial health disparities and promote practices to combat the needs of the community. Communication and service delivery should also be inclusive to the family and or family members in order to eliminate conflicts. As a CHW/service coordinator at a health center, I experienced working with a Micronesian family who embraced a social norm different from my culture. The male patient barely spoke, which led me to think that communication and language could possibly be a barrier in receiving the quality care he deserves. After asking several questions, I noticed the patient continued to stare at me with a flat affect. He then gazed at his wife, who would answer. As his CHW, I offered translation services, which the patient declined. However, after further assessment, I learned in their culture, the female usually speaks on the family's behalf or in this case, the patient's behalf.

While ensuring and adhering to the patient's rights and privacy, it is the health center's policy to have a written consent in order for the patient's spouse to speak on his behalf. The patient did not understand why his wife needed to sign paperwork in order for her to speak but after explaining the guidelines to him, they fully understood. This experience had made me realize that a common practice in society may not always align to individuals of a different culture.

—Ashley Corpuz, Service Coordinator

These three stories again describe the importance of assessing language and communication ability of clients and their cultural norms via cultural humility and competency. This requires the utilization of appropriate assessment tools, interpreters, cultural resources, etc. Lastly, these assessments necessitate putting aside personal assumptions and biases based on different ethnicities, race, culture, and language.

12.2.5 Community Assessment

In contrast to individual assessment, which focuses on identifying the needs of one particular person, community assessment refers to examining the needs, gaps in service, and resources of a community—including policies, systems, the environment, barriers, needs/problems, etc.—to identify areas for improvement. After the assessment, communities can create a plan or intervention for health improvement by creating strategies to make positive, sustainable changes (Centers for Disease Control and Prevention, 2013).

On the island of Maui, CHW Chasity Cadaoas of Maui AIDS Foundation describes a project CHWs helped conceptualize that serves incarcerated community members, which included assessing the needs of a particular community:

> The Hepatitis C Virus (HCV), a "silent epidemic," for over a decade has infected numerous people, unaware of their status, who have gone unrecognized and/or untreated for years. HCV affects the liver and, if left untreated, can lead to liver damage and swelling, cancer, and death. Hawai'i has the highest rates of liver cancer in the U.S. due to Hepatitis B and C. Incarcerated persons have a much higher risk than the general population for HCV, partly because 16% of U.S. State prisoners are serving for drug offenses—which drug abuse is a risk factor for HCV. In Hawai'i, substance abuse has affected an estimated 80% of our prisoners.
>
> As a non-profit organization centered on promoting sexual health and well-being to all members of our community, the Maui AIDS Foundation (MAF) along with Hawai'i's Department of Health (DOH) and CHWs, conducted an assessment. Assessment results suggested MAF's HIV and Hepatitis-C educational and testing services could positively impact our incarcerated population. MAF drafted a project proposal and received a grant to plan and implement the program.
>
> CHWs play a vital role in the planning and implementation of programs such as MAF's Corrections Project. During the planning process, along with MAF's administrators and finance department, Maui Community Correction Center's (MCCC) Warden, Programs Director and Clinical Administrator, an experienced CHW facilitated groups in correctional settings to help establish a feasible program. The wealth of knowledge and insight gained by having a CHW highly engaged in this process brought a different perspective to the table and fostered a better understanding of the setting and target population. The vision of this program at its beginning looked much differently after planning, due in large part to the insights and ideas of the CHW. The end result of the planning process tentatively, became, a 3-part series: Day 1: HIV/HCV Education and Inmate medical request; Day 2: HIV/HCV Rapid Testing; Day 3: Results and individual counselling (format depended on the number of participants and test results).
>
> Once we had our action plan, MAF hired a CHW to develop, coordinate, and implement the program. Due to the uniqueness of this program, MAF knew we needed to find a non-judgmental member from the Maui community that could relate to this population, assess clients' needs, and deliver information to large groups. Once we found the right fit, the next part of the process consisted of creating a simple educational presentation for inmates to understand, a risk-assessment intake form, program assessment forms and other documents evaluate the success of the program.
>
> Since the program's initial start in March 2018 at MCCC, MAF has successfully met the goals of its Corrections Project. In four months, the project educated 56 inmates of MCCC (males and females) and tested 40 of those for HIV and Hepatitis C—with a return of 10 positive results for Hepatitis C. Due to the non-judgmental and easy nature of the CHW, after asking what was liked most about the class, one inmate stated, "Information. No shame- could ask any question."
>
> The workings of a CHW can be very complex. CHWs need to have the ability to wear different hats, be resourceful, and be able to adjust quickly to both the needs of their community and the environment. One of the challenges presented to the CHW of MAF's Corrections Project is the lack of a classroom setting and not knowing where she/he would be teaching a class. Since starting, the education piece of this program occurred in a dorm setting, which can create many obstacles for a facilitator. The dorm setting is often noisy, distracting with inmates and guards coming-and-going, and lacks classroom tools such as

a board to write on. In order to overcome some of these obstacles, our CHW coordinated with MCCC to ensure adequate supplies such as a dry-erase board to conduct class. This CHW also kept the audience engaged, focused, and on track through interactive educational presentations. The capability of a CHW to assess his/her clients' needs through observation, empathy and awareness of potential program barriers, and possessing the skills and resourcefulness to overcome barriers is a unique strength of CHWs.

CHWs remain critical to the process of assessing, planning, and implementing programs meant to make positive impacts on communities. The information and vision they can provide is priceless. The success of MAF's Corrections Project is the result of our CHW's passion and the need of services in MCCC. "I can learn information that can help me in the future so I can prevent getting HIV/Hep-C," said an MCCC inmate participating in MAF's Corrections Project.

—Chasity Cadaoas, CHW and Director of Education and Prevention,
Maui AIDS Foundation

This example highlights the key role CHWs played in first assessing the needs of the broader community related to HCV, which identified the need to provide HIV and Hepatitis-C educational and testing services for incarcerated populations. CHWs actively participated in the development of the project and served as the facilitator/trainer in the project. To meet the incarcerated community's needs, the CHW conducted group sessions and used motivational interviewing to assess their collective needs and potential solutions, which the program then addressed through tailored education and testing. A key principle of assessment here is that CHWs have the capability of a CHW to assess community needs through observation, empathy, and awareness of potential barriers, which they then help mitigate through resourcefulness and a multitude of other skills including communication, organization, and interpersonal skills.

12.2.5.1 Utilizing Assessment Results to Meet Client Needs

Another exciting project highlights the crucial role CHWs play in assessing and understanding community needs within their service area. A 14-year veteran CHW from Kaua'i's community health center, Ho'ola Lahui Hawai'i, describes a unique approach to identifying a community-wide need and then addressing that need through collaboration. Here's June's story about how they met their clients' needs after assessing the needs in the community:

On the island of Kauai, we set up regular community outreach locations where we piggy back on existing food pantries. These established sites spread throughout the community serve a wide range of individuals and families from kupuna to keiki (older adults to children), veterans, disabled and the homeless. We assist clients in filling out SNAP and Medquest medical applications—which fits well in serving our community. Local churches host these pantries around the island, from Kekaha to Hanalei; the churches welcome our outreach efforts and provide us with needed tables and chairs. In addition to applications and business cards, we distribute information about our Federally Qualified Community Health Centers and other current health programs and activities on Kaua'i.

We have found that having regular outreach makes everyone more comfortable and approachable and helps build trust, which allows us as CHWS to work best to address our clients' needs. We expand outreach by inviting other community partners to join us, such as

Agency on Elderly Affairs, Project Vision (providing vision screens/glasses); Child and Family Services; Public Health Nursing with the Department of Health (conducting free blood pressure checks); Wilcox Hospital (providing flu immunizations); Legal Aid; Catholic Charities; and others when available. This gives those attending the pantries access to other services and makes for stronger community building. Along with our partners, we have also set up Community Resource Fairs in our local housing communities on Kaua'I, like Lihue Court Townhomes, Kaniko'o Elderly Housing and Hanapepe Salvation Army. All our activities come from assessing our community's needs.

We love our island home, and building stronger communities is possible when we all can reach out, connect, and work together with one another … aloha is the key!

—June Munoz, CHW, Ho'ola Lahui, Kaua'i

Next, a CHW from Kaua'i shares her personal experiences with individual assessment and how she applied the results from assessing clients' needs to create action plans to improve their health and well-being:

On March 5, 2018, I received a call from Lihue Medicaid office asking if our (HLH) west side case manager could assist someone in reapplying for Medicaid. His Medicaid was terminated in February because his mail was returned. He is homeless, wheel-chair bound, receiving dialysis treatment, and is physically unable to check his general delivery mail on a timely basis. I knew who this person was by the description because we visited him occasionally at the beach park.

Unfortunately, our west side case manager was unavailable, so I drove to Waimea and completed his application at West Kauai Dialysis. I was concerned about this recurring situation and asked if he could use another mailing address, and he said no. I had an 'Aha!' moment. An awesome homeless advocate allows some clients use her personal post office box. A call was made (she was on vacation), we explained this person's situation, she kindly allowed us to use her mailing address, and his Medicaid was reinstated within 3 days!

Here's another story:

Imagine being told you have colon cancer. Now, imagine being told you have colon cancer with metastasis and being houseless. As CHWs, we have the opportunity to meet the community where they gather, such as food pantries and community lunches. United Church of Christ in Hanapepe serves a weekly lunch (healthy, hot, homemade) for their entire community–not just the homeless. We sit, eat, and share stories with this community on a weekly basis and have established a unique rapport and trust. At this luncheon, I had the pleasure of meeting a humble, soft-spoken Hawaiian gentleman. He shared his hanabata (childhood) stories of growing up on the west side of Kauai and his life experiences, which included not seeing a physician.

One day, he told me he was having pain and asked for help in re-establishing care with Ho'ola Lahui Hawaii health center. After many weeks of tests, he received the diagnosis: Stage IV colon cancer. The noisy church hall seemed to go silent, and the world stopped for a moment as I experienced a flashback from hearing my own cancer diagnosis. As I shared my story, his eyes lit up; he had someone who understood what he was going through.

I helped him connect to other resources. Most importantly, he finally accepted housing through HUD-VASH (a program for homeless veterans) because he needed a clean and safe place while hooked up to a chemo pump. Another CHW sewed curtains for his place. He even invited me to walk the survivor's lap at Relay for Life, which I gladly accepted. However, as his cancer metastasized, he refused more chemo and eventually went into hospice. We visited him one last time at the hospital before his passing in December 2017.

—Susan Oshiro-Taogoshi, Ho'ola Lahui

These stories emphasize the importance of going beyond assessment—which is the first step. CHWs then work collaboratively to identify and/or create solutions to address identified needs. When CHWs identify a need, they work together to come up with creative solutions. In June's story, CHWs identified the need in their community for residents to access several types of health and social services at one time, at one location. Their solution to this need was outreach locations that capitalized on existing food pantries. In Susan's first story, after she assessed the barrier of a lack of a mailing address that resulted in the cancellation of Medicaid benefits, she worked to find a solution, which included drawing on her social networks and resources. In Susan's second story, she described how she helped meet identified needs of a homeless veteran with stage IV cancer. She shared her personal experience with cancer via motivational interviewing techniques to encourage the client to accept help, and she continued to assist him through the end of this battle with cancer. The applicable lesson here is to take assessment findings and work with others within the community to find solutions: *Aloha* is the key!

12.2.6   *Conclusion*

CHWs in Hawai'i join their colleagues across the United States and around the world in providing excellent, dedicated services to their communities. CHWs employ their unique perspective as being firmly based on their communities while working in the public health system to participate in community assessments as well as conducting individual assessments. As so eloquently shared by several members of our CHW community in Hawai'i, CHWs have unique qualities and skills that equip them to assess both individual and community needs—which is often the first step in improving health status. This section discussed different types of individual assessments, including barriers, health needs, psychosocial needs, social determinants, financial status and need, eligibility requirements, language and communication needs, and cultural norms/values. Further, the section highlights community assessments, which involve the identification of needs, gaps, and resources with the end goal to create a plan or intervention to improve community health. Additionally, the section described various types of assessment methods, such as motivational interviewing; need identification and prioritization; assessment tools (surveys, checklists, forms); screening tools; guided discussions; and focus groups. Lastly, the CHWs shared the qualities and skills needed to assess individual and community needs; a few include self-assessment; establishing rapport and building relationships; empathy; trust; active listening; ability to put people at ease; clear communication; a non-judgmental spirit; and *me ka mahalo 'ana kekahi i kekahi* (valuing each other).

Some of our lessons learned and recommendations for conducting assessments include:

- Consider when this type of work sometimes occurs (depending on clients' availability), and offer flexibility in work schedules and locations.
- Provide extensive training so that CHWs can confidently carry out the assessment role (including activities learning techniques, role play, participant observation, etc.).
- Gain buy-in from your entire team to engage CHWs in this role (including CHWs, supervisors, support staff, primary care providers, and administrators).
- Equip supervisors with the skills to effectively support CHWs in doing assessments.
- Allow CHWs the freedom and flexibility to make decisions in the field.
- Allow your mission and vision to drive your assessment practices.
- Respect and value the perspectives CHWs bring to the table—particularly in regard to individual and community assessment.

In closing, we leave you with these words of wisdom from the kupuna (elders and ancestors) of Hawaiʻi that our CHWs reflect and strive to fulfill in their work and in life.

E hele me ka puʻolo
(Make every person, place, or condition better than you left it)

Hoʻohanohano
(To honor the dignity of others, conduct yourself with distinction and cultivate respectfulness)

E ʻopu aliʻi
(Have the heart of a chief—the kindness, generosity, and even temperedness of a chief)

E kuahui like i ka hana
(Let everybody pitch in and work together)

References

Centers for Disease Control and Prevention. (2013). *Community needs assessment*. Atlanta, GA: Centers for Disease Control and Prevention.

Hawaiʻi Appleseed Center for Law and Economic Justice. (2019, April 16). *The effects of boosting Hawaii's minimum wage*. Hawaiʻi Appleseed Center for Law and Economic Justice. Retrieved from https://hiappleseed.org/wp-content/uploads/2019/04/17-by-2024-press-release-4-16-19.pdf.

Hawaiʻi Health Matters. (2014–2018). Demographics dashboard. *Hawaiʻi health matters*. Retrieved from http://www.hawaiihealthmatters.org/indicators/index/dashboard?alias=demographics.

Kaholokula, J. K., Okamoto, S. K., & Yee, B. W. K. (2019). Special issue introduction: Advancing native Hawaiian and other Pacific islander health. *Asian American Journal of Psychology, 10*(4), 306–306. https://doi.org/10.1037/aap0000170

Mokuau, N., DeLeon, P. H., Kaholokula, J. K., Soares, S., Tsark, J. U., & Haia, C. (2016). *Challenges and promise of health equity for native Hawaiians. Discussion Paper* (p. 6). Washington, DC: National Academy of Medicine.

Office of Disease Prevention and Health Promotion, HRSA. (2020a, May 27). *Access to health services*. Retrieved from HealthyPeople.gov: https://www.healthypeople.gov/2020/topics-objectives/topic/Access-to-Health-Services.

Office of Disease Prevention and Health Promotion, HRSA. (2020b, May 27). *Social determinants of health*. Retrieved from HealthyPeople.gov: https://www.healthypeople.gov/2020/topics-objectives/topic/social-determinants-of-health.

Puku'i, M. K. (1983). *'Olelo No'eau: Hawaiian proverbs & poetical sayings*. Honolulu, Hawai'i: Bishop Museum Press.

Smith, S. A. (2008). Chuukese patients, dual role interpreters, and confidentiality: Exploring clinic interpretation services for reproductive health patients. *Hawai'i Journal of Medicine & Public Health: A Journal of Asia Pacific Medicine & Public Health, 77*, 83–88.

Spock, R. N. (2013). *Evaluation summary from a CHW meeting on Hawai'i Island*. Hawai'i Primary Care Association. Unpublished report.

Spock, R. N. (2016). *Personal notes from CHW focus group discussions on "essential qualities of a CHW," held on Hawai'i, Maui, O'ahu, and Kaua'i*. Hawai'i Primary Care Association. Unpublished.

U.S. Department of Health & Human Services. (n.d.). *Think Cultural Health: Culturally and Linguistically Appropriate Services (CLAS)*. Retrieved from U.S. Department of Health & Human Services: https://thinkculturalhealth.hhs.gov/clas/what-is-clas.

United States Census Bureau. (2019, July 1). *QuickFacts, Hawaii*. Retrieved from United States Census Bureau: https://www.census.gov/quickfacts/HI.

12.3   Assessments: More Than a Piece of Paper[2]

Dominique Lucas, Wes Warner, Melanie Apodaca, Roshni Biswa,
Deborah White, Rebecca Anderson, and Dennis Dunmyer

KC CARE Health Center (KC CARE) is a Federally Qualified Health Center in the urban core of Kansas City, Missouri. Serving the community since 1971, KC CARE is formerly the Kansas City Free Health Clinic. KC CARE began employing community health workers (CHWs) over 15 years ago in a peer support model for individuals living with HIV. In 2011, KC CARE started deploying CHWs to coordinate the care of patients with chronic conditions and with social barriers to health. KC CARE CHWs complete a CHW curriculum endorsed by the Missouri Department of Health and Senior Services.

Today, CHWs at KC CARE work with patients of the health center and many people in the community that do not have a regular source of medical care. KC CARE CHW clients come from many different communities within the Kansas City region. Some KC CARE CHWs are embedded with our primary care delivery team, and some are embedded on-site at partner organizations, such as hospitals, clinics, and other faith- and community-based organizations.

Based on a client-centered care planning system, KC CARE adopted a locally modified version of the Arizona Self-Sufficiency Matrix (ASSM). CHWs use this tool to assess their clients along a continuum of self-sufficiency in 14 life domains. The results of this assessment drive the goals of a care plan that is developed to guide the work of the CHW with each client. Working with Intraprise Health, an innovative patient engagement and care coordination technology, KC CARE embedded this assessment into the Care Navigator™ database to increase efficiency to drive care planning, documentation, workflow management, and referral coordination.

CHWs bring a unique perspective to a healthcare team because of their connection to the community. This shared life experience helps CHWs build rapport with clients where other healthcare professionals may struggle to build this level of trusting relationship. This unique ability of CHWs plays itself out in the assessment process where we see CHWs able to gain knowledge of clients and their life circumstances that adds to the care team's ability to serve those clients. In adopting the ASSM, KC CARE created a standard tool and workflow for CHWs to assess their clients. This helps to ensure that CHWs gather a similar set of data for care planning and for quality management. Nevertheless, a few years down the road from adopting the ASSM, each CHW obviously still brings his/her own personal perspective to the assessment process and builds rapport in his/her own way, despite this standard protocol. KC CARE has found that this tool creates a framework for CHWs to leverage their strength in knowing the community to create workable and realistic goals for each client. Despite the standard questions in the tool, CHWs ask intuitive

---

[2] With contribution by Tom Miras Neira, KC CARE Health Center, Kansas City, MO, USA

questions based on their experience and their life experience that might not appear on the tool. What follows are five examples of how this manifests in daily practice of KC CARE CHWs.

12.3.1   Similar Interests

My name is Dominique Lucas, and I am a 26-year-old Black American woman. I am a CHW who works in the Emergency Department (ED) of a hospital system. I meet with patients in the ED that are uninsured and not established in primary care. My role is to assist and empower clients to navigate the health and social service systems for follow-up care. The ED visit is my first but not my last encounter with clients; I meet them at home or at a public space in the community. Before I enroll clients into the program, I complete an assessment to determine their needs and establish goals to work on. Once enrolled in the program, these clients have a list of mutually agreed upon goals to improve their health and overall well-being.

Ashley,[3] a 52-year-old Caucasian woman, came to the ED for a severe migraine and chest pains. She was uninsured, unemployed, and not established in primary care. Ashley was feeling overwhelmed from taking care of everyone else. She recently lost her grandmother. Soon after, her daughter was admitted to the hospital for GI issues. When I assessed her for mental health needs, Ashley reported that she struggles with anxiety and asked for assistance with finding free or affordable yoga and meditation centers—not the doctor-recommended solution. Ashley did not want to use medication, which is something that I could relate to. We talked about how she copes with her stress, and Ashley reported that she watches yoga and meditation demonstration videos on YouTube and listens to ambient music to calm her racing thoughts. I suggested that Ashley continue to do what is working for her and gave Ashley a list of community mental health resources for meditation and mindfulness. In addition, while in the ED, I attempted to discuss establishing primary care, but Ashley wanted to wait until her daughter was out of the hospital.

I met with Ashley at a home she shares with a friend. During this visit, I continued to assess Ashley's mental health and initiated another conversation about stress management and good sleep. Ashley shared that she learned and practiced home remedies passed down in her family for self-healing, but since her grandmother's passing, she did not have the motivation or the guidance to do these practices. She wanted to get better and feel better, but she preferred natural medicines over Western or conventional medicines and treatments. I shared with Ashley that there was a possibility she could use herbal medicines in conjunction with prescribed medicine, if she had a conversation with a medical provider. Ashley had a light bulb moment: she did not know she could talk about herbal remedies with a doctor. Ashley thought

---

[3] With the exception of the authors' names, all other names have been changed to protect privacy and confidentiality.

most doctors "in white coats" frowned upon herbal medicines and non-conventional treatments. I could tell Ashley was opening up to me as I reinforced her values and beliefs, allowing me to help her navigate the health system in a way that aligned with those values.

Ashley was able to accomplish many goals during our time together. She attended two appointments with her new primary care physician who is treating Ashley for fibromyalgia and severe migraines, enrolled in therapy and counseling for anxiety and depression, completed the Social Security Administration physical and mental health evaluations for disability benefits, and self-reported improvement in overall health and well-being.

Before clients are enrolled in the program, I assess their needs and interest in receiving assistance from a community health worker. Before engaging with a client, I review his or her charts in the hospital electronic medical record to see if a primary care physician is listed and for history of recent visits. I check demographic information to see what part of town the client resides in so I have an idea of what resources are available to him or her. I assess clients using the ASSM assessment tool that identifies medical needs, social needs, and other barriers. While I use the assessment tool, I assess for the client's motivation and capacity to complete his or her goals through motivational interviewing. I communicate to the client that his or her involvement in the CHW program is a partnership and that while I will assist him or her, he or she is ultimately responsible to achieve his or her goals.

Every time I enroll a new client, I am reminded of why I am a CHW. Because of shared experiences with those I serve, I am able to relate to my clients and make an impact that others cannot. The eldest of 4 girls and eldest of 15 grandchildren, I was raised by my parents, my grandmother, and my aunts in a multifamily household. From my grandmother, I learned how to take care of my health with home remedies and herbal teas and the importance of caring for others. With the exception of food and seasonal allergies, as a child I rarely ever got sick, so when I was diagnosed with asthma and more severe allergies, I was afraid of the treatment. Like Ashley, I, too, struggled with anxiety and depression on at least two occasions. This occurred when I felt overwhelmed and unable to find my voice and independence from my family because I believed I needed to take care of everyone and be everything to everyone. Seeking counseling took time due to stigma and fear of my family's response. In my community, fear and distrust in the health system is prevalent and frequently a reason many do not go to primary care or seek help from mental health services. I always keep this in mind as I am assessing clients.

What makes CHWs the relatable and trusted individuals they are is the fact that CHWs are aware of the challenges and barriers within individuals through past experiences and trauma. CHWs are best at pulling from their own experience to better assist with navigation of these systems. As a result, their assessments are like gold because they hold evidence other care team members are not always able to capture.

12.3.1.1   Building Trust (Wes Warner)

The work I do fills my days with purpose. My work is funded by a Centers for Disease Control and Prevention (CDC) grant called the High Impact Men's Movement (HIMM) Project implemented in Kansas City, Missouri. This grant allows me the opportunity to work with HIV-negative males to access Pre-exposure Prophylaxis (PrEP), a daily pill to reduce their risk of contracting HIV.

As a KC CARE CHW, I conduct an assessment with clients to identify what their concerns are and we set SMART goals to accomplish them. I strive to meet my clients where they are and listen to their story. We discuss a range of topics with sexual history being an important focus, so it is vital to establish trust. The importance of being able to relate to the client cannot be understated. Utilizing the "SMART" (Specific, Measurable, Attainable, Relevant, and Timely) goals is one way to help ensure client success. Once we have identified a goal to work on, we begin the process of completing the SMART worksheet. I believe that for many clients, the act of writing the goal out and seeing how to accomplish the goal helps them to succeed.

Nick attended an HIV testing/outreach event at a local bar. During this event, he indicated that he would like someone to contact him about PrEP. I called him and explained what I do as a CHW and set up a time to meet him to complete the ASSM. I prefer to meet my clients in person and conduct the assessment using a conversational style. This helps in setting ground rules and boundaries. This is an important part of connecting and establishing trust with your client; they need to know program expectations to be a successful self-sufficient graduate.

Our conversation covered a range of topics, and I was able to highlight a few areas of concern. We discussed setting goals, and he picked three: PrEP access, dental care, and mental health. We briefly discussed available resources for mental health services and how to enroll. Nick was hesitant to access mental health services and asked for general information on KC CARE clinic services. Providing resources and letting clients know when they are ready to work on a goal is important.

A week later Nick reached out to me via text message stating that he ranked "8" out of "10" on a scale of 1–10 for depressive suicidal thoughts. I called my client and spoke with him about his text. I learned during our conversation that he did not intend to act on his suicidal thoughts. I connected Nick with a counselor who further assessed his suicidal thoughts and set him up for long-term counseling. I worked with Nick for a few more months to accomplish the other goals he set. The use of SMART goals to frame what he wanted to accomplish was beneficial for him in the long run. This allowed him to make his goals manageable and enforced that he is ultimately in control.

Nick graduated from the program after accomplishing several of his goals. Once a client leaves the program, he/she has the option to enroll again in the future, but you hope the client does not need you again. Nick was out of the program for the better part of a year. Then 1 day, he sent me a text stating that he was not in a good place. I called him. I learned Nick was skipping his therapy appointments due to cost, felt like a burden to friends, self-imposed himself in isolation, and was not happy with who he was. Nick did not mention the last three statements explicitly, but I was able to infer that from our conversation. He had mentioned never speaking to others about his problems because others come to him with theirs'. He does not feel it is right to do that to them. He also referenced numerous times that you cannot put "lipstick on a pig" and how he does not get invited to parties anymore. Those last two sentences got me thinking. Being gay is hard enough with the world around you turning their back on you, but add to that the pressure to live up to unrealistic ideals in your community and you are destined to fail.

I have some insight into these unrealistic ideals of body image and what that does to you. I used my personal experience to hear what Nick was *not* saying. I had an idea as to what was going on, but first I needed to ensure Nick was able to access care, or he was not going to get better. The next day I spoke with a financial counselor about Nick, and by that afternoon, he was on a payment plan that he could afford for an extended period of time.

I met with his therapist to discuss him reaching out to me after so many months and my concern that he had not disclosed to her what he had to me. I translated to her what his issue was—summer time and in gay culture that means your body needs to be perfect for pool parties and being shirtless. Those that are not able to reach their cultural "ideal" image only see the impact of their failure staring right back at them every time they look into a mirror. His counselor said he had avoided discussing body image in the past, and they had been discussing other things before he stopped coming to his appointments.

Being a part of my client's community helped me to identify something that his counselor was not able to see. This partnership with your client is an opportunity to lift up another person. Your clients need someone in their life to be there for them, tell them they can do it, and show them ways to accomplish the goals they set so they are successful. This is something I do as a CHW to positively impact my client's life.

12.3.1.2   Older and Wiser (Melanie Apodaca)

My name is Melanie Apodaca. As a CHW, I work with older adults. My referrals come from a regional agency funded through the Department of Aging.

When I meet clients for the first time, I often start by just talking to them, asking questions, and building trust, because in the long term, this will allow me to assist them in better ways. If I were to go straight into the assessment without building a bond, I would not get as much information from the client. The assessment I use consists of 14 domains; once we have discussed all 14 domains, the assessment is over. That is when the client and I determine on what goals to work. Most of the clients I serve have Medicare. When performing the assessment, normally I ask the question: "What type of Medicare do you have?" If the patient is not on Medicare, then we discuss and explore insurance options. During the formal assessment, the most frequent needs for the older adult population are medication cost, medication management, and household management.

During and after the initial meeting, besides assessing our clients, we also visit their homes. A visual home assessment gives the CHW a better perception of living conditions and barriers. While performing the home visit, we check on the condition of the home—is the home clean and safe, do they have stairs, how does the client navigate the home, are clients hoarding, etc. Understanding their daily life can provide a deeper knowledge of the barriers to health and how to better address them.

As a CHW for older adults, considering that their habits and routine have existed for a long time is important, and therefore, we must empathize and relate to them. We need to meet them where they are at and listen in a non-judgmental way. We must also have a humble attitude and not come in and try to save the day. We need to assist our clients to set up goals that are achievable. Luckily, connecting older adults to resources can be easier than other populations; there are social structures set up from which they can benefit. Knowing the most up-to-date senior resources in the community is vital in assisting the older adult population. Things like senior centers, programs for home repair, home-delivered meals, adult day care programs, senior housing, and transportation are necessary. Being able to network and have quick access to these programs is helpful.

In addition to having a visual assessment of the home, information about the client's family structure can put the whole puzzle of the situation together. Assessing family structure can give the CHW insight on how the older adult is supported, if at all. It can also give understanding to challenges and personality characteristics that may have been barriers to having family involved.

As with most populations, continued reassessment and follow-up is vital as the relationship with the client strengthens. Here is an example: Jane had been admitted to the hospital in a diabetic coma. I met her bedside and started a conversation with her to see what brought her into the hospital. I waited until the client felt more comfortable to perform the assessment. We initially talked about how she was unaware that her sugar levels were out of control, and she could not see her primary care physician because of an outstanding balance. We also spoke about the life-changing event of her son being killed on Super Bowl night in a car accident and how traumatic this event was for her. The son left behind six children and was the patriarch of the family structure. The grief from the loss of her son had been gradually debilitating, leaving Jane in a deep depression that led to her leaving her job and going on disability. The depression and disability resulted in a strained financial situation, which cascaded into the uncontrolled diabetes and, ultimately, the diabetic coma. She also indicated at our initial meeting that she had visited a counselor for grief, but that it was no longer helpful. At this point in our meeting, I had an idea of what her goals would be without even performing the formal assessment. I went on to complete the formal assessment, which also revealed an issue with her bank, a need for dentistry, need for mental health services of a different type, and a new primary care physician.

Of note, we know CHWs do not work in isolation and are part of a larger care team; another support she had was the social worker at the hospital who applied for Medicaid and food stamps for Jane. When Jane left the hospital, she was connected with home health care and set up with a new primary care physician. I was able to follow up with her about the bank issue during our next home visit and make a plan to decide how to move forward. We were also able to start the conversation about grief support groups and possibly a therapist. We also visited the farmer's market, to demonstrate the Double Your Bucks program for food stamp recipients.

After some time, I was able to come back around to the need for some grief support. At this point after a conversation with Jane, she agreed that it was essential for her to receive counseling. I was able to connect her with a community center for older adults with a variety of services. Jane attended a grief support group which not only provided Jane the support and encouragement she needed but also gave her a new group of friends to socialize with outside of the center. Jane has also connected with a social worker at this center who was able to help her with utility bills and taxes. This social worker has become a secondary case manager for Jane.

At this point, I thought the time might have come to graduate Jane, but this has not been the case. Jane has struggled with food instability, issues with her property owner, family relationship issues, and problems with transportation. All this emerged from our ongoing home visits and phone calls. Despite all these emerging issues, Jane continues to be empowered, and she is still working toward positive goals, like getting a part-time job and a more affordable place to live.

Working with older adults is a matter of learning to recognize the small successes, whether it be affording medications or making new friends, and also being able to encourage them when dealing with big challenges and guiding them on how to overcome those barriers. Empowering someone in the final years of life is very rewarding.

12.3.1.3 Madam (Roshni Biswa)

My name is Roshni Biswa; I am 26 years old, born and raised in Nepal. I grew up in a missionary family surrounded by love, support, and respect. I received my education in India, where I learned discipline and core values. Being raised in a refugee camp and not knowing how life could be out of the camp made me become a strong and powerful person. Despite the political environment, I always wanted to assist and advocate for those who could not speak for or help themselves.

On June 11, 2009, we received an opportunity to move to the United States. We considered ourselves fortunate because many families did not have this privilege. I was 17 years old when we arrived in Kansas City, Kansas, to a world that we were not familiar with. Like other refugees that moved to another country, learning, adapting, and moving forward in a new country was very challenging. As new arrivals, we struggled to comprehend new health and social systems. Language, culture, and transportation were some of the barriers with which we dealt. As the time went by, we became our own advocates, and once ready, we advocated for the new refugees going through a similar process. The more I saw my community thrive, the more motivated I was to become a CHW. I felt like I was a lighthouse for those who needed guidance and a touchstone for those who needed reassurance.

As a CHW, I use my knowledge, my expertise, and relatability to bridge the cultural gap between the refugee community and the health and social systems in a caring, passionate, and structured way. I connect my clients to resources and accompany them in the community to medical visits or governmental offices appointments. This is because they mirror themselves in me that I am able to relate to them, build trust, and find out the needs they have, even the unspoken ones they do not verbalize.

One of my long-term clients is a Nepali woman who moved to Kansas City from Houston 2 years ago. The client was referred to me after being seen at an Emergency Room because of her frequent high blood sugar levels. When she answered my first phone call, I could sense her fear and concerns, as I had similar experiences every time I got a phone call when I first arrived in the United States. All her feelings promptly went away when she heard me talking in Nepali. I was able to hear a smile in her voice.

I introduced myself as a CHW, and I explained my role and how was I going to help her. I could tell she trusted me. She shared her confusion regarding her ER visit. She knew that something was wrong with her health but didn't know what the next steps were.

During my first home visit, I performed an assessment and discovered the needs that she had. I did not stop there though; I continued to ask further questions because, as a refugee, I knew that some of the needs would not be captured just with the assessment. Only someone who experienced what it means to be a refugee could empathize with the client and ask the right questions. Besides, there is no translation in Nepali for many of the English concepts that we use on our daily basis. However, I was able to use words that convey similar concepts that the assessment was trying come up with. We decided to connect her with a provider who could speak our language and address some issues with her diet. I also accompanied her to a diabetes education class to assist her on learning and retaining the information to manage her diabetes and be compliant with her regimen.

As I kept working with my client, she shared more concerns and needs. She was struggling to follow up with her scheduled appointments because of not being familiar with the area. She was not able to complete all the paper work correctly. I had to address the language barrier and act as an interpreter several times until she understood how to request an interpreter, not only for the medical appointments but also for any other type of appointments. Her facial expression and tone of voice told me that her fears lessened, and she became more comfortable and confident with herself as time went on.

Our next step was to identify and reassess for new tasks and objectives. My client wanted to apply for Child Support, receive assistance with SSI application, and follow up with her doctor regarding medication and other recommendations. She also wanted to develop a prevention plan where an ER visit will not always be necessary when her sugar levels are unbalanced. She was able to accomplish all of these goals. During all this time while working with my client, we have established trust with each other. She continues to call me to thank me, as well as to share some of her emotions and successes with me.

Most of my refugee families see me as a role model, as a mentor, and as a support figure. They feel like I listen carefully to their needs and empathize with them and help them address all the barriers they encounter. Once I build trust with them, they share in a genuine and sincere way what they are really thinking, feeling, and doing. Sometimes they call me "Madam," which is a respectful term in my community that means leader. Hearing all this makes me feel humbled and grateful. I am the light and translator of my people. I assess their needs and help them accomplish their goals, only truly knowing them because I have walked the same path.

12.3.1.4   Busy and Pregnant (Deborah White)

My name is Deborah White. I am over 50 years old. All four of my children are adults and no longer live at home. I work in the city I was born in, and I have never lived anywhere else. I have an affinity for my city.

I work with the pediatric population and their parents. One day a social worker in the specialty clinic called me with a referral. The specialty clinic is where children with special developmental needs are seen.

I was told that there was a mom in the clinic who was pregnant but had not received any prenatal care. The social worker did not know how far along the pregnancy was, but to her estimation, she suspected her to be 8 or perhaps 9 months along. The social worker told me that when she tried talking to her about the pregnancy, she became evasive and elusive. I had to figure out how to broach what was obviously a delicate subject with a perfect stranger.

After receiving the referral, I called the mom on the phone explaining who I was and why I was calling. English was not her native language, but we understood each other, and more importantly, I had not offended by calling about such a delicate matter, so she talked to me. She mentioned that she had no idea how far along she was in her pregnancy but thought perhaps the end of 8 months, or maybe even 9 as she had been having contractions for the last few days.

This was her fourth child. Her eldest son had many special needs, and she was "too busy with him," to focus on herself. So I asked her, "If something happened to you and someone else had to take care of your children, would they do as well as you?" She was quiet on the phone. We continued the conversation, and I learned some details to provide the clinic when I called to get her prenatal care before delivery of the baby.

Upon calling the prenatal unit at the hospital where she had her two youngest children, they gave me unorthodox advice to pass on to her. They wanted her to come to the Emergency Room as soon as possible, as that would be the most expedient way to get services going. It seemed that this mother's circumstance was not a rarity.

I called her back and told her to meet me in the ER ASAP. I went there and waited, but she never showed up. When I called her afterward, she mentioned that she had to get her son off the bus, but she promised she would go once dinner was done, the children were fed, and all her duties were done. "OK" I told her. "Can I call you tomorrow morning to see how it turned out?" I did not want to push too far or too hard, because I was afraid she would not engage with me.

The next morning, I called her. She had gone to the ER as promised, and they were going to take care of her. She had seen a social worker in the ER, she was going to get Medicaid for expectant mothers, and the baby would be covered when he/she was born. This opened the door for me to ask her about insurance. Her other children already had Medicaid. Her husband worked full time, but the insurance was so high they could not afford insurance for him or her. The social worker who referred the client to me had given me a case of powdered milk to give to this family, and I offered to take the milk to the family. After asking my client, she told me I could bring the powdered milk "today."

Upon stepping on the porch, I noticed a pile of shoes pushed to one side. I had worn easy slip-on sandals that day. The mother opened the door; I kicked my sandals off and to the side as if I was a guest in their home. I handed her father the case of milk, walked in the house stepping over toys and two teen girls laying close together on a couch pull out bed and sat down at the kitchen table to talk. The young pregnant mother sweetly introduced me to the teenage girls who turned out to be her sisters. Her two small children introduced themselves to me by climbing unto her lap to get her attention as we talked, and I did an assessment of her needs.

I understood her delay in getting prenatal care: she had done this three times and, therefore, she knew the drill. She was also overwhelmed. I watched how attentive and gentle she was with her two children as they climbed in and out of her lap commanding equal attention. I asked her where 'E', her special needs child, was. She told me he was asleep with her husband who worked nights.

While I was at her home, the clinic called to set up her sonogram and doctor's appointment. Without asking, she put them on speakerphone so that I was included in the conversation. They strongly admonished her not to miss a single appointment. I was the amen corner to the woman on the phone from the hospital setting up her maternity care.

After the call, we continued the assessment. The mom was resourceful. She knew about WIC. Her other children were on WIC already. She was going to get on it herself at the kids' next appointment. When I asked about food insecurities, she hesitated. She knew they could not get food stamps as their income made them ineligible. I mentioned pantries. Her face and body said, "No." So I told her about mobile food pantries that supply fresh produce. She liked that better, and I instantly supplied her with a list of their drop sites and times. I finished the assessment and stood up to leave. Her father came back through the living room, and this time his wife accompanied him. They were struggling to carry a large piece of furniture through the house and up the steps leading to the second story. I looked at the multitasking teen girls who did not move to get up and help. "Y'all need help?" I asked out of habit more than anything else. They stopped and looked at me. The father, who I had mistaken for her husband when I entered the house, smiled at me. By making the mistake of asking if this were her husband, I was already in his good graces. He was ageless. He told me that this was his wife. He also told me that they did not need any help with the dresser.

I announced my departure, and the father's eyes traveled down to my pink, orange, green, and white floral skirt and then traveled to the skirt his wife was wearing and announced, "That is the kind of skirt our people wear." His wife's skirt was floral as well. I was wearing a skirt I rarely wore. It made my bigness look even bigger, but this morning for no reason my rational mind could think of, I wore it. "I am your people" I told him. The father smiled; his wife seemed a little embarrassed. I wanted to hug the mother when we got to the front door. I told her she was doing an amazing job. And, I could relate to this mother: I was 6-month pregnant when I started prenatal care with my last child. This mom only needed a nudge to get her to shift courses and include prenatal care in her busy life.

12.3.2 Conclusion

KC CARE, like many other health centers, benefits from assessment tools like the ASSM. Our CHWs are able to use the ASSM as a way to understand the needs of clients and help them create goals that are Specific, Measurable, Attainable, Relevant, and Timely. Upon referral, this assessment can give others on the care plan team a formal understanding of a client as well. The ASSM is a snapshot of a client's life that has proven to be valuable, especially to CHWs. Many times, however, assessment for CHWs is much more than just the questions on the paper. Assessment is learning what interests and background a client has. It is observing their home's condition and understanding their domestic, familial, and personal relationships. It is listening to a client and understanding where his or her motivation derives from. Through this informal assessment, CHWs form a better understanding of their clients and open a window for successful partnership.

Informal assessment alone does not produce outcome. Other characteristics of the CHWs are key to improving their work with clients. CHWs' relatability enables them to form a trust that positively drives clients to work on SMART goals and stay committed to the CHW program. The CHWs with KC CARE show an empathy that their clients appreciate and makes them feel that they are not alone. CHWs use their understanding of clients and their situations to empower and encourage them, leading them to self-efficacy. Because CHWs are from the community, they have a knowledge of resources in their clients' neighborhoods. CHWs then provide their clients with that knowledge leading them to greater independency. The time a CHW takes to work with a single client varies. Some clients can complete a number of goals in just a couple months; others are in delicate situations or have pasts with trauma that call for an increased duration of time in the program. CHWs are sensitive to such barriers and take the time needed to show clients that they are a true ally, there to provide support and encouragement, even in minor ways. These qualities of

CHWs offer clients an advantageous relationship that help them become healthier and thrive as a whole. Assessment continues even after the first few contacts a CHW has with a client and aides a CHW with perspective on how to effectively present each of these qualities with each of his or her clients. Informal assessment is an ongoing process that gives CHWs the ability to capture what the ASSM could not. Simply, assessment is imperative to maximizing the accomplishment in clients' lives and grows the relationship between CHWs and clients.

Chapter 13
Conducting Outreach

**Caitlin G. Allen*, Gabriela Boscan, Gregory J. Dent, Amy Elizondo,
Catherine Gray Haywood, Gail R. Hirsch, Teresa Mendez, Laura McTighe,
Katharine Nimmons*, Janice Probst, Floribella Redondo-Martinez,
Carl H. Rush, David Secor, Myriam Torres, and Ashley Wennerstrom***

13.1 Introduction

Caitlin G. Allen, Carl H. Rush, Gail R. Hirsch, and Floribella Redondo-Martinez

Conducting outreach includes the following subroles: case finding and recruitment of individuals, families, and community groups to enroll in and utilize services and benefits; follow-up on health and social service encounters; doing home visiting for multiple purposes such as education, assessment, and social support; and making presentations at local agencies and community events. This role was newly introduced during the C3 Project. Participants in C3 were surprised when they recognized that outreach had not previously been described as a top-level role. Earlier assessments of community health worker (CHW) roles may have taken for granted that outreach was part of the very definition of the CHW and therefore did not need to be delineated as a specific role.

Authorship is organized alphabetically in ascending order by surname.

C. G. Allen (✉)
CGA Consulting, Charleston, SC, USA
e-mail: caitlin.gloeckner.allen@emory.edu

G. Boscan · A. Elizondo · D. Secor
National Rural Health Association, Washington, DC, USA

G. J. Dent · T. Mendez
Northwest Georgia Healthcare Partnership, Dalton, GA, USA

C. G. Haywood
Louisiana Community Health Outreach Network, New Orleans, LA, USA

G. R. Hirsch
Massachusetts Department of Public Health, Boston, MA, USA

© Springer Nature Switzerland AG 2021
J. A. St. John et al. (eds.), *Promoting the Health of the Community*,
https://doi.org/10.1007/978-3-030-56375-2_13

Case finding was originally a subrole in 1998 National Community Health Advisor Study.[1] All other subroles under conducting outreach are newly defined. When describing outreach, the roles are diverse and varied, with CHWs working across the range of outreach (from recruitment through individualized post-service follow-up). Increasingly, outreach can be part of the identification of individuals needing further assistance such as care coordination or navigation. This newly recognized diverse and evolving role is an example of the ways that CHWs are continuously engaged with their community. As a new role, conducting outreach will continue to evolve.

The two sections on this role demonstrate concrete methods of CHW outreach, including the importance of building relationships in some foundational CHW work in Louisiana and engaging CHWs and technology to provide more in-depth health education and outreach to promote better health outcomes in a project in rural Georgia.

---

[1] https://crh.arizona.edu/sites/default/files/pdf/publications/CAHsummaryALL.pdf

---

L. McTighe
Department of Religion, Florida State University, Tallahassee, FL, USA

K. Nimmons (✉)
Public Health Sciences Department, Texas A&M College of Dentistry, Dallas, TX, USA
e-mail: knimmons@tamu.edu

J. Probst · M. Torres
University of South Carolina, Columbia, SC, USA

F. Redondo-Martinez
Arizona Community Health Workers Association, Douglas, AZ, USA

C. H. Rush
Community Resources, LLC, San Antonio, TX, USA

A. Wennerstrom (✉)
Department of Behaviorial and Community Health Sciences, LSU School of Public Health;
Center for Healthcare Value and Equity, LSU School of Medicine, LSU Health Sciences
Center New Orleans, New Orleans, LA, USA
e-mail: awenne@lsuhsc.edu

13.2 "You Have to Build a Relationship": Reflections on a CHW's Career of Outreach in Communities of Color

Ashley Wennerstrom, Catherine Gray Haywood, and Laura McTighe

In late Spring 2016, Women With a Vision's (WWAV) co-founders, Catherine Haywood and Danita Muse, gathered with the organization's current staff and board members for a multiday strategic planning retreat. The meeting had a packed agenda: boldly aiming to honor the model of street-based outreach that Catherine and Danita had pioneered in 1989 in some of the darkest days of the AIDS epidemic, and to carry that history forward to the organization's present and future as one of the leading national voices on Black women and criminalization in the South. Critical to realizing that temporal bridge was the training of several new members of WWAV's staff in the methods and principles that grounded the organization's work for nearly three decades.

Catherine had already been working closely with WWAV's newest outreach worker, Raven Frederick. In the short time she had been with WWAV, Raven demonstrated the precision with which she could translate the WWAV mission for different audiences. The challenge now was to apprentice Raven (and others) to the methods of "doing the work."

The conversation had been running for about an hour, bouncing from person to person around a large circle as Catherine, Danita, and several of the more senior WWAV staff pieced together the strength of conviction with which the WWAV foremothers had always moved in and through community. Raven added to the cipher: "But times have changed." After a few minutes, the group circled back to reflect on how WWAV's presence in post-Hurricane Katrina New Orleans compared with its past. The facilitator asked Raven to elaborate on what exactly had changed. "Like, how you say that you could walk through the community and get that respect," Raven offered. "Now you can't do that... And then the communities that you worked with are no longer there. The people are no longer there." Several of the newer staff nodded in agreement, affirming the bitter reality of how nearly 100,000 native New Orleanians—most coming from the communities that Catherine and Danita originally worked with—had been willfully and permanently displaced through policies of organized abandonment after the storm.

Catherine, however, was growing restless. As the consensus surrounding the "new" New Orleans began to build, she interrupted, "You're killing me. I'm sorry. I love you, but you're killing me. The thing says that 'you have to build a relationship regardless.' Once you build that relationship... Me, in the St. Thomas Project? I'd just go out and sit on people's porch. And they'd say 'What you doing here?' And I'd say, 'I'm sitting here, but my name is Catherine and I'm doing this...' At that point, I didn't even try to give them or try to educate them. I just told them what I was doing. And then after a couple of weeks or so, it was good. I could go in, and do what I do. And I think this same thing holds for now... It's not impossible. If you build that relationship, then you're good to go."

In that moment, Catherine not only passed on the method of "doing the work." She also called Raven into a relationship, so that together they could figure out how to use the principles Catherine had developed in the context of street-based harm reduction outreach and adapt them to the current WWAV issues and priorities.

* * *

Catherine Gray Haywood has been a community health worker (CHW) in New Orleans for over 30 years. Although she has had a wide variety of job titles, workplaces, and health areas of interest, her career has always centered on supporting and building the capacity of communities of color to address health and social concerns. Known to her closest friends as "Lady," perhaps Catherine's most defining characteristic is her ability to build complex, trusting relationships across neighborhoods, social classes, and professional sectors. Catherine is undoubtedly the beloved matriarch of her family, often referring to her three children, daughter-in-law, grandchildren, and great grandchildren as simply "my people."

Writing this section without acknowledging the relationship between Catherine and her co-authors is impossible. Catherine first met Laura McTighe, an HIV and anti-prison activist and scholar, in 2009. Laura came to New Orleans to facilitate a coalition meeting surrounding the criminalization of street-based sex work at the invitation of Catherine's eldest daughter, Deon. Shortly thereafter, Laura became a board member of WWAV, a nonprofit organization Catherine co-founded in 1989 (incorporated in 1992) and for which Deon serves as executive director. Laura conducted an extensive ethnographic research project with WWAV over the course of several years, which aimed to document the histories, methods, and practices that have guided the organization's decades-honed work and to excavate the tradition of southern Black women's organizing of which WWAV is a part. In the process, Laura became a member of the extended Haywood family. Ashley Wennerstrom, a university-based public health professional focused on community health, met Catherine in 2010 after conducting a survey of New Orleans CHWs. Catherine attended a community conference at which Ashley presented the results of the study to the participants, and Catherine immediately expressed interest in collaborating on efforts to support the local CHW workforce. The two, with support from Kristina Gibson, Dana Feist, and Renee Jenkins, collaborated to co-found the Louisiana Community Health Outreach Network shortly thereafter. Finally, in 2015, Catherine sent a one-line introductory email to Laura and Ashley suggesting that the two should meet. Unclear on the professional purpose of the meeting but knowing that one does not say "no" to Catherine, both agreed to a lunch date. An initially awkward conversation rapidly turned into the realization that Laura and Ashley had an eerily similar, life-defining experience that few others understood. The two became fast friends, now referring to one another as "chosen family," or "my sister from another mister." When Ashley later asked Catherine whether there had been a particular professional goal for the encounter, Catherine looked at her incredulously and said, "No, I just thought you'd be friends." United by Catherine's unique knack for bringing people together, the authors write this piece collectively as friends, colleagues, confidantes, and proud New Orleanians.

New Orleans, Louisiana, which celebrated its tri-centennial in 2018, is a city racked with beauty and complication. Several confederate monuments, including a statue of Robert E. Lee (Wedland, 2017), have recently been removed, and the first woman mayor, an African American, (Adelson & Williams, 2018) was inaugurated in 2018. An argument could be made that the city has entered into a new era of equality.

However, the vestiges of white supremacy remain. Until this year, Louisiana had the highest rate of incarceration in the world (Prison Policy Initiative, 2018), with a highly disproportionate representation of Black men under state control (Mauer & King, 2007). At the infamous Angola prison, a former slave plantation just 2 h from New Orleans, some incarcerated people are forced to work in the fields for a wage of two cents per hour (Benns, 2015). Voting rights for formerly incarcerated people in Louisiana were only returned in 2018 as a result of advocacy conducted by grass-roots community organizations (Crisp, 2018).

For decades, New Orleans has had the dubious distinction of being a national leader in per capita murder rates, currently falling just behind St. Louis, Baltimore, and Detroit (CBS News, 2018). Discussion about violence became so blasé that in 2007, a local church developed a "murder board" that lists the names of all of the city's murder victims to call attention to their humanity (Kaye & White, 2007). Violent crime has undoubtedly played a role in shaping the chasm between life expectancies in different neighborhood, which range from 55 in Central City, the Seventh Ward, and several other predominantly Black communities to 80 in wealthier, Whiter neighborhoods such as Lakeview (RWJF, 2013). Other social determinants of health also play an enormous role. Racial economic inequality has worsened in recent years (City of New Orleans, 2017). Over a third of renters in New Orleans are considered "rent stressed," paying at least half of their income in rent, and public housing is insufficient to meet the needs of many low-income individuals and families (La Rose, 2016). The public transportation system service is only about half of its pre-Katrina levels, and many low-income communities have long wait times (Ride New Orleans, 2017). Schools remain primarily segregated, with the majority of white families sending their children to private schools, while 85% of public school students are Black (Weixler, Barrett, Harris, & Jennings, 2017).

13.2.1   It All Began with a Relationship

Most of these issues have existed for decades. This reality birthed WWAV more than three decades ago. In the early days of the organization's work, Catherine and the other co-founders were on the move and responding to crisis: trying to stop the disappearance of their community members from AIDS-related illnesses, drug overdose deaths, poverty, mass criminalization, and a host of other structural issues that had not yet been captured under the framework of "social determinants of health." There just was not time to document their daily work of street-based outreach people involved with sex work and injection drug use. There was barely enough time to *do* the work.

As the years progressed, the WWAV foremothers have been able to pause to build an archive of their knowledge and methods of pioneering outreach work in partnership with co-author Laura McTighe. This documentary process was also born out of crisis. The "Born In Flames" oral history project was so named to commemorate the bone-deep work of surviving a nearly fatal arson attack on WWAV's offices in 2012 following a tremendous victory against the criminalization of street-based sex work. That evening, all records of WWAV's work went up in flames. Since then, Laura has been working with everyone in the WWAV family to put the stories of the organization and of the women who crafted them into permanent record.

As the story goes, Catherine and Danita Muse, both Black women raised in multigenerational New Orleanian families, linked eyes across a crowded health department conference room in the height of the AIDS epidemic. Catherine was 8 years Danita's senior, born in 1949 to Danita's 1957. Catherine was the oldest child of three and also old enough to remember life in segregated New Orleans. She explained it to Laura like this during her life history interview:

> "I've lived through some segregation. I remember where I have to ride in the back of the bus. I also remember when my daddy couldn't take me in the store on Canal Street to use the bathroom, so I had to go behind a car, right? I remember the first time that we were allowed to ride in wherever on the bus and I sat in the front and a little white woman got up and I basically just looked at her. Because I thought as old as she was, if you were going to stand up because I'm sitting here, you go for it."

Catherine got married right after high school and had her first child, Deon, shortly thereafter and two more children, Dawn and Charles, about a decade later. During that time, she worked as a nursing assistant and a barmaid, in a laundry, and at a bed and breakfast. Her entry into community work came when she went to work for the National Council of Negro Women with a program to train high school dropouts in housekeeping skills to work in the hotels. From there, she moved to the Children's Pediatric AIDS Program and was working to find people who used injection drugs and bring them in for HIV testing. When her supervisor saw the deftness with which she moved through community, she told her, "I need you to meet this woman called Danita."

Danita was already making waves in the city's health and human services arena. When Laura worked with Danita on her life history interview, Danita talked about how "I've always wanted to help people." She graduated from Southern University in New Orleans in 1978 with degrees in psychology and sociology and went on to get a master's in social work from Tulane soon after to make her passion legible and employable:

> …I've always wanted to help people that most people didn't want. Because that's how I saw black people. People really didn't want to help us. They just helped us because they felt sorry for us. And that was probably why I was interested in drug addiction treatment because those are the people who people *really* don't want to help. They don't want them—

they don't want them to have nothing; they don't want them to be with nothing. They just don't want them with *nothing*. So I was drawn to them.

She laughed herself into an addendum to that story, "Beside the fact that I got a job offer. Always helpful when you get a job offer. You're drawn to people where you can get a job."

That job was with the state of Louisiana—first in a ward for people with severe mental health issues and head traumas, then with child protective services, and then with the Office of Substance Abuse, which is now called the Office of Behavioral Health. From that post, she started to work with the community. From her "good government job,"[2] Danita ran groups with people struggling with addiction, which put her in a position to be the drug and alcohol representative to some of the earliest white-led HIV response efforts in the city. These efforts, she learned, were willfully *not* reaching out to poor Black people in the city's ten public housing projects; they were targeting the bars. That decision was deadly for Catherine and Danita's community. Danita explained the situation to Laura like this: "All of these people kept coming up HIV positive, and they *knew* that the intravenous drug users were not necessarily the gay people; they were just regular Joes out of the housing projects. They knew that."

And so Danita began to try to recruit other women who saw what was going on and were just as pissed off as she was. She met several in meetings at the Office of Public Health. Myra was a quick typist; Marion was a good bookkeeper. What she was missing was a partner for community outreach—a partner in doing the work. And then Danita met Catherine at yet another meeting at the Office of Public Health. For Catherine, of course, Danita's reputation preceded her.

This fateful meeting at the Office of Public Health had been called because the City of New Orleans had gotten an influx of funds to address a surging syphilis epidemic. And this time, the outreach maps were following the epidemiology. When the city's zip codes were called out, Catherine and Danita claimed the ones to their uptown neighborhoods, including the public house developments called St. Thomas, Magnolia (officially "C.J. Peete"), Melpomene, and Calliope. That spawned their relationship. They drove throughout the city—Catherine in her car and Danita in her truck—to make deliveries. The health department simply wanted them to take boxes of condoms and drop them at barrooms, grocery stores, beauty shops, and laundromats. After a few weeks, Catherine and Danita figured out that the people who ran these businesses were selling their *free* condoms for $1.50 apiece. So, they quit "bulk dropping" condoms and started figuring out how to get them into people's hands for free. That was when the work started. That syphilis outreach funding dried up, and the epidemic in their community got worse. Catherine and Danita decided to shift from traditional work hours to after-work—from their vehicles to front porches.

---

[2] Later in her interview with Laura, Danita explained how she needed a job with security ("my check would come every month") and protection ("they'd have to go through civil service to get rid of me") when they started WWAV.

13.2.2   Creating a Nationally Recognized Model of Community Outreach

Front porches are where Catherine and Danita gathered with Catherine's family to make harm reduction and wellness packs for late-night outreach. Front porches are where they sat talking with members of their community who had at best been forgotten and at worst had been left to die. Front porches are where they brought their community members into care and hope. Front porches are where they pioneered a model of community-driven outreach that continues to guide public health research today. Catherine explained the process to Laura like this:

> We didn't have an office. We would work from home, my porch—and my poor little mama would do condom packets and she'd say, "Ssshhhh! I'm not getting paid from Women With A Vision!" …because she didn't. I mean… But, you know, *everybody* did condom packets—the children, my sister, my nieces, my mama. So, that's how we did. And we did that for a while…
>
> But, how we did outreach, right? My thing is: you just can't go in somebody's house—in their neighborhood, in their house—and just start talking. So for weeks almost, I would go and sit in the St. Thomas. I would find a porch and just sit there. You need to get to know me before I start walking up and down your street, right? …And then people ask you what you were there for and you're like, "I'm trying to build a relationship with you."

After the first year, Catherine and Danita had built a network of what they called "gatekeepers" to disseminate vital health information and supplies to those they did not touch directly through street-based outreach. A gatekeeper could be a person who ran a drug shooting gallery, or an experienced drug user who taught younger drug users how to inject safely, or a barkeep, or someone who kept a lookout for cops, or just someone everybody liked. Using gatekeepers maximized the impact of WWAV's outreach; this also affirmed the power of the enduring strategies communities used to care for themselves. Amid constant surveillance, survival depended on carefully and methodically concealing of the intricacies and intimacies of everyday life. Gatekeepers in the 1990s got harm reduction tools into the hands of people WWAV would never see on the streets and also into the hands of people WWAV would never know were using.

Gradually, WWAV's presence in and with community gave them a rare understanding of precisely how systemic poverty and targeted criminalization were driving vulnerability to HIV/AIDS and a whole host of other health issues. A few years in, Catherine and Danita started surveying the country to find networks for learning from and with other people working in community like WWAV was doing. That search landed them at the first National Harm Reduction Conference in Oakland, California, in September of 1996. And that conference then propelled WWAV into new networks. Gradually, people across the country started to recognize WWAV and depend on Catherine and Danita for their expertise in *doing* community outreach.

Even though the model they were teaching was lifesaving, the model was not always well received. One of their more infamous stories was presenting at a "little hole in the wall in Texas." There, they were meeting with mostly white-led service organizations and funding agencies. By the mid-1990s, there was a lot of money to "target" Black people and other people of color for treatment and care because of disparate rates of HIV and other health issues. However, the white-led organizations (and the people who funded them) were not getting the numbers they promised to deliver. Catherine and Danita were bearing witness to how the organizations had started to blame people of color for not going in! But both women knew that their community was not to blame. The people providing services were. These providers did not know how to reach the community—how to *do* community outreach. And most of these organizations did not have a single person of color working for them.

At this conference, as with countless other meetings, Catherine and Danita refused the gaze on their community and on themselves. They did this through their dress, through their conversation, and through their work. They showed up in that "little hole in the wall in Texas" in their African garbs, because they were pissed off. They told the burgeoning network of HIV educators and funders that they were *wrong*. Then, they demonstrated having a massive impact on health and well-being was possible by respecting the long-standing patterns of community caretaking already established by Black women in their communities.

13.2.3 Building Institutional Capacity for Community Engagement

Although Catherine loved her work at WWAV, there was insufficient funding to support a consistent full-time salary for her. Throughout WWAV's history, Danita had always maintained her "good government job," which kept her social work license active and provided her with the steady income and protection that came from being a civil servant. That job provided Danita the freedom to work with WWAV without straining the organization's scarce resources. A decade in, Catherine made a similar move for job security, but one that would also dramatically expand the terrain of her relationship-driven community outreach work. In 1999, she took her skills to a type of institution that has historically failed to partner with and build capacity of communities of color—a university.

Catherine was initially hired to work on a study focused on lead poising prevention and abatement among children in New Orleans and several other South Louisiana communities. Catherine already had solid relationships with many community leaders and well-respected agencies in New Orleans from her previous work, but she was not as familiar with the landscape in other areas. She and colleagues would travel to rural communities in an RV and spend time developing partnerships with health and social services agencies in those areas. Ultimately, taking this time allowed Catherine to reach families and provide them with education and support.

Over the course of the following 5 years, she worked on several other research projects to which she contributed vital insight. For example, one HIV prevention initiative involved setting up a storefront in a community that, even today, has a life expectancy of 55–56 years. The idea was to attract community residents, including people who used injection drugs, by providing basic necessities such as food and toiletries at no cost. When people came to pick up supplies, Catherine would offer them education about HIV prevention. Catherine quickly realized and reported back to the research team that their efforts were not reaching the intended population because "drug users don't wake up at 8 o'clock!" The team changed the store's operating hours to better accommodate the needs of the people they wished to reach.

When hurricanes Katrina and Rita struck in 2005, Catherine's home was flooded. She moved in with Deon and Deon's now wife, Shaquita Borden, for several months while she searched for a new place to live. Knowing firsthand the experience of being displaced gave Catherine unique insight into the challenges that so many New Orleanians were facing in rebuilding their lives. So when the researchers with whom she worked began addressing issues related to supporting disaster recovery, she was precisely the person to continue doing the work of building relationships with hard-hit communities.

Catherine and her colleagues began conducting outreach to people living in temporary housing funded by the federal government, known locally simply as FEMA trailers. Over the course of several months, they worked across several South Louisiana parishes conducting surveys, "mostly just to see how people were doing and what they needed," and assessing mental health. Catherine also helped with mold remediation for residents whose homes had flooded. "I didn't like that work at all because you had to wear a suit and it was hot!" she said. But she did the work nonetheless to help her fellow community members.

When the post-disaster work began to taper off, Catherine became affiliated with one of the university's research centers that focuses primarily on physical activity and healthy living. One of her early experiences at the center involved a colleague taking her to a meeting with fellow health professionals, and "he told me not to say anything." But she refused to be silent about issues related to community needs. In that moment, her colleague was upset with her for speaking up, but after that she says, "he got it." He began to understand the value of Catherine's input, as her insights were informed by the true lived experiences of the communities whose health he hoped to improve.

Since then, Catherine has been involved in a wide variety of activities including supervising staff collecting surveys in under-resourced neighborhoods, leading cooking classes, developing a robust neighborhood health ambassador program, creating and leading a community advisory board, and doing door-to-door outreach to "listen to the needs of the community." Based on what she heard, Catherine says, "I've worked on blight, planted trees, and cleaned drains. If it's a need and I can help, then here we are."

Catherine is a passionate advocate for true community engagement. One of the most important roles she consistently plays is to question why she is treated as a single representative for communities to the university, often asking the question, "why isn't the community at the table?" when decisions are being made about research and funding. Her outspokenness has led the university to invite more community partners to be involved in designing and executing research. She also serves on the community advisory board for a multi-institution research collaborative in Louisiana, constantly encouraging investigators to address community-identified concerns.

Catherine is particularly outspoken about the importance of researchers and community members developing meaningful relationships and together using community-partnered participatory (CPPR) research methods to improve the lives of people experiencing health disparities. She has provided multiple trainings to university-based researchers and students about how to conduct CPPR, and she knows firsthand how to do this. From 2014 to 2017, she and Ashley served as dual principal investigators on an NIH-funded study on a topic that Catherine suggested was a major area of interest for Black women in New Orleans—intimate partner violence (IPV) (Wennerstrom et al., 2018). Catherine organized a community coalition and focus groups of men and women to gather insight into causes of and solutions to IPV. The data gathered are now being used to inform a future intervention. Catherine also serves as a co-investigator on two CPPR projects funded by the Patient-Centered Outcomes Research Institute (Arevian et al., 2018). Both aim to improve mental health among marginalized populations in New Orleans and Los Angeles. Catherine's major role is to make linkages and support community involvement throughout the research process.

13.2.4 Supporting the Next Generation of Community Health Workers

Finally, Catherine's skills in building relationships have been valuable for improving not only community health but also the CHW workforce. Catherine began conducting outreach to unite CHWs nearly a decade ago when she became involved in an informal CHW support group. From 2008 to 2010, Ashley managed the REACH NOLA Mental Health Infrastructure and Training (MHIT) project, a community-academic partnered effort focused on building capacity to improve mental health service delivery in post-Katrina New Orleans (Springgate et al., 2011). One component of MHIT involved training CHWs and other frontline social service providers on how to do or conduct outreach, education, screening, and referrals for depression services (Wennerstrom et al., 2011). For many training participants, addressing behavioral health was completely novel, so the program convened monthly support meetings to provide space for participants to discuss successes and challenges and share resources.

Although MHIT was coming to a close when Ashley and Catherine met at a community conference in August of 2010, Ashley hoped that the outreach group could still convene in some capacity, as the participants seemed to find the support it provided helpful to their work. Catherine agreed to attend the next meeting to learn more. On the agenda was a discussion of whether the group wanted to continue to meet after project funding ended that fall and, if so, how the group would survive without funding, space, or support staff. Catherine immediately recognized the potential value in creating a structure for CHWs to gather on a regular basis and began attending meetings regularly.

Within a few months of months of her involvement, the group began to grow. As new participants began to show up for gatherings, each would explain that they knew Catherine from previous work and that they'd come based on her invitation. As newcomer Dana Feist expressed, "You don't say no to Catherine."

In 2011, the regular members of the group decided to develop a more formalized structure under which to operate. Various agencies had been offering meeting space, which often created confusion for participants who were unsure of where the next monthly gathering would take place. Catherine recognized the value in having a more permanent space and offered to the group, "Well, we could always meet at Women With A Vision." Shortly thereafter, members of the group engaged in a self-facilitated strategic planning process at WWAV. Participants came to consensus that group would be known as the Louisiana Community Health Outreach Network (LACHON) (LACHON, 2018) with a mission of supporting and developing the CHW workforce, as defined by the American Public Health Association. A five-member board was selected to lead the group.

Catherine became the chair of LACHON in 2012 and made a commitment to growing the organization. One of her main priorities was to create an inclusive environment for CHWs to share their professional struggles and support one another. Catherine often says, "What I like about our monthly LACHON meetings is that you can vent. You can say whatever, and you know it's not going to go anywhere." In addition to being a safe space for CHWs to express challenges, LACHON has also become a source of support and mentoring for newly hired CHWs such as Raven. Perhaps most importantly in a community that was affected heavily by a disaster and slow to benefit from Medicaid expansion, LACHON became a place for CHWs to share resources and information with one another.

In 2013, LACHON hosted its first annual conference, bringing together about 60 CHWs around New Orleans. Subsequent conferences have included CHWs and allies from several other areas of Louisiana who highlighted their programs. Another of Catherine's goals has been fundraising for the organization. With WWAV as its fiscal sponsor, LACHON began to collect member dues in 2014. These funds have been used to send CHWs to participate in state and national professional development opportunities.

LACHON sponsored Catherine to attend the APHA meeting in 2014 to present about the organization's work. At that conference, Catherine made connections with several other CHWs and allies that led her into supporting the CHW profession on a national scale. For example, shortly after the meeting, she was invited to serve as one of just two CHW fellows on the Community Health Worker Core Consensus (C3) Project (C3, 2018) through which she lent her skills and expertise to creating a nationally agreed-upon set of skills, roles, and competencies that the workforce embodies. She was also invited to participate in interpreting the results of the 2014

National Community Health Worker Advocacy study, which was the largest study of CHWs ever undertaken (Sabo et al., 2015). Her growing national reputation earned her an invitation to serve on the founding board for the National Association of CHWs.

Back home, although LACHON has continued to operate with no paid staff, Catherine's leadership has helped the organization come to be recognized as an important voice for Louisiana CHWs. In 2017, the state Office of Public Health collaborated with LACHON to conduct a CHW needs assessment and invited LACHON to participate in CHW workforce development technical assistance initiative offered by the Association of State and Territorial Health Offices.

Catherine's current focus is expanding LACHON to reach a larger segment of Louisiana's CHWs. Through her recent participation in a project that aimed to help Baton Rouge communities recover from the Great Flood of 2016 (Keegan et al., 2018), Catherine established new contacts in the state's capital city. She is meeting with CHWs and allies monthly to establish the structure for the Baton Rouge-based chapter of LACHON.

13.2.5 Conclusion

Catherine Haywood has undoubtedly had a noteworthy career as a CHW. Her work in conducting outreach has addressed a host of health issues from HIV to obesity, through which she has touched the lives of countless individuals and communities. Perhaps what is most impressive, though, is that she has made her work the work of others. By thinking expansively about the relationships she already had, she brought her family and friends into the work of conducting outreach to highly marginalized populations. By maintaining a consistent message about the importance of community involvement, she has pushed her university-based colleagues to more equitably involve the community residents they aimed to serve. And by developing local and national CHW networks, she has ensured that grassroots community health professionals will have the sustainable sources of mentorship and support they need to facilitate their efforts to improve community health. Catherine's model is not only inspiring but also completely replicable: **focus on building relationships and bringing community to the table**. In closing, she offers the following advice on building relationships: "When conducting outreach, know your community or communities you're working with. You have to gain their trust, and you have to trust them. Always be respectful and non-judgmental, and know what you're talking about. If you don't have the answer to a question, let the person know that you'll come back with it and make sure that you do. If someone won't talk to you, don't try to force a conversation. Just try another time."

References

Adelson, J., & Williams J. (2018, May 7). *'It's gotta be we.' LaToya Cantrell ready to move New Orleans forward, together, as city's new mayor.* Retrieved from https://www.theadvocate.com/new_orleans/news/article_188008a2-5208-11e8-bc76-a7a13f24afcc.html.

Arevian, A., Springgate, B., Jones, F., Starks, S. L., Chung, B., Wennerstrom, A., … Wells, K. B. (2018). The community and patient partnered research network (CPPRN): Application of patient-centered outcomes research to promote behavioral health equity. *Ethnicity & Disease, 28*(2), 295–302.

Benns, W. (2015 September 21). *American slavery, reinvented.* Retrieved from https://www.theatlantic.com/business/archive/2015/09/prison-labor-in-america/406177.

City of New Orleans. (2017). *City of New Orleans Annual Data Report 2017.* Retrieved from https://data.nola.gov/stories/s/6a26-q6dq/.

Community Health Worker Core Consensus (C3) Project. (2018). *2016 Recommendations on CHW roles, skills, and qualities.* Retrieved from https://www.c3project.org.

Crisp, E. (2018, May 31). *Gov. John Bel Edwards signs law restoring felon voting rights after five years.* Retrieved from https://www.theadvocate.com/baton_rouge/news/politics/legislature/article_8f432008-6515-11e8-a42c-4f773f2862c5.html.

Kaye, R. & White, J. (2007, August 29). *Names of victims fills 'murder board.'* Retrieved from http://www.cnn.com/2007/US/08/28/murder.board.nola/index.html.

Keegan, R., Grover, L., Patron, D., Sugarman, O. K., Griffith, K., Sonnier, S., … Wennerstrom, A. (2018). Case study of resilient Baton Rouge: Applying depression collaborative care and community planning to disaster recovery. *International Journal of Environmental Research and Public Health, 15*(6), 1208.

La Rose, G. (2016, January 15). *New Orleans ranked 2nd worst housing market for renters.* Retrieved from https://www.nola.com/news/business/article_3ca10da3-8dcd-57a3-a3ca-d2d927d5d6f4.html.

Louisiana Community Health Outreach Network. (2018). Retrieved from https://www.lachon.org/.

Mauer, M. & King, R.S. (2007, July 1). Uneven Justice: State Rates of Incarceration by Race and Ethnicity. The Sentencing Project. Retrieved from https://www.sentencingproject.org/publications/uneven-justice-state-rates-of-incarceration-by-race-and-ethnicity/.

Prison Policy Initiative. (2018, June). *States of Incarceration: The global context.* Retrieved from https://www.prisonpolicy.org/global/2018.html.

Ride New Orleans. (2017). *The state of transit in 2017: Creating our transit future.* Retrieved from http://rideneworleans.org/wp-content/uploads/2017/08/SOTS-2017-FINAL-PDF.pdf.

Robert Wood Johnson Foundation. (2013, June 19). *Metro Map: New Orleans, Louisiana- infographic.* Retrieved from https://www.rwjf.org/en/library/infographics/new-orleans-map.html.

Sabo, S., Wennerstrom, A., Phillips, D., Haywood, C., Redondo, F., Bell, M. L., & Ingram, M. (2015). Community health worker professional Advocacy: Voices of action from the 2014 National Community Health Worker Advocacy Survey. *The Journal of Ambulatory Care Management, 38*(3), 225–235.

Springgate, B., Wennerstrom, A., Meyers, D., Allen, C., Vannoy, S., Bentham, W., & Wells, K. B. (2011). Building community resilience through mental health infrastructure and training in post-Katrina New Orleans. *Ethnicity and Disease, 21*(3, Suppl 1), 20–29.

Wedland, T. (2017, May 20). With Lee statue's removal, another battle of New Orleans comes to a close. Retrieved from https://www.npr.org/2017/05/20/529232823/with-lee-statues-removal-another-battle-of-new-orleans-comes-to-a-close.

Weixler, L.B. Barrett, N., Harris, D. N., Jennings, J. (2017, April 4). *Education research alliance. Did the New Orleans school reforms increase segregation?* Retrieved from https://

educationresearchalliancenola.org/files/publications/040417-Bell-Weixler-Barrett-Harris-Jen-nings-Did-The-New-Orleans-School-Reforms-Increase-Segregation.pdf.

Wennerstrom, A., Haywood, C., Wallace, M., Sugarman, M., Walker, A., Bonner, T., … Theall, K. (2018). Creating safe spaces: A community health worker- academic partnered approach to addressing intimate partner violence. *Ethnicity & Disease, 28*(2), 317–324.

Wennerstrom, A., Vannoy, S., Allen, C., Meyers, D., O'Toole, E., Wells, K. B., & Springgate, B. (2011). Community-based participatory development of community health worker mental health outreach role to extend collaborative care in post-Katrina New Orleans. *Ethnicity and Disease, 21*(3, Suppl 1), 45–51.

13.3 Case Study: Diabetes Outreach in Rural North Georgia

Katharine Nimmons, Gregory J. Dent, Teresa Mendez, Amy Elizondo,
Gabriela Boscan, David Secor, Janice Probst, and Myriam Torres

13.3.1 Introduction

This section tells the story of a community health worker (CHW) team that implemented an innovative outreach program in rural northwest Georgia to engage CHWs and technology in response to rising rates of diabetes. With a population of less than 40,000 people and 22.4% of that population living under the federal poverty level, Murray County, Georgia, residents face a set of socioeconomic challenges that make access to education, employment, and healthcare difficult. Neighboring Whitfield County shares similar rates of poverty (over 20%), rates of uninsured adults (over 30%), and rates of adults living with type II diabetes (11%).

Disparities related to social determinants of health are common across rural America. Rural populations experience poor health outcomes at higher rates than other communities. On average, they have relatively more older adults and children; unemployment and underemployment; and poor, uninsured, and underinsured residents. Rural communities also suffer from an uneven distribution and relative shortage of healthcare professionals. An estimated 62 million of the United States' population lives in areas considered rural or nonmetropolitan (Hart, Salsberg, Phillips, & Lishner, 2002).

To address these disparities, many health programs have turned to CHWs for their unique ability to connect patients with healthcare services (University of Arizona & Annie E. Casey Foundation, 1999). This is especially true in rural and underserved areas of the country. CHWs are uniquely qualified as connectors because they live in the communities in which they work, they understand what is meaningful to those communities, they communicate in the language of the people, and they recognize and incorporate cultural buffers (e.g., cultural identity, spiritual coping, traditional health practices) to help community members cope with stress and promote health outcomes (Wilson, Brownstein, & Blanton, 1998). This was the case in North Georgia where the National Rural Community Health Worker Patient-Centered Diabetes Management Program (referred hereafter to as "the Program") incorporated best practices for CHW-led outreach to address diabetes in their rural community.

13.3.2 Team Members

The Program was a collaboration between two organizations: the National Rural Health Association (NRHA) and the Northwest Georgia Healthcare Partnership (NGHP).

The NRHA first began engaging CHWs in 2011, when they engaged with partners to train 100 CHWs along rural areas of the US-Mexico border. The NRHA is a nonprofit membership organization with over 21,000 members around the country and a mission to provide leadership on rural health issues through communications, education, research, and advocacy. Past collaborators have included the Community Anti-Drug Coalitions of America (CADCA), the Dentaquest Foundation, the Livestrong Foundation, the National Eye Institute, the Office of Minority Health, the US-Mexico Border Health Commission, the Appalachian Regional Commission, the Federal Office of Rural Health Policy (FORHP), and state Offices of Border Health. These partnerships have helped fund the training of over a thousand CHWs along the US-Mexico border and the state of Georgia. This national experience was helpful when designing, implementing, and assessing the Program.

The Northwest Georgia Healthcare Partnership (NGHP) is a regional collaborative effort between healthcare organizations, business and industry groups, local government, educators, and public health stakeholders. The 501(c)(3) organization, founded in 1992, aimed to create fundamental changes in the delivery of health services in Murray and Whitfield Counties. For almost 30 years, the organization has facilitated a strong community commitment to improve overall health status while controlling costs, improving accessibility, and promoting high-quality care. Part of this mission is to identify sustainable solutions to significant health issues via innovation, benchmarking, and application of best practices. Not driven by just one or two local entities, the NGHP is truly a community-oriented collaboration that addresses issues related to the topic of health. This long-standing relationship with the people and organizations of North Georgia enabled NGHP to successfully lead the Program described in this section.

Together, the NRHA and NGHP identified, hired, and trained six CHWs to implement the 3-year program. Three CHWs were already employed by NGHP, and three new CHWs were recruited and hired. For this project, the team sought CHWs that met the following criteria: understanding of type II diabetes, the ability to educate patients on best practices to improve their diabetes-related health outcomes, knowledge of local resources and services available to patients, basic comfort level with technology being used in the program (i.e., tablets, Fitbits, and glucometers), proficient in Spanish and English, and strong organizational and interpersonal skills.

13.3.3 Project Initiation

The Program was established in 2014. The NRHA, with funding from the Verizon Global Corporate Citizenship and the Appalachian Regional Commission, proposed to develop a new technology-based CHW training. They envisioned a way to help patients achieve two goals: to use technology to manage their type II diabetes and other chronic diseases and to increase their physical activity. The technology used in this program included tablets, activity trackers, and glucometers. Over the course of the program, the 6 CHWs from the Northwest Georgia Healthcare Partnership served 300 patients living in Murray and Whitfield Counties. Researchers from the University of South Carolina (USC) collected and analyzed program data as part of a study of this program.

The inclusion criteria for participants in this pilot study included (1) age 18 years or older; (2) clinical diagnosis of type II diabetes; (3) residence in Murray or Whitfield Counties, Georgia; (4) commitment to follow doctor's visit schedule and willingness to share selected study-related medical information such as blood sugar and hemoglobin A1c (HbA1c) levels through medical records; and (5) willingness to take part in the study through its timeline. After consenting to participate, each participant was randomly assigned to 1 of the 3 study arms, each consisting of 100 participants. All patients completed the same questionnaire at the beginning and at the end of the program to assess knowledge on nutrition and type II diabetes. A description of each group follows:

Group 1: Participants received standard clinical diabetes care. Participants completed a baseline and an exit survey assessing their diabetes-related knowledge and self-efficacy in disease management during the 12-month study period. While these patients did not receive CHW support during the observation year, CHWs engaged with them following the initial period.

Group 2: Participants received an educational intervention delivered by CHWs. Each CHW in this group received training to deliver standardized diabetes education and maintained weekly communication with the participants.

Group 3: Participants received both the CHW-delivered educational intervention and electronic devices (tablet computers, Fitbits, and glucose meters) to help them keep track of their type II diabetes. The tablets were equipped with Fuze software, which allowed for HIPAA-compliant communication between the participant and the CHW assigned to that participant. The TelCare glucose meters are connected to the tablets and recorded the three glucose readings per day. Patients in Group 3 received lancelets and test strips, required for use with the TelCare glucose meter. Fitbits given to participants in this group assisted them in keeping track of their physical activity and sleep patterns. Participants in Group 3 and their assigned CHWs received an additional educational training on how to properly use the technology.

The NRHA submitted the program materials to the Institutional Review Board (IRB) at USC in March 2015, which was approved in June 2015, allowing the project team to collect and analyze data from program participants.

While waiting for IRB approval, the project team planned a training session for the CHWs and prepared materials to assist with patient recruitment. The NRHA collaborated with the National Community Health Worker Training Center at Texas A&M University to develop the CHW training session. This collaboration produced a CHW curriculum focused on chronic disease management, intervention strategies, and building trust within a community at risk. Additionally, NRHA acquired and delivered the Samsung Galaxy tabs, the Fitbits, and the glucometers for the Northwest Georgia Healthcare Partnership. On May 11, 2015, staff conducted a training involving team-building exercises, role-playing, and chances for the CHWs to share their own experiences. The training also included the technology training to set up the Samsung Galaxy tabs, the Fitbits, and the video conferencing application, Fuze.

The first patient enrolled on June 30, 2015. Enrollment continued steadily in July, as the CHWs attended health fairs, disseminated literature, canvassed neighborhoods, and contacted clinicians in the area. Initially, the recruitment process took over an hour per patient, but based on CHW feedback, USC streamlined the pretest and the recruitment process accelerated. From June 30, 2015, to December 16, 2015, the NGHP recruited the target number of 300 patients, enrolling 100 into each group.

Challenges with recruiting patients included the long distances between residences in Northwest Georgia, community skepticism of yearlong academic projects, and language barriers during outreach efforts and the enrollment process. While Spanish-speaking patients received a Spanish-language pretest, many community members still found the pretest poorly worded and confusing, slowing enrollment during the initial weeks. Additionally, many of the area's residents had not previously had local access to care, making answering questions about their health history difficult. The CHWs worked with dialysis clinics to help overcome some of these challenges. With the help from the Advisory Committee, CHWs expanded the geographic scope of the project to a neighboring county to reach more potential patients. Additionally, the NGHP escalated its grassroots strategies of canvassing neighborhoods; disseminating literature in English and Spanish at health fairs, churches, schools, and local stores; and spreading awareness of the project through word-of-mouth. With formal collaborations with dialysis clinics, local providers, and national partners, as well as a strong grassroots strategy in an expanded geographic scope, the CHWs met the enrollment targets.

13.3.4 CHW Feedback on Outreach

As CHWs enrolled the 300 total patients, they created a working document to informally identify any stories, challenges, problems, or best practices they uncovered throughout the process. One CHW noted, "one patient is very excited about receiving a Fitbit and challenges himself to hit 10,000 steps every single day." Another patient was listed as "happy that the CHWs were able to provide the tools to routinely check their glucose levels." This indicates that participating community members gave the CHWs positive feedback about the program and incentives. CHWs also appreciated the support from community organizations. As an example, a CHW wrote she was "excited to collaborate with the Ingles grocery store to provide 'healthy protein-rich nutritional meals' to families in Murray County." The connections CHWs have with community residents and businesses are critical for implementing a yearlong outreach program. Finally, the working document describes success stories. One patient in Group 3 successfully lost 91 pounds and lowered his A1C level from 11.6 in December, a reading well above the normal range, to 6.1 in March, within the treatment range for people with diabetes. The CHW supporting this patient was pleased by the transformative effect of the program.

13.3.5 Participant Impact: In Their Own Words

USC program staff conducted focus groups with 18 study participants and 3 CHWs. The purpose of the focus group sessions was to assess the experience of being in the research project and, secondarily, to see how faithfully the intervention was implemented within a small rural community. Key findings from the focus groups are summarized by category.

13.3.5.1 Outreach

Most of the participants learned about the study at a health fair or at a festival at a church; a few learned from a CHW directly. One participant said he at first turned down a request to participate until his wife told him to participate. All were glad there was a study like this because "… *most of us never think about [diabetes]. …. Until it comes to your own family. My wife – she passed away. This September it'll be two years. And the doctor said it was because of her diabetes…. And so about three months later or so, [I also] became a diabetic.*"

13.3.5.2 Knowledge of Study Design

Participants seemed to know the group to which they had been assigned. Those who had the Fitbit and tablet were very pleased. We asked participants if they knew other people participating in the study but assigned to different groups—most said they did not know other participants. One man said his son-in-law got the tablet and the Fitbit, indicating an awareness of the differences between groups of the study.

13.3.5.3 Relationship with CHWs

Participants receiving CHW assistance without technology expressed that they were very satisfied with the visits: "*it's not like you are a burden to them, they answer everything you ask…. It's been amazing for me.*" All participants whom had a CHW said it was very beneficial to talk about diabetes, exercise, healthy diets, and medications. Most of the positive comments from participants were related to diet and diabetes guidance.

13.3.5.4 Impact of Program

Participants from both groups (CHW alone or CHW + electronic devices) reported they had lost weight and reduced their blood sugar levels. Other participants mentioned that the program helped them to being aware about their diabetes and about its symptoms.

13.3.5.5 Access to Care

The participants were ambivalent about local care access and quality. Several participants mentioned they had a long wait at a specific local provider's office and complicated scheduling that required one visit to see the doctor for tests and a second visit to learn about the results. One participant said, *"Sometimes they [local healthcare providers] are good and sometimes they are bad. They change the doctors so often."* Another stated, *"They'll set you up an appointment and at 8:00 you're supposed to go in there and get a blood sugar and then … sit there and wait until 11:00, 12:00."* Though some participants described positive experiences obtaining care locally, one person added, *"This program was better for me than my own doctor."* Someone else said, *"I believe the problem is the doctor."* Finally, a participant stated that *"I don't have health insurance and I have to pay a lot of money for my meds and stuff,"* indicating that even if the quality of healthcare is acceptable, cost is an access barrier.

13.3.5.6 Technology

Many participants liked their devices and were using them, even beyond the initial 12-month program. These participants mentioned their devices have helped them to lose and maintain their weight. One person said, *"It [the Fitbit + tablet] was a motivator. After you eat you sit down and enter your food. It made me aware of what I put in my body."* Other positive feedback included: *"I got the tablet and the Fitbit...I have to exercise but now I don't have to go to the gym … I do it right there on my TV in my living room on that tablet."* Another participant said he is using the tablet to look for information about diabetes and *"help my cousins and those in my family who are also diabetic."*

There were reports of challenges using the devices. One person in this group said that her work does not allow any type of jewelry like a Fitbit, so she had to limit its use for evenings and weekends. One participant said the devices work *"if you pay attention."* Additionally, several participants reported that the devices provided through the study were broken. One participant said: *"the Fitbit lasted for about a good year but then, it was broken."* Another respondent noted that the Fitbit was bothering his arm "*because I am diabetic.*" Another person said the Fitbit was counting more steps "*than what I was taking.*" Three different participants had lost devices at the hands of teenagers: "*a 14-year-old messed up with my tablets and broke two of them.*" A second stated: "*Don't let a teenager get ahold of it. That's what happened to mine. Mine's messed up.*" The third added: "*That's just exactly what happened to me. I let my daughter-in-law stay with me, and her 14-year-old son. And every time you turned around, you'd have to tell him, 'That's not yours. You have no business touching it.' But before they left, it was already broken.*" Finally, an additional participant said "*my stepmom didn't understand what she was supposed to do,*" adding that, for older people with dementia who want to participate in a program like this, they need more user-friendly apps.

Unexpectedly, several study participants reported having received devices outside of the study: "*They've started a new program through my insurance with the Fitbit. [And it takes] your blood pressure rating, the steps, [unclear]. … Have to write down what I eat, how many calories in and out. Put it in the – it's got a little smart book with it, telephone.*" A second respondent had a similar program through a different insurer: "*I have United. And they have a watch that does your heart, your blood pressure, and the steps you take. And it's a new insurance to me 'cause I was with Humana for years.*" The effect of this unforeseen access to devices on the study results is unclear.

13.3.5.7 Problems People with Diabetes Face

Several participants mentioned difficulties maintaining diet and exercise. Some participants even mentioned not having the right medication or the correct dosage. Another participant said he did not encounter any problems because, "*I look for information on the internet.*" When discussing the main problems patients with diabetes face, participants talked about the cost of medicines and the cost of healthy foods. A consistent theme throughout the discussion was that people with diabetes have a hard time changing unhealthy eating habits, particularly those acquired when young. Dietary change was acknowledged to be both necessary and difficult. Many participants implied that these changes meant a change in culture, because "*when we grew up, if you didn't eat what was in your plate, you would be in trouble.*" One person talked about the importance of reading labels but noted confusion over portion sizes (e.g., bottles that show the calories of a single portion but actually contain three portions). Another noted that lots of foods do not advertise the calories in their products, such as bakeries.

13.3.6 CHW Perspective

The focus groups with the CHWs revealed that the survey was very long and difficult to administer, particularly with several people who could not read. In addition, recruiting 300 participants was noted as a challenge for a single agency in a small rural community. Some participants acquired Fitbits even though they were not assigned to that research group, which may have compromised the results of the study. One CHW said, *"I think the awareness of word of mouth – it's huge. Because this person might know this other person that we had no idea they knew each other. So "I got the Fitbit." "I want the Fitbit, too, so we can compete against each other." So I think that's how it starts. And the awareness – and, "Okay, let me go ahead and go and buy one because it's counting how many steps I'm doing" "or whatever."*

The CHWs reported that they answered questions equally for anyone, regardless of the group to which the individuals were assigned. From the conversation with the CHWs, assigning persons to a control group was problematic, because CHWs wanted to help all the participants. One CHW stated: *"And I think that's where [as] promotoras – our mentality comes in. Yeah, they were in group one or two, but if somebody called us for a question…it is different when it's on paper than when you're working with actual people. Yeah, if they have a need, then obviously our heads – even your hearts – it's like, 'Hey, I'm gonna help you. Even though I know I'm supposed to leave you alone, it's just, I'm gonna help you.'"* CHWs emphasized they related well with the participants because they took time to visit with clients and answered their questions and also because CHWs are people just like the participants.

13.3.7 Program Impact

Data collected throughout this study included survey data and clinical data. Self-reported data was collected using a paper-based survey instrument. The pre-survey completed at entry into the study and post-survey completed at the 12-month point assessed diabetes-related knowledge, attitudes, and self-efficacy in disease management. Additionally, the survey included questions related to sociodemographics (e.g., age, race, ethnicity, education, employment, marital status, annual household income, insurance, etc.) and other relevant information (e.g., nutrition, physical activity, etc.). Clinical data consisting of HbA1c levels were retrieved on all 300 participants from their medical records at 3 points in time: at baseline, at 6 months, and at 12 months.

Data analysis evaluated the efficacy of each educational intervention approach and compared that to the standard clinical care in improving participants' knowledge related to diabetes and self-efficacy in disease management. All statistical analyses were conducted using SAS version 9.4 at 95% confidence level ($\alpha = 0.05$). Univariate and bivariate analyses were performed to describe the overall sample and group characteristics. Multivariate analysis was performed to examine the impact of the two educational approaches on three outcomes of interest: (1) diabetes-related knowledge, (2) diabetes-related self-efficacy, and (3) HbA1c levels compared to the standard clinical care. Results for the HbA1C tracking were as follows: among participants in Groups 2 and 3, there was a decline on the values taken after the intervention was implemented; however, none of those differences was statistically significant. Group 1 had a minor decline (-0.03) when comparing the final to the initial measurements; but the remaining comparisons show an increase in HbA1c values (not seen among Groups 2 and 3). In general, all participants in every group increased their knowledge about diabetes, but the change was not statistically significant. Among insulin users only, we found that the increase in knowledge was significantly higher among the group that had standard care compared to the other two groups. Our study was not able to find any consistency with the results measuring self-efficacy. None of the score differences between pre- and post-intervention was found to be statistically significant. However, in general, the data showed that those participants assigned to Group 3 (CHW + electronic devices) started and ended with higher scores on all of the items measuring self-efficacy. The study did not find a clear pattern of change in knowledge, HbA1c, or self-efficacy scores among groups and between pre- and post-intervention in any of the groups.

Beyond the initial 12-month program, there was an additional 6-month sustainability phase. This phase allowed the project team to further study the impact that technology has on type II diabetes and CHW/patient interaction. In this phase, CHWs recruited patients from the original Groups 1 and 2 and taught them how to use technology they already owned to help them track their health. Staff created a CHW training curriculum on the use of technology by patients to help them manage their diet, physical activity, and type II diabetes. The training incorporated the use of applications for smartphones and tablets that help its users track calorie intake, water consumption, steps taken throughout the day, and specific applications to help patients educate themselves on type II diabetes and track their glucose levels. The main findings of this additional phase were that the additional time patients had with CHWs was encouraging, but due to limited data plans and the limited access to broadband in rural communities, the technology was not used as frequently and, therefore, not as successful in managing the patient's health.

13.3.8   Reflections on Barriers to Outreach

The CHWs acknowledged county characteristics as barriers to enrolling as many individuals as quickly as they had hoped. For instance, the census indicates a growing Hispanic community and many homes with Spanish as the first language. The NGHP team found that many of the program materials did not translate for these community members and that many residents were not familiar with or did not feel comfortable with a yearlong academic study. In some instances, residents would not talk to CHWs for fear that the NGHP was connected to federal authorities.

Other persistent challenges involved access to care and preferences; some patients did not want to enroll if they would not receive visits from a CHW, and other patients did not have reliable A1C readings, receiving their care either in Mexico or through the emergency room. In spite of this, the grassroots strategies and the formal collaboration with local clinics eventually succeeded.

As expected, problems with technology persisted for some patients. After providing technological trainings in the beginning of the program, staff continued to troubleshoot issues related to unresponsive Fitbits, Samsung Galaxy 4 tablets, and glucometers, including replacing defective devices, recharging nonresponsive batteries, and finding alternative strategies for fraying charging stations. In one instance, an elderly patient's wrist was too large to use the Fitbit, despite his initial enthusiasm in enrolling in the project. Staff looked through a number of possible solutions to keep the patient engaged, eventually replacing his Fitbit Flex with another Fitbit product that clips onto clothing, rather than fastens around the wrist. Throughout the program, staff kept these kinds of tools and flexible responses available so that no participant became deterred or disengaged because of technology.

Overall, about 28% of participants recruited to the study were lost to follow-up, including 22% of participants from the group who received the CHW + electronic device intervention, approximately 26% of those receiving the CHW intervention, and 34% of those receiving the standard care. Even though these differences were not statistically significant, we should note that, as expected, the participants who had the electronic devices added to the CHW intervention returned for the surveys and measurements in greater proportions.

13.3.9 Lessons Learned

For similar projects engaging in CHW outreach with a research component, planners may wish to assign groups by place, rather than within the same small community. While adjusting analytically for differences across communities is necessary, using geographically separated populations may serve to mitigate knowledge leak across participants. This will also spare CHWs the ethical dilemmas that arise when a "control" individual asks for their assistance. Conversations with participants and CHWs revealed several threats to the integrity of a "three separate groups" research strategy. Each of these would have reduced differences between the three different groups, by giving "control group" members equipment or services similar to those in the most intensive intervention group. These included knowledge transfer across groups, which provided "control" persons with additional information; implementation of similar strategies by health insurers (i.e., provision of a Fitbit to persons with diabetes); and CHW reluctance to deny services to persons in need. It is known that CHWs have great relationships with communities, and they may feel they had to support all patients regardless of the group they were assigned. Follow-up may allow for identification of any activities with participants who were supposed to be receiving a different type of care.

Some changes, such as a higher increase in diabetes knowledge among insulin users in Group 1 (standard care), were unexpected. How much knowledge health providers had of the study is unknown. However, if providers knew which patients were not receiving the extra education and assistance from a CHW and/or the electronic devices, they may/could have strengthened their diabetes education.

Overall, the focus groups found that both the CHW alone and the CHW + device interventions were viewed favorably by participants. Participants of the focus groups agreed that the CHWs were a key factor influencing their successes in dealing with diabetes. The CHWs spend time with their clients, listen and answer their questions, and are dedicated to them. We found that participants were very knowledgeable about diabetes and factors related like diet and exercise. Participants were also very savvy when using their tablets and/or computer equipment. Even if they were not assigned to the intervention with electronic devices, several participants knew a lot about looking for information on the Internet and apps that could assist with diet.

There are many unknowns relating to the project outcomes. Even though the group assignments were dictated by a random number that the table provided, the groups varied greatly in composition. The role other factors may have played in the assignment to groups is uncertain. Follow-up interviews with the CHWs may clarify this. There were problems with retention of participants, especially in the "standard care" and "CHW-alone" groups. How the loss of follow-up might have affected the results is also not known. There were also some staff changes during the study, and the change of CHWs may have affected the intervention outcomes. In-depth follow-up interviews or focus groups with patients and providers could assess these potential confounding factors.

Altogether, the lessons from this outreach project will help staff design future CHW and technology-based programs supporting rural residents with diabetes. Support with managing their disease and improving quality of life could be a game changer. Chronic medical conditions such as diabetes take a tremendous toll on communities, especially for those people who already experience barriers to accessing healthcare and other support services. Engaging CHWs and technology tools through outreach activities can help address rural-urban disparities in access to care, healthcare service delivery, and health outcomes.

References

Hart, G., Salsberg, E., Phillips, D. M., & Lishner, D. M. (2002). Rural health care providers in the United States. *The Journal of Rural Health, 18*(S), 211–231.

University of Arizona & Annie E. Casey Foundation. (1999). *The National Community Health Advisor Study: Weaving the future*. Tucson, AZ: University of Arizona Press.

Wilson, K., Brownstein, J. N., & Blanton, C. (1998). Community health advisor use: Insights from a National Survey. In *Centers for Disease Control and Prevention, Community Health Advisors/Community Health Workers: Selected Annotations and Programs in the United States* (Vol. 3). Atlanta: Centers for Disease Control and Prevention.

Chapter 14
Participating in Evaluation and Research

Caitlin G. Allen*, J. Nell Brownstein, Olveen Carrasquillo, Tamala Carter, Irene Estrada, Jill Feldstein*, Durrell J. Fox, Alexander Ross Hurley, Shreya Kangovi, Carmen Linarte, and Brendaly Rodríguez*

14.1 Introduction

Caitlin G. Allen, Durrell J. Fox, Alexander Ross Hurley, and J. Nell Brownstein

The final role, participating in evaluation and research, was newly identified during the analysis undertaken by the C3 project in 2015. The three sub-roles include engaging in evaluating community health worker (CHW) services

---

Authorship is organized alphabetically in ascending order by surname.

C. G. Allen (✉)
CGA Consulting, Charleston, SC, USA
e-mail: caitlin.gloeckner.allen@emory.edu

J. N. Brownstein
Texas Tech Health Sciences Center El Paso, El Paso, TX, USA

O. Carrasquillo · C. Linarte · B. Rodríguez (✉)
University of Miami, Miami, FL, USA
e-mail: brendaly.rodriguez@cvesd.org

T. Carter · I. Estrada · J. Feldstein (✉)
Penn Center for Community Health Workers, Penn Medicine, Philadelphia, PA, USA
e-mail: Jill.Feldstein@pennmedicine.upenn.edu

D. J. Fox
JSI Research and Training, Inc., Atlanta, GA, USA

A. R. Hurley
University of North Carolina, Chapel Hill, NC, USA

S. Kangovi
Perelman School of Medicine, University of Pennsylvania and Penn Center for Community Health Workers, Penn Medicine, Philadelphia, PA, USA

© Springer Nature Switzerland AG 2021
J. A. St. John et al. (eds.), *Promoting the Health of the Community*,
https://doi.org/10.1007/978-3-030-56375-2_14

and programs; identifying and engaging community members as research partners; and comprehensive involvement throughout the evaluation and research process (e.g., development of research questions, design methods, data collection and interpretation, sharing results, and taking actions on findings).

Inspired in part by community-based participatory research and citizen science, this role reflects growth in the field and support for employing CHWs in academic and clinical settings, where research is primarily occurring. Community-based participatory research is an approach to research that emphasizes equitable involvement of community members, organizational representatives, and researchers throughout the research process. Citizen science falls into a similar vein where community members (i.e., citizens or the public) engage in scientific research. While these two approaches to research take place across several research domains, they are particularly well-suited for research related to public health, health care, and health disparities/inequities. These efforts and emphasis on community-engaged research are further supported by a national focus on patient engagement and funding announcements that promote patient-centered care and community advisory boards. CHWs serve a unique role as a member of these boards, partners in research, case finding, and shaping research agendas.

Evaluations of programs and services involving CHWs have also grown in sophistication and volume over the past decade. Program evaluations, unlike sponsored research, appear less frequently in peer-reviewed journals, but they are equally important to making the case for sustainable financing of CHW positions in public health and health care. Organizations that employ CHWs and funders of evaluations increasingly see the wisdom of engaging CHWs earlier in the evaluation process—both to increase understanding of the relevance of evaluation to CHWs' daily practices and to benefit from CHWs' understanding of what may work best in connecting both study design and data collection practices to the real-world experience of community members and CHWs alike.

Although there have been many advances to the roles of CHWs in research, few programs exist to develop CHW skills in the research enterprise, and states generally have not included research skills as an entry-level requirement for CHW employment or certification. However, we may soon see substantial growth in CHW training in evaluation and research as a result of the growth of this evaluation and research collaboration role by CHWs.

The following two sections further depict opportunities for CHWs in research activity by describing a program that has developed multiple randomized controlled trials in a clinical setting and a training platform/project for CHWs to engage in patient-centered research.

14.2 How Patients and Community Health Workers Helped Design the IMPaCT CHW Model: Nothing About Us Without Us—And Make Sure It Doesn't Go into the Cabinets and Collect Dust!

Jill Feldstein, Tamala Carter, Irene Estrada, and Shreya Kangovi

14.2.1 Introduction

Research is a complicated word. As with most words in the English language, research is loaded with history and meaning—what you hear depends on where you sit. A high school student might hear *research* and start dreading his next term paper. A physicist might hear *research* and start thinking of ideas for her next lab experiment. Unfortunately, a middle-aged African American might hear *research*, particularly in the context of health care, and automatically flash to the Tuskegee Experiment of the mid-twentieth century, when the US Public Health Service intentionally left syphilis untreated in poor southern Black men in order to study how the disease affected people. Even after penicillin became widely available as the standard of care to treat syphilis, researchers did not provide this cure to hundreds of men in the Tuskegee study (Reverby & Foster, 2010). While the Tuskegee study may be the most famous, the study serves as just one of many examples of research that harmed and exploited marginalized communities in the United States and across the world.

So the legacy of healthcare research in the Black community is fraught, to say the least, and those tensions are naturally heightened when large institutions are involved. The University of Pennsylvania has cast a long shadow in Philadelphia, a city with a significant Black population for much of the last few decades. As the second largest private employer in the state, the University generates a staggering $30 million *a day* in local economic activity (University of Pennsylvania, 2016). The University's Health System, Penn Medicine, is a big driver of that engine, employing 20,000 individuals and generating $500 million in construction projects in a single year.

As a physician at the University of Pennsylvania, Dr. Shreya Kangovi was familiar with the legacy of Tuskegee and the role of the University and its health system in the surrounding neighborhoods of West and Southwest Philadelphia. Kangovi, a researcher interested in reducing health disparities, was passionate about finding ways to improve health outcomes for lower-income patients, and she felt like she had an opportunity moment she couldn't pass up.

14.2.2 Designing a Program Based on Research With and For Patients

14.2.2.1 Seizing an Opportunity

The origin of that opportunity came from 150 miles away in Washington, DC. The year was 2010, and Congress had just passed the Affordable Care Act (ACA). The ACA, most well-known for expanding Medicaid and providing subsidies to purchase insurance through state-run exchanges, also laid the groundwork for sweeping changes in funding health care. The ACA introduced penalties for preventable readmissions and prioritized value-based purchasing over traditional fee-for-service reimbursements (Kaiser Family Foundation, 2013). As a result, payments to healthcare providers in the post-ACA environment are increasingly based on *how well* providers care for their patients (e.g., the quality of patient outcomes) rather than on *what* providers do for their patients (e.g., ordering a CAT scan or completing an office visit). The ACA also required nonprofit hospitals like Penn Medicine to conduct a community health needs assessment and implement a plan to address the concerns they uncovered (Shaw, Asomugha, Conway, & Rein, 2014).

These changes created a new landscape where health systems like Penn Medicine were incentivized to better understand and meet the needs of their patients, particularly lower-income individuals who often fared worst on value-based metrics such as primary care access, quality of care, and hospital readmissions. Kangovi and her mentors, Drs. Judith Long and David Grande, both experienced health disparities researchers, saw this policy and financial landscape as an opportunity: health systems needed to understand and improve outcomes in lower-income populations. These researchers felt the timing was right to build an effective, financially sustainable program for caring for lower-income patients at Penn Medicine and perhaps beyond. They wanted to make sure that whatever program they developed was informed both by the best available science *and* by the perspectives of the people the program was intended to benefit.

14.2.2.2 Assembling the Team

What is the best way to include the insight and expertise of a community in a research working group? This is a vast topic with a rich history. Community-based participatory research (CBPR) is one approach. As defined by Barbara Israel et al. (2010), CBPR is "a partnership approach to research that equitably involves community members, practitioners, and academic researchers in all aspects of the process, enabling all partners to contribute their expertise and share responsibility and ownership." Frequently, CBPR is operationalized through community advisory boards who work with researchers to inform and guide studies (Newman et al., 2011). These boards are often made up of leaders of local organizations that have deep roots and histories within the community.

CBPR has many advantages: community members can make sure that research questions get at issues that matter to the people most affected, help ensure that research is conducted ethically, and spread the word about the study and its results. However, there are limitations to conducting CBPR through a community advisory board.

First, these boards are usually made up of a small number of people who are often put in a position to speak for "the community." These individuals can have different socioeconomic backgrounds from the majority of community members. This is partly driven by logistics: attending a meeting requires that you aren't working at the time it's scheduled, have a way to get there, and can find someone to watch your kids. Second, communities are complex and heterogeneous and considering them otherwise could be an oversimplification. A 30-year-old mother who comes to the Emergency Room with panic attacks after her son died from a stray bullet in the neighborhood will have a different perspective from the 40-year-old father of four admitted to the hospital with shortness of breath after picking back up his pack-a-day habit when he unexpectedly lost his job and the bills started to pile up.

The best way to capture these nuances, the team concluded, was to conduct in-depth qualitative interviews. Surveys are great if you want feedback on a specific idea. Discussion at community meetings works well to brainstorm and build on people's ideas. However, if you want to understand the main challenges in people's lives, the best approach is to talk to folks one-on-one, through what researchers call "qualitative interviews." There are many types of qualitative interviews, but health research often uses in-depth, semi-structured interviews, where an interviewer uses a set of "predetermined but open-ended questions" to learn about an individual's experiences or opinions (Given, 2008). According to Irving Seidman (2006), the purpose of in-depth interviewing "is an interest in understanding the lived experience of other people and the meaning they make of that experience." The goal of these conversations is to identify common themes and patterns.

There are two secrets to successful qualitative interviews. First, the interviewer needs to quickly establish trust. People are not going to open up if they do not feel comfortable. One of the quickest ways to establish trust is to be able to say, "You and I are from the same community. We share the same life experiences and speak the same language." To find the right community member to conduct interviews, the research team circulated an easy-to-read job description throughout the neighborhoods adjacent to Penn Medicine. The job announcement described the project and the ideal applicant: a long-time resident of the neighborhood with good knowledge of community resources and prior experience in outreach or interviewing.

If the first ingredient of a successful in-depth interview is quickly building trust, the second ingredient is creating a space for people to talk. The best interviews unfold as more of a guided individual reflection than a conversation. That requires someone who is naturally a good listener, who is present enough to keep the conversation going but who does not take over the dialogue. That quality is impossible to assess by reading job applications or resumes, so Kangovi met with applicants in person to get to know them. One of the people she met was Tamala Carter, who at the time was working as part of a street outreach team at a local community organization. A lifelong resident of West Philadelphia, Ms. Carter was familiar with the needs and resources in her neighborhood through her work organizing community events and canvassing door-to-door in the community educating residents about services. When she met Carter face-to-face, it was clear there was an immediate fit. "Carter is the type of person you want to tell your life story to," says Kangovi. "Her friendly face and thoughtful demeanor immediately puts you at ease."

Carter was also drawn to the project, as she recalls, because it showed that "someone was actually interested in what was going on in the community." Additionally, the project's research focus reminded Carter of her high school experience more than 20 years before. As a young woman, she would go to the local library to seek out literature written by African American scholars about black life and culture. As she recollected, "I had an interest in Black studies, because of me being Black. I felt like I wasn't exposed enough to my culture in school." At the library, Carter found writers like James Baldwin, Maya Angelou, and W. E. B. Du Bois. The job announcement reminded her of Du Bois, who had been hired by the University of Pennsylvania in Carter's own backyard in the late nineteenth century to interview African Americans about many facets of their daily lives. He went door-to-door in the neighborhoods, personally talking with more than 5000 people about their health, education, social connections, family lives, and more, situating their responses in the context of segregation and discrimination. The resulting collection, *The Philadelphia Negro*, challenged common perceptions of Black Americans' social and economic challenges and is credited as one of the foundational building blocks in the field of sociology.

14.2.2.3   Identifying the Questions to Answer

Carter joined Dr. Kangovi and Dr. Richard Shannon, then-chair of the Department of Medicine and a health system leader who brought expertise in designing a financially sustainable program, to form the core research team. The group discussed and debated the questions they wanted their study to answer, ultimately settling on why lower-income patients visited the hospital instead of their primary care providers and what could improve their access to and experience with primary care. Carter's role on the team at this time was critical. From Dr. Kangovi's perspective, Carter's participation in the study design was essential. "Since it was a community based initiative," Kangovi recalls, "there needed to be a community member co-leading it."

Carter also saw the value she brought to the project. "Coming from an academic background, you are taught certain things," she says, recalling her initial meetings with her research colleagues. "You are taught about people from different environments, different cultures, and different economic backgrounds. My job was to bring reality to what they believed." Part of her role was raising subtleties that can be missed when looking at statistics about race and poverty. Too many people, Carter knew, wanted to "make where I come from define me," and her role on the project was to bring more nuance to the picture of her community.

The team worked with Penn Medicine's data specialists to analyze hospital read-missions and primary care use across the entire health system. They identified five contiguous zip codes in West and Southwest Philadelphia that accounted for more than one out of every three readmissions occurring less than 30 days after the patient had been discharged from the hospital. These neighborhoods also had some of the lowest rates of access to primary care in the entire city.

14.2.2.4 Going to the Source

With the primary research questions and patient population of focus identified, Carter and Kangovi set about to write an interview guide. They reviewed scientific articles of studies that had used qualitative interviews with lower-income patients, using these as the basis for an interview guide they co-developed. Many of the inter-view guides were overly academic, remembers Carter, and she worked to "chop them off and talk in language that people can understand."

The guide she and Kangovi ultimately developed was semi-structured; in other words, the guide included a set of questions but also kept things open enough for patients to take the lead in telling their own stories. For Carter, this format was an important part of carrying on the oral traditions in the African American community. As she recalls, "it's part of our culture to pass down stories from one generation to the next. This tradition is rooted in wanting to ensure that our stories are told. And these are stories told in our own voices, with our own words, which is part of making sure that we are heard."

Interview questions in hand, Carter started going to the hospital every day, knocking on the doors of patients who lived in one of the selected zip codes. She described the goals of the study and asked them if they would like to participate. Once people said they wanted to participate—which most people did—Carter pulled up a chair and asked her first question, which set the tone for the format of the entire conversation. "Tell me," Carter asked, "what makes it hard for you to stay healthy? Not just medical issues but life issues?"

Carter remembers the quizzical looks she often received from the doctors, nurses, and social workers on the floors where she interviewed patients. Clinicians are used to their colleagues from Quality Control passing out surveys asking, "How satisfied were you with your treatment and care today?", but this was something altogether new. This was someone from the community, sitting with patients at their bedside, saying "I want to understand about your life outside of this place. What are you dealing with when you're *not* here?" To boost her confidence when dealing with skeptical doctors and nurses, Carter made sure to pass by the W.E.B. Du Bois College House, established on Penn's campus in 1972, on her way home after a day full of interviews. The building has a plaque commemorating the work of Du Bois, which contains a quote from his 1903 book, *The Souls of Black Folk*. "It is a peculiar sensation, this double-consciousness, this sense of always looking at one's self through the eyes of others…." Communing with Du Bois at the end of the day boosted Carter's spirits. "I would walk past his building," she recalls, "and feel like I was standing on the shoulders of my ancestors."

Carter's interviews with patients convinced her that the team was onto something—it felt as though people had been waiting for someone to want to hear what they had to say. With someone sitting in their living room, who looked like them, whose body language said, "I have all the time in the world – tell me what's going on," the stories came pouring out. People talked about becoming the "black sheep" in the family after experiencing sexual abuse; their struggles to make their meager salaries stretch to meet all their family's needs; and the disconnect they felt from doctors and social workers, who, as one patient told Carter, "can give you advice like 'here's the medicine you need' but don't really know what it's like in the real world."

14.2.2.5 Designing a Program Based on Patient Feedback

As Carter completed interviews, research assistants reviewed the written transcripts from her conversations and used a software program to identify common themes, a process called "coding." As they worked, Carter would review their analyses to make sure that the research assistants, who weren't from the same communities as the patients, accurately captured patients' perspectives and experiences. Carter was able to expand on quotes, correct things that were not clear, and, perhaps most importantly, clarify the intent behind certain words or phrases that might pass by someone who was not as familiar with the community and culture.

When Carter and the rest of the study team reviewed the transcripts, three overarching themes emerged. First, patients frequently talked about feeling disconnected from typical healthcare personnel and yearned for support from someone more relatable. Second, patients talked about being "set up to fail" when given a set of to-dos to complete after they got out of the hospital. From patients' points of view, these tasks were confusing, not aligned with their priorities, and/ or unrealistic given their limited financial resources or how few people they could turn to for help. Third, patients experienced so many obstacles getting to their primary care doctors that they preferred visiting the emergency room when they needed care.

These three themes helped form the basic structure of what would become the IMPaCT (Individualized Management for Patient-Centered Targets) community health worker (CHW) model: hiring natural helpers from the local community to join existing care teams; talking with patients to discover and prioritize patient-selected goals; and ensuring that patients found a long-term source of support, including a primary care provider they liked, before the program ended.

With the basic outline in place, the study team drilled down on the most common problems identified by patients during Carter's interviews, identifying the implications for:

1. What community health workers should do with and for their patients
2. What qualities to look for when hiring CHWs
3. What kind of training CHWs would need to prepare them for the role

As one example, patients talked about feeling rushed and confused during hospital discharge—they felt like the nurse read required medication lists and follow-up appointments at 100 miles per hour, rushing through unfamiliar prescription names and specialist doctors while the housekeeper hovered at the door to prepare the room for the next patient. To improve this experience, CHWs needed to be in the room when patients talked to nurses before they left the hospital. They needed to deliberately slow things down, inserting a "teach back," or a time when the patient could repeat what they heard to ensure everything made sense. Adding a third person into the nurse/patient dynamic requires a nuanced balance of skills and qualities—CHWs need to be confident enough to speak up and say, "Excuse me, Nurse John, but do you mind letting Mr. Alexander repeat back what he just heard?" *and* do so in a way that doesn't ruffle any feathers. This also requires teaching CHWs about things like drug formularies, so they can recommend that doctors identify less expensive generic medications when their patients can't afford co-pays.

Table 14.1 summarizes the main themes that emerged from Carter's interviews, along with illustrative quotes (Kangovi et al., 2014). This also shows the process the research team used to figure out what CHWs need to do (e.g., the intervention); who CHWs need to be (e.g., what to screen for in the hiring process); and what CHWs needed to know to be successful in their role (e.g., topics for what became IMPaCT's month-long, college-accredited CHW training).

14.2.2.6 Finalizing the Intervention

As Carter was interviewing patients, W. E. B. Du Bois and *The Philadelphia Negro* were largely a source of strength. But there was one aspect of Du Bois's experience that made her cautious. From Carter's point of view, *The Philadelphia Negro* did not help spur change for Blacks in Philadelphia—or the United States—when it was published. Although the book eventually received accolades, Carter recalls that, "my fear at the beginning of this project was that, just as Du Bois' research has been stored in a cabinet, I feared this, too, would go into the cabinets and collect dust. The research would be in vain!"

Thankfully, Carter's initial concern was unfounded. The team was able to secure funding to hire two CHWs to pilot the program. With all the pieces in place, Carter called each patient she had interviewed to share the news. She told them how what she learned from the interviews helped to design the IMPaCT CHW program. Patients were delighted to hear from her and even more excited that this was not just research for research's sake—there was actually something to point to, a new program, for people from the neighborhood, to help them with life's challenges. The program had an additional tangible benefit: new jobs for people from the community who became IMPaCT CHWs.

One of the first things Carter, Kangovi, and the two newly hired CHWs did was codify CHWs' day-to-day workflow in an easy-to-read manual that included a step-by-step guide for how CHWs should work with patients. Carter and the CHWs provided input into the manual's graphic design, including how to make

Table 14.1 Translating patient interview themes into CHW program elements (Adapted from Kangovi, Mitra, et al., 2014)

Theme	Illustrative quotes	What CHWs need to do	Who CHWs need to be	What CHWs need to know
Relationships: Patient wanted to establish a relationship with a healthcare provider—someone who they relate to—during hospitalization	• "I need to share with somebody that can share with me, like I been there, I know where you're at" • "[I'd like to work with someone] from the neighborhood…I think it would be a wonderful thing They're able to help you and people bond together like that"	Meet and establish a connection while patients are still in the hospital	• From the community • Discreet • Non-judgmental • Reliable	• Privacy training • Certified once training is complete
Goal setting: Patients felt that healthcare personnel didn't take time to understand their perspective or their personal goals	• "When patients are in the hospital, ask them what they might need [after discharge]. They can get them prepared for those issues" • "Just talk to the patient and see what they might need and help them with that"	Help patients create an individualized action plan for each goal they have related to their health/life	• Someone who listens more than they talk • Insightful • Able to solve problems • Organized	• Qualitative interviewing • Goal setting theory • Action planning

Theme	Quotes	Intervention	Characteristics	Resources/Training
Alignment: Patients felt like the things providers were telling them to do were confusing, weren't realistic, or weren't their top priority	• *Not realistic:* "[The doctor] tells me I need to lose weight by exercise. But [my] job is home care and that is 24/7. So it's difficult for me to leave her by herself and, you know, go for a walk or anything as I would like to do for the exercise" • *Not their top priority:* "I went back [to work], because...we have to work. But it wasn't in my best interest to go back because of my injuries" • *Confusing:* "[Discharge] is a scary experience...they need to give you some time to think, calm down and figure out what's going on, before they actually throw you out"	Helps align patients and the care team on what needs to happen after discharge	• Confident • Respectful	• Low-cost formularies • Project BOOST's Patient Pass to help patients stay organized about appointments and follow-up care
Support: After discharge, patients often felt abandoned by social and health system supports, just as they began to face a variety of "real-life" barriers to recovery. What they needed were different kinds of *help*, not information	• "The [hospital social worker] was telling me something about a transportation service that I can have. I have to call them ten days prior or something to that nature. And it is something that I am not use to, so did not use it. Maybe somebody could go set it up with you the first time to make it more feasible" • "Right now the doctor is doing all the prescriptions and appointments, but once I go home...it would be nice to have someone helping me get this done"	Provide tailored one-on-one support to help patients achieve their goals via home visits, phone calls and text messages	• Creative • Calm • Knows limits • Not directive • Compulsive about getting the best for people	• Training to address the main problems patients shared: (a) psychosocial, (b) health system navigation, (c) neighborhood, (d) access to resources, (e) health motivation
Primary care follow up: Their own doctors, many of whom worked in local health centers, weren't connected to their hospital care. Also, there were too many barriers to going to the doctor—It was easier to just "tough it out" and go back to the hospital if things didn't get better	• "Some [doctors] ... you gotta wait at least two months. If you miss it, he's gonna tell you 'hey, I don't know when I'm going to be able to see you.' So you schedule an appointment for two months after that. And half the time, I forget it by then" • "But [my doctor] don't spend all that time with me either"	Help patients prepare for doctor's appointments and ensure the clinic has info about recent hospitalizations and the patient's goals	• Pushy • Polite • Punctual • Able to end relationships and transition responsibly	• Doctor's appointment checklist and prep • How to schedule appointments

patient-facing handouts easy to read and understand. They also helped develop the safety protocol and home visit training for CHWs, which included recommendations on how to move safely through communities and be respectful when visiting people's homes.

The team used what they learned from patient interviews to build the structure of the IMPaCT model and create tools that help CHWs do their best work. For example, Carter's interviews revealed some commonalities among people with shared experiences or characteristics that affected their needs. This helped the IMPaCT team create a shorthand of patient "profiles" or types that would allow CHWs to effectively support patients with different needs. The first of these patient types, referred to as "Profile A" patients, are people who have experienced some type of traumatic event (e.g., abuse, assault, or time spent in jail) and often have strained or non-existent relationships with family members. In contrast, "Profile B" patients have supportive ties. In fact, they are often the backbone of their family or friend networks. When their loved ones are sick or have problems, Profile B patients tend to take care of them, providing financial, logistical, and/or emotional support, which means they tend to put their own health or life concerns on the backburner. Over time, as CHWs have worked with more patients, they have recommended the creation of additional profiles, including those for patients nearing the end of their lives and patients who have a high degree of independence.

Carter's interviews also helped the team decide where to invest small, but impactful, dollars. Given patients' desire for personalized, hands-on support, IMPaCT established a petty cash fund so CHWs could buy unique gifts to jumpstart patients' goals and tangibly demonstrate that their CHW was there to help them. Examples of patient gifts include garden plants for veterans with post-traumatic stress to relieve stress by cultivating flowers; a funky, colorful water bottle for a patient who needed to drink water, instead of soda, to control her diabetes; and crochet materials for a homebound senior citizen who needed a hobby to occupy her time. These expenses work out to just $2.67 per patient.

Patient interviews also helped Carter and Kangovi create tools to help clinicians more effectively bridge the doctor/patient divide, which is often exacerbated by socioeconomic differences. As one patient said: "I've got to lift furniture all day. [Doctor] sits in his chair in front the computer all day, so he don't lift no heavy stuff. I'm blue collar, okay? He's white collar. He doesn't understand me." To bridge this chasm, Carter and Kangovi worked with Penn's School of Medicine to create the IMPaCT Teaching Service, a month-long elective where medical students apprentice to a CHW. This structure is a complete inverse of the typical doctor/CHW relationship, where the doctor sits at the top of the hierarchy. In the IMPaCT Teaching Service, the roles are reversed—the CHW supervises and evaluates the medical student.

The course is "an opportunity for future doctors to understand what life is like for patients they serve," said Cheryl Garfield, a Lead CHW who has trained more than a dozen medical students. "A lot of them have never rode a city bus before, have never been into these neighborhoods before. They get to see firsthand what it's like being in the community. They get to see how people are living and learn how to not pass judgment, because you don't know what got them there." Students taking the course have stood in line with uninsured patients at 7 a.m. before the health center opens to guarantee they'll be able to see a doctor and witnessed firsthand the stress of a young mother trying to get back home to relieve the baby-sitter after a doctor's appointment, only to be told by cab driver after cab driver, "I don't take people to that neighborhood."

From Carter's perspective, the course gives soon-to-be doctors a better understanding of patients and the communities they come from. "With this course, they're able to spend time one-on-one with patients and get them to open up as a person – their background, what they've been through, and what's going on for them," Carter says. For example, a Teaching Service student initially had an unfavorable impression of a 30-year-old uninsured patient who was taking street Xanax. Her perception shifted when she saw the woman open up after talking with her CHW. The student noted, "My whole impression of her changed from this really difficult patient to just a sweetheart." Carter has seen this time and time again with the course, as medical students "are able to see patients from a different perspective, which helps them understand them at a different level."

14.2.2.7 Testing the Model

Since IMPaCT was a new program, the team wanted to test it in a clinical trial with the same level of rigor applied to evaluating a new drug. However, unlike a drug trial, which can cost millions of dollars, the team was interested in a more pragmatic approach to evaluation. They raised $60,000 in grant funding to set up a two-armed study: an intervention arm comprised of patients who worked with CHWs and a control arm of patients receiving usual care. Patients were randomly assigned to either the intervention or control group. The team hired research assistants who were blinded to patient assignments. In other words, when assistants collected outcomes data from patients, they did not know if they were talking to an intervention or control patient. If the research assistant was really invested in, for example, the idea that CHWs improve the quality of primary care, he or she might unwittingly ask about patients' experiences of care differently to intervention versus control patients in a way that influenced people's responses. Blinding the assistants reduced the likelihood of this bias.

Over 400 patients participated in the initial study of the IMPaCT model. The study team based the trial's primary outcome of interest on patients' highest priority: improving access to primary care. Research assistants also collected data on additional outcomes like patient engagement and hospital readmissions. The findings of the initial study were exciting and revelatory—compared to patients who did not work with a CHW, IMPaCT patients were 12% more likely to see a doctor after they were hospitalized; had a 13% increase in the quality of communication with their providers; saw improvements in their mental health and level of engagement with health care; and had 25% fewer hospital readmissions (Kangovi et al., 2014). The findings spurred the University of Pennsylvania Health System to invest in the

Penn Center for Community Health Workers as a nexus for CHW research, patient care, and dissemination in 2013.

In the intervening years, the Center has grown to 60 full-time staff, the majority of whom are CHWs. More than 12,000 patients have benefitted from working with an IMPaCT CHW. The Center has developed tools, training, and technology used by more than 1000 organizations, helping CHWs across the country get the kind of support they need to do their best work. The model has been continually refined and tested: two additional clinical trials have shown improvements in mental health, quality scores, and chronic health conditions, along with a 65% reduction in hospital days (Kangovi et al., 2017, 2018). Analysts have quantified the financial impact of these improvements, determining that Penn Medicine has received $2 in savings for every $1 invested in the program (Morgan, Grande, Carter, Long, & Kangovi, 2016). Beyond expanding the evidence base for effective CHW programs, these outcomes give CHWs confidence in the IMPaCT approach and methodology. As Lead CHW Irene Estrada notes, "I love the fact that we asked patients what they wanted, then we did it, then we studied it, and saw that it works! As a Community Health Worker, having data that says this works motivates me to stay on track with the training that we're given."

14.2.3   Creating Systems to Support, Evaluate, and Improve CHW Work

Once the IMPaCT model became part of routine care at Penn Medicine, the focus shifted to developing systems and process for three key elements of day-to-day operations: (1) helping new CHWs master the core elements of the work, (2) designing an evaluation system that would work for everyday needs, and (3) creating a feedback loop so that CHWs' experiences with patients help the program continually improve. While *patients' experiences* were the main sources of information to design the intervention, both *patients' and CHWs' experiences* served as the design source for these process elements.

14.2.3.1   Core Competency Certification

When the Center was created in 2013, Penn Medicine provided funding to hire 30 CHWs. Hiring and training so many people at once required IMPaCT to develop a structured way to determine when CHWs had mastered the main elements of the position. After IMPaCT CHWs are hired, they complete a month-long college-accredited CHW training. The topics for that training, which include everything from Motivational Interviewing to maintaining privacy, were chosen based on Carter's original patient interviews. However, training alone isn't enough to guarantee that new CHWs are ready to work independently. As Carter notes, "the month-long training is a lot to absorb, so you need a way to test absorption once CHWs are actually working with patients."

The team thought about the most important elements CHWs needed to demonstrate *and* the best way to demonstrate them, ultimately settling on a set of checkpoints that includes:

- Shadowing a Senior/Lead CHW for a few days
- Learning how to stay organized by using tools like to-do-lists and appointment calendars
- Following the safety protocol from the manual
- Explaining their role to other members of the care team
- Observation and sign off by various team members, including a Senior/Lead CHW, manager, and the program director

These checkpoints reinforce key elements about the work, like ensuring CHW safety. Having experienced CHWs play a role in certifying new CHWs helps reinforce these core values in a peer-to-peer format. Estrada notes that, "as Senior CHWs, we have an obligation to make sure that things go the way they should. One example of this is safety. New CHWs might not see the importance of that. I can step in and frame that for them: 'This is not a game. This is safety. Real things can happen.'"

These checkpoints also give CHWs time to develop and practice new habits, like writing a daily to-do list. As Carter notes, "Habits are really hard to do ... and really hard to break," so it's helpful to have time to practice them. They also allow each new CHW to develop a relationship with a Senior CHW, who serves as an informal mentor while they learn all the facets of the job. "Each checkpoint focuses on a different area that make sure CHWs are prepared to handle different circumstances," Estrada notes. "Every organization should have something like this so CHWs are prepared for all the experiences they're going to have: in the clinic, in the home, in the community – it prepares them for all of that."

14.2.3.2 Performance Assessment

The three randomized clinical trials—the gold standard of research—proved that the IMPaCT model worked. However, clinical trials take enormous resources and time and aren't practical for determining that an ongoing program is staying on track. Once the IMPaCT model became part of routine care, the focus shifted to designing an evaluation system that would work for everyday needs and could be easily implemented as the program rolled out across the health system. Kangovi and Carter assembled the Center's team of CHWs and their managers to design these processes.

Early on, the team nixed the idea of having CHWs collect outcomes data themselves. The reason for this was twofold. First, the group wanted to keep CHWs' workloads manageable and their focus on patient care. Second, there is an inherent conflict of interest in asking someone to evaluate their own work. For example, a patient might not feel comfortable telling his CHW, with whom he has a strong relationship, about a negative experience he had with his care or suggested areas for improvement. As mentioned previously, to avoid this potential bias during the clinical trial, the research team decided to have blinded research assistants evaluate outcomes. In routine care, however, blinded evaluators are *too* removed from day-to-day workings to collect performance assessment data.

CHW managers, on the other hand, are close enough to the work to understand the ins-and-outs, share CHWs' passion for improving patients' lives, and are in the best position, when the data reveals a problem, to help CHWs do something about it. The team therefore decided to incorporate a large quality control function into the manager's role.

To figure out what types of data to collect, the team thought about different ways to know if the program was working. They did not want to rely solely on one source of data, preferring a holistic approach that combined multiple sources. First, the group started with what patients said was important to them. Many things that patients told Carter fit nicely into the Institute for Healthcare Improvement's Triple Aim framework (Berwick, Nolan, & Whittington, 2008), including wanting to lose weight or improve their diabetes (the Triple Aim's *better health*), having positive interactions with doctors and nurses (the Triple Aim's *experience of care*), and going to the hospital less (the Triple Aim's *reductions in cost*). The team rounded out this list by including other things patients said were important, such as achieving goals that patients—not doctors—said were priorities.

The team also thought going directly to patients for feedback on how the work was going was important. They also wanted managers to get out from behind their desks on a regular basis—in other words, not just look at data and talk with patients but also see the work firsthand in homes, in clinics, and in the community. Estrada remembered a time when her manager joined her on a visit to a patient struggling to control his diabetes. When the patient revealed his father had recently passed away, Estrada did not offer condolences and move on. Instead, she asked him: "how has that been for you?" The patient shared that his dad, also a diabetic, had called him every day to remind him to check his blood sugar and nudge him about eating right. With his dad no longer around, the patient had slipped. What he needed most was a new person—and a new set of routines—to replace the stable presence his father had been for him. Estrada was able to help the patient identify his cousin as a motivational buddy to fill the role made empty with his dad's passing. Her manager was able to see how Estrada used open-ended follow-up questions to better understand her patients' experiences.

With all of these performance management goals in mind, the team created a recurring series of data to collect. One week each month, managers:

1. Call patients to get feedback on the program, including their likelihood to recommend IMPaCT to a friend or family member
2. Observe the work directly (e.g., accompany a CHW on a home visit or call; join a daily huddle in the doctor's office)

3. Read all CHW notes for one patient from beginning to end, observing areas where the work is going well and offering suggestions for improvement
4. Review Triple Aim outcomes for patients

These processes share a common thread: the data is collected and reviewed *while* CHWs are working with these patients. In other words, managers do not wait until the end of the program to ask patients about their experience because by then, it would be too late to make any changes. For example, after a manager does an in-depth review of chart notes, he can follow up with the CHW to say, "Mr. Burns seems like he is slow to trust new people. He mentioned that he used to love going to the casino – what do you think about inviting him to play cards with you next week? It would give the two of you some relaxed time together where you could just talk."

Given that displaying data in ways that are useful for people can be difficult, the team worked with a designer to design different "dashboards," or views, in HOMEBASE, an application co-designed by CHWs specifically for IMPaCT. The CHW dashboard (Fig. 14.1) functions as a patient-level to-do list. This at-a-glance snapshot summarizes patients' goals and progress, which CHWs appreciate as it helps them stay organized and on track. "I like that this is already programmed for me," Carter says. "It's an easy way to see what I have done and what I still need to do." In contrast, the director dashboard (Fig. 14.2) is organized by CHW and includes time trend analyses, allowing program leaders to spot improvements or declines over time.

# a2 James	Discharge: 2018-01-04	Meds Filled
PCP: Dr. Carols, 215-630-3945	Target Close Out Date: 2018-01-18	Followup Appt Not Completed
Root Cause: Doesn't want to admit he is depressed		Home Care Not Completed
Roadmap 1 -	Next Steps	Resolved:No
Get patient a new primary care doctor that he likes	[x] 1/3 CHW and patient will call pts insurance and get a list of primary care doctors in his area, pt will choose one	
	[x] 1/3 CHW and patient will call to schedule an appointment and change PCP on patient's insurance card	
	[ ] 1/14 CHW will remind patient of his new primary care appt with with Dr. Carols on 1/5 at 1:30pm and plan to attend with him	
Roadmap 2 Addresses Root Cause	Next Steps	Resolved:Yes
Go bowling to get some fun in patient's life	[x] By 1/4 CHW and patient will go bowling on discount tuesday	
Roadmap 3 -	Next Steps	Resolved:No
Attend a counseling appointment to talk about loss of mom	[ ] CHW and patient will call to schedule therapy appointment by 1/11	
	[ ] CHW will meet patient at his home and travel to appointment with him	

Fig. 14.1 CHWs can track their patients' goals and progress via the CHW dashboard, which helps them stay organized and on track

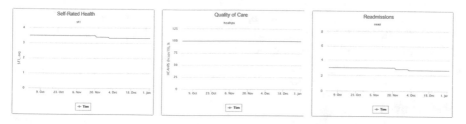

Fig. 14.2 Directors use this dashboard to monitor individual and team performance over time. This allows them to easily track progress on program goals related to patient health, cost, and quality

14.2.3.3 Program Improvement

CHWs also play an important role in evaluating how IMPaCT is working. One of the practices the IMPaCT team uses is affectionately called a "design jam." CHWs come to the jam with ideas for how to improve the program, based on their experiences working with patients.

At one design jam, the team heard the story of a 70-year-old patient that Estrada had worked with who wanted to improve her diabetes. One of Estrada's suggestions was that the patient give up certain foods. After some time, the woman hadn't made any changes to her diet and her relationship with Estrada started to strain. Later, Estrada learned the patient grew up, as she described it, "dirt poor." When she was a kid, the woman recalled, her goal in life was to buy and eat whatever she wanted. And now here comes Estrada recommending she *cut* certain foods from her diet! The very idea ran counter to her notions of success.

How could Estrada have learned this earlier on, she wondered? The answer lay in the initial meeting with new patients. This first CHW/patient interaction is guided by the Meet-the-Patient Interview, a semi-structured interview guide that CHWs use to meet and set goals with their patients. During the design jam, Estrada and her CHW colleagues looked at the interview guide's questions with fresh eyes. The first question, "tell me about your health," now seemed overly medical. What they really wanted to ask was, "tell me who you are." CHWs started firing off the kinds of details they would want to know: What was it like growing up? Who are the most important people in your life? What kinds of things do you like to do for fun?

In real time, the team reworked the interview guide, replacing "tell me about your health" with "tell me a little bit about yourself" and then listing the CHW-generated questions as prompts. The revised interview guide has improved CHW work with patients, enabling them to more effectively tailor their work and approach.

14.2.4 Conclusion

Research is still a loaded word. The complicated legacies of Tuskegee and *The Philadelphia Negro* remain part of our country's past and present. Yet Carter is amazed and humbled by how far the IMPaCT program has reached. "I was skeptical of the research project in the beginning," she recalls. "I knew that studies like this had been done before but no one listened. So the big question for me back then was, 'Will they listen?' And it turns out the answer was yes."

References

Berwick, D. M., Nolan, T. W., & Whittington, J. (2008). The triple aim: Care, health, and cost. *Health Affairs, 27*(3), 759–769.

Given, L. M. (2008). *The SAGE encyclopedia of qualitative research methods* (Vol. 1-0). Thousand Oaks, CA: SAGE.

Israel, B. A., Coombe, C. M., Cheezum, R. R., Schulz, A. J., McGranaghan, R. J., Lichtenstein, R., … Burris, A. (2010). Community-based participatory research: A capacity-building approach for policy advocacy aimed at eliminating health disparities. *American Journal of Public Health, 100*(11), 2094–2102.

Kaiser Family Foundation. (2013). *Fact sheet: Summary of the Affordable Care Act.* Retrieved from http://files.kff.org/attachment/fact-sheet-summary-of-the-affordable-care-act.

Kangovi, S., Grande, D., Carter, T., Barg, F. K., Rogers, M., Glanz, K., … Long, J. A. (2014). The use of participatory action research to design a patient-centered community health worker care transitions intervention. *Healthcare, 2*(2), 136–144.

Kangovi, S., Mitra, N., Grande, D., Huo, H., Smith, R. A., & Long, J. A. (2017). Community health worker support for disadvantaged patients with multiple chronic diseases: A randomized clinical trial. *American Journal of Public Health, 107*(10), 1660–1667.

Kangovi, S., Mitra, N., Grande, D., White, M. L., McCollum, S., Sellman, J., … Long, J. A. (2014). Patient-centered community health worker intervention to improve posthospital outcomes: A randomized clinical trial. *JAMA Internal Medicine, 174*(4), 535–543.

Kangovi, S., Mitra, N., Norton, L., Harte, R., Zhao, X., Carter, T., … Long, J. A. (2018). Effect of community health worker support on clinical outcomes of low-income patients across primary care facilities: A randomized clinical trial. *JAMA Internal Medicine, 178*(12), 1635–1643.

Morgan, A. U., Grande, D., Carter, T., Long, J. A., & Kangovi, S. (2016). Penn Center for community health workers: Step-by-step approach to sustain an evidence-based community health worker intervention at an Academic Medical Center. *American Journal of Public Health, 106*(11), 1958–1960.

Newman, S. D., Andrews, J. O., Magwood, G. S., Jenkins, C., Cox, M. J., & Williamson, D. C. (2011). Peer reviewed: Community advisory boards in community-based participatory research: A synthesis of best processes. *Preventing Chronic Disease, 8*(3), A70.

Reverby, S. M., & Foster, H. W. (2010). Examining Tuskegee: The infamous syphilis study and its legacy. *Journal of the National Medical Association, 102*(2), 148–150.

Seidman, I. (2006). *Interviewing as qualitative research: A guide for researchers in education and the social sciences* (3rd ed.). New York, NY: Teachers College Press.

Shaw, F. E., Asomugha, C. N., Conway, P. H., & Rein, A. S. (2014). The patient protection and affordable care act: Opportunities for prevention and public health. *The Lancet, 384*(9937), 75–82.

University of Pennsylvania. (2016). *University of Pennsylvania: Powering Philadelphia and Pennsylvania.* Retrieved from http://www.evp.upenn.edu/strategic-initiatives/community-and-economic-development/economic-impact-on-pennsylvania-and-philadelphia.html.

14.3   Community Health Workers as Stakeholders in Research: Training Community Health Workers in Patient-Centered Research and Their Impact on Clinical Trial Interventions[1]

Brendaly Rodríguez, Carmen Linarte, and Olveen Carrasquillo

"Titi" Carmen
My aunt "Titi" Carmen was the first promotora ("Community Health Worker" in Spanish) I met. As the youngest of six siblings, her "old school" father encouraged her to drop out of school to take care of her aging family members. She did both – completed high school and fully dedicated herself to take care of her parents. Subsequently, she also took on the role of health advocate and champion for others in her extended family and neighborhood. Through self-teachings from various sources (doctors' visits, radio programs, health-related materials, prescriptions instructions), plus her own experience as a patient and a family caregiver, "Titi" Carmen navigated the healthcare delivery system for us. She was motivated to serve and rewarded with the appreciation and trust of all those around her. Since then, I have met many other Titi Carmens. From Australia to Ecuador, and in the U.S., I have worked with CHWs in numerous research and evaluation projects, and for 10 years leading a CHW statewide organization. In all these settings, I still see in CHWs what I first saw in my Titi Carmen – despite formalized healthcare training, they had utmost commitment and caring for the well-being of others. They provide health education and emotional support, make calls, fill out paperwork, go with someone to their doctor's appointment, and link people with community resources. They see themselves as having a key role in contributing to the health of their families and their communities. Indeed, they do.

–B. Rodriguez

14.3.1   Introduction

As detailed in other chapters, community health workers (CHWs) serve as connectors between healthcare consumers and providers to promote health among groups that have traditionally lacked access to adequate care. They provide members of the community who traditionally lack access to quality health care with information and support from a culturally competent point of view that they can understand (Rosenthal et al., 2010; U.S. Department of Health and Human Services, Health Resources and Services Administration, Bureau of Health Professions, Community Health Worker National Workforce Study, 2007).

One specific area CHWs have shown great promise is in reducing health disparities (Community Health Resources, 2007). Addressing diseases related to health disparities requires innovative approaches to both prevent disease and illness and also to improve healthcare access and quality in underserved communities. Requisite in

[1] The work described in this section was partially funded by two Eugene Washington Engagement (EAIN) Awards from PCORI (UMIAMI #2219, 2015–2017 and in FL UMIAMI #7239, 2017–2019).

formulating such approaches is the meaningful engagement of the communities affected by such conditions to meet our nation's commitment to eliminating health disparities. This has been a niche CHWs are well equipped to occupy. Not surprisingly, there is considerable amount of scientific evidence of support of CHWs in addressing the needs of diverse and disadvantaged populations across a variety of health conditions (Kim et al., 2016; National Center for Chronic Disease Prevention and Health Promotion, 2015). Although there still remain gaps in knowledge of the most optimal approaches for utilizing CHWs, many programs aimed at addressing disparities employ CHWs in various roles, including outreach and direct service provision.

14.3.2 Training and Certification of CHWs

One long-standing challenge to integration of CHWs into the healthcare delivery system as lay healthcare workers had been their lack of formalized training (O'Brien et al., O'Brien, Squires, Bixby, & Larson, 2009; Ruiz et al., 2012; U.S. HHS HRSA, Bureau of Health Professions Community Health Worker National Workforce Study, 2007). Employers such as health delivery systems, public health programs, and other health organizations have expressed concern that without CHWs having any recognized credentials or training pathway, including such workers as part of their healthcare workforce would prove difficult (Witmer, Seifer, Finocchio, Leslie, & O'Neil, 1995). In contrast, other voices felt that by providing formalized training and certification, CHWs would no longer retain the qualities that served them best. Such standardized training and professionalizing of CHWs would take away the flexibility and out-of-the-box thinking that made CHWs unique in the healthcare workforce (Catalani, Findley, Matos, & Rodriguez, 2009). Early attempts to have CHWs trained by hospital-based nurses in areas such as diabetes, for example, created CHWs who ended up sounding and acting like traditional members of the healthcare delivery system. In such cases, CHWs may compromise their access and credibility and damage the trust with community members. This had become a particularly recognizable concern when CHWs were trained in settings by staff with little or no connection to the community. This eroded the trusting relationship which had been the essence to the CHW-community connection and usually the very quality for which CHWs were originally sought out.

Despite these concerns, there was increasing consensus that CHWs do need some form of formalized training. Key to appropriate training for CHWs was the need to be done through contextually appropriate means and channels (e.g., not only available online, accessible literacy levels, interactive formats rather than self-guided instruction, etc.). With such training, the end result would be well-equipped and qualified CHWs who can contribute to the public health research support workforce (Florida Center for Nursing, 2016; Witmer et al., 1995). Several states, such as Texas and Florida, began initiatives to formalize process and procedures for a standardized CHW training framework. This movement was further accelerated when the CHW role was codified in a national context as part of the Affordable Care Act in 2010.

14.3.2.1 Certification of CHWs in Florida

According to the 2012–2016 US Census American Community Survey 5-year estimates, Florida is our nation's third most populous state with 22 million people, and 45% of the population is made up of minorities (U.S. Bureau of the Census, 2016). The state of Florida is highly diverse, with Hispanics and Black/African Americans comprising 24.1% and 17% of the population, respectively. Further, by 2035, the percentage of Hispanics is projected to increase to 50% of the state population. Some areas already have a particularly large concentration of Hispanics, such as Miami-Dade County, where 66.4% of residents are Hispanic, and Central Florida, where Hispanics make up 27% of the population (before migration due to Hurricane Maria). The state also houses great numbers of other ethnic groups, with 252,000 Haitians living in Florida, who make up 47% of all Haitians in the United States (U.S. Bureau of the Census 2012–2016). These demographics make Florida an ideal state for CHWs to play a role in the healthcare workforce (Florida Center for Nursing, 2016). However, until recently Florida did not have a formal CHW training or certification pathway. As a result, many organizations employing CHWs were using homegrown training approaches, often unaware of the existing theoretically and evidence-based structured training programs.

To address the need for a formalized training program for CHWs in Florida, a multi-stakeholder taskforce formed. Originally supported by the Florida Department of Health, the working group ultimately incorporated as the Florida CHW Coalition (FLCHWC) and now is a statewide partnership dedicated to the support and promotion of the CHW profession in Florida. Operating as a volunteer organization, the Coalition conducted outreach and met with relevant healthcare professional groups such as nurses and social workers. The group framed the need for CHW credentialing in Florida as a common ground, healthcare workforce development cause, in alignment with national trends (U.S. HHS, HRSA, Community Health Worker National Workforce Study, 2007). Other key partners included the University of Miami (UM) and other departments in the Florida Department of Health.

After several years of working towards its goal, in 2015, the FLCHWC was successful in creating formalized standards and training pathways that would lead to credentialing of CHWs by the Florida Certification Board (FCB). As reported by B. Rodriguez at the ninth Annual FLCHWC Summit in Orlando, by 2019, there were 573 certified CHWs in the state. In fact, the Florida Center for Nursing recently identified the first of the top six priority occupations for Florida as that of a CHW and called for "academic programs to draw on practitioner input, competency development, and experiential learning…" (p. 22) to develop training programs for emerging occupations like CHWs (Florida Center for Nursing, 2016). This is also reflective of current trends in Florida's healthcare job market that call on existing occupations to evolve with redefined competencies and become more interdisciplinary, specifically in allied health professions.

Getting a certificate

At the end of every CHW training event I lead, when the certificates are distributed, CHWs rush to commemorate the moment by taking pictures with their certificates, proud of having achieved CHW certification. From their comments, I learned that for many this is a formal recognition for their hard work and may serve as a stepping stone in their careers. For others, it is self-realization of their own abilities, the value of their experiences, and their impact in improving health outcomes.

–B. Rodriguez

14.3.3   Community Health Workers in Research

14.3.3.1   Part 1: Our Group's Experience with CHWs in Healthcare Research

Over the last 20 years, in New York City, Atlanta, and now in Miami, our group has worked to address health disparities, with particular attention to the Hispanic/Latino communities, African Americans, and Haitians. With community input, our group has developed and tested community-based research strategies to advance the health of minority communities in a variety of disease areas including diabetes, cardiovascular disease, HIV, and cancer (Carrasquillo et al., 2017; Carrasquillo et al., 2018; Carrasquillo, Patberg, Alonzo, Li, & Kenya, 2014; Chang et al., 2018; Ilangovan et al., 2016; Kenya et al., 2013, 2016; Kobetz et al., 2018; Lebron, Reyes-Arrechea, Castillo, Carrasquillo, & Kenya, 2015). Our teams include medical doctors, epidemiologists, statisticians, project managers, community engagement specialists, research coordinators, and research assistants. A central component to all of our work has been incorporating CHWs in our community-engaged disparities research projects. We have trained and deployed CHWs to deliver various interventions and have demonstrated that CHWs can improve healthcare outcomes for these groups (Carrasquillo et al., 2014; Carrasquillo et al., 2017; Carrasquillo et al., 2018; Chang et al., 2018; Ilangovan et al., 2016; Kenya et al., 2013, 2016; Kobetz et al., 2018).

In these projects, CHWs have been trained to actively participate in research processes. CHWs have helped to design the intervention and refine and deliver the intervention; assisted the team in analysis of the data; written or co-authored some of the published papers, posters, and presentations; disseminated results and findings; and engaged stakeholders on implementation of study findings. In the following section, we provide several specific examples of how CHWs have contributed to and improved our community-based research studies. These descriptions exemplify the dedication, impact, and valuable input CHWs bring to a research team.

14.3.3.2   Examples of the Impact of Community Health Workers as Stakeholders in Research Interventions and Clinical Trials

Human Tissue Plastic Bag Replacement   The first example comes from our South Florida Center for the Reduction of Cancer Health Disparities (SUCCESS). SUCCESS was a randomized controlled trial of 600 minority women in 3 communities of Miami-Dade County, who were between the ages of 35–60 and had not completed a cervical cancer screening within the past 3 years. The intervention used a novel cancer screening method which involved having women themselves collect vaginal samples with a cotton swab using a home self-sampling kit. The sample was placed in a bag and submitted by the CHW to the laboratory for analysis. The overall study finding was this CHW intervention increased cervical cancer screening (Carrasquillo, McCann, et al., 2014; Ilangovan et al., 2016; Kobetz et al., 2018).

In the study, one of our CHWs, Valentine Cesar, expressed concerns about the image stamped on the small plastic bag that the laboratory provided to transport the specimen after collection with the self-sampling kit. The bags had a commonly recognized red and black image on the front of the bag that means biohazard. She explained to the research team that she had spent additional time with research participants to help alleviate fears and address their concerns associated with the symbol on the bags. Participants were concerned that the red and black toxic symbol meant poison was being brought into their homes; this negative connotation also contributed to possible delays and lack of participation with data collection during the home visit.

Upon discussion with the research team and laboratory staff, regular commercially available transparent plastic bags were incorporated to the study protocols to transport the plastic container with the body tissue sample back to the lab. This small change in replacing a bag was significant in that this reduced a perceived barrier to participation in the clinical trial. Furthermore, this demonstrated the CHW's ability to engage in a trusting relationship with the community members, utilize both oral and nonverbal communication skills, and address the concerns of the research participant. This also removed unnecessary barriers during patient education on study procedures and briefing.

Test Sample Check Boxes The next three examples come from our Health in Your Hands (HIYA II) study (Carrasquillo et al., 2020), where a multi-modality strategy for the early detection and/or prevention of four priority health conditions was tested utilizing some of the latest technologies for home-based screening. They include human immunodeficiency virus (HIV) through oral buccal swab testing; hepatitis C virus (HCV) through finger-stick testing; colorectal cancer (CRC) through home fecal immunochemical testing or FIT; and cervical cancer (only women) through self-sampling for human papillomavirus (HPV).

In the study, the CHWs had to determine which test each participant needed. However, at the beginning, it was difficult for the CHWs to easily determine and record which test was needed for each participant. The need of a consistent and standardized use of the recruiting tool (screener) by CHWs was imperative for efficiency in data collection. Since this study was being implemented at three separate clinical sites across diverse South Florida communities, the team needed to prepare a systematic way to collect and enter information on screening tests in the same format. At the time of screening, CHWs review all criteria questions and verify what test is needed by marking the appropriate test sample(s) according to participants' classification. After CHW Ana Rendón had begun recruiting and screening patients, she suggested the idea of adding *check boxes* onto the last page of this tool which we were using to determine if participants met study eligibility criteria. After this suggestion was implemented, CHWs could recruit and follow up with participants by selecting appropriate test sample(s) using the newly modified test sample check boxes. This add-on of the four check boxes facilitated follow-up for the required test samples to be collected at the home visits. They were also incorporated into the *Intake Questionnaire* which research assistants are now also using. Thanks to Ana Rendón's idea of visually including check boxes, data collection has been streamlined, and future data analysis planning can be better implemented from the beginning. This example shows how CHWs can be integral to the development of the tools and how CHW input can save practical time and effort in research design, especially since many of them are also collecting data.

Rapid Test Form In HIYA II, all three CHWs do community-based rapid testing for HIV and hepatitis C screening that involves a multistep process including referral for confirmatory testing for samples that test positive. At study onset, there were no forms being used to capture the detailed steps in this process. The CHWs brought the idea of having a form where information on completion of these steps could be tracked. This new form they helped develop has enhanced the systematic documentation of these procedures and enhanced study fidelity. The document captures specific information to the data entry specialist so that it can be codified into the online database associated with the research project called Research Electronic Data Capture (REDCap). The form also allows for the study physicians to easily review, monitor, and sign off on the test results. This allows for checks and balances in the protocols and the procedures. This also provides the advantage of having a hard-copy form document to accompany the electronic version A in case backup documentation is ever needed.

Kit-Tracking Database Feature As noted above, in HIYA II the data is entered and stored in an online database called REDCap. All three CHWs were asked to provide feedback on potential enhancements that would facilitate and ease the process of CHW follow-up with participants. Based on that initial feedback, a Kit-Tracking feature was included in the online database as a prominently visible tab. This enhancement included adding specific day(s) and time for all four tests (to obtain an average time frame of how samples were processed) and assisted in streamlined analysis of how many tests were completed by each participant, how many kits were returned, and how long it took. This also assisted CHWs in following up with those that needed to be contacted. This REDCap formatting feature also allowed both CHWs and their supervisors to crosscheck and confirm results.

This example highlights the importance for all team members to be a part of the development of tools in that those in the field have experience and insight that are essential to such research procedures. The contribution of CHWs, their experiences in data collection processes and incorporating their perspectives, has helped shape and improve study procedures and protocols in HIYA II to be better tailored to the study needs for structured data collection and interpretation.

Welcome Video The next three examples of CHW contributions to research and evaluation come from the Hispanic Secondary Stroke Prevention Initiative (HiSSPI), a randomized controlled trial of 200 Hispanic/Latino stroke patients at high risk for having another stroke (Carrasquillo et al., 2018). CHWs were part of the intervention arm of the study called CARIÑO (Care, Attention, Resources, Information, Nutrition and Optimism), which educated and monitored study participants after a stroke. Through the CARIÑO program, CHWs offered services such as one-on-one home visits (that often included other family members); support through phone calls and texts; immigration referrals; housing and food assistance; mental health referrals; disability referrals; and companionship during medical appointments and health fairs. The program also a text based mobile technology system, as a two-way communication engagement opportunity. Study participants received scheduled messages for documenting their home blood pressure readings, reminders for medical appointments, and health education messages on nutrition, physical activity, and sleep.

Something new that was implemented to the program was filming a welcome to CARIÑO Initiative video from the doctor (Welcome to CARIÑO Initiative; retrieved from https://www.youtube.com/watch?v=OQ-jxsWGcaw). The idea of creating a welcome video from the doctor for participants came from CHWs as a way to promote an immediate connection into the program. In this 10-minute video, the study Principal Investigator, Dr. Olveen Carrasquillo, introduced himself in Spanish, welcomed the participant to the program, and provided information about stroke, stroke risk factors, and stroke prevention. More importantly, the video explained the role of the CHWs and how they were there to provide social support during this life-changing event. The feedback received from participants about this video introduction was extremely positive. Participants felt connected to the CHWs, and they saw the program as a great benefit. The use of the video also had a positive impact during the visits with the CHW. The participants remembered specific statements from the video and reiterated phrases like: "As the doctor said in the video…," "I know when to call 911," and "like the doctor said, I need to stop smoking." Participants expressed that the video was informative, straight to the point, pleasant, and clear.

With the addition and implementation of the video into the program, this presented an opportunity for an immediate conversation on stroke prevention. The video served as a low-cost strategy that greatly impacted and enhanced entry into the program. For example, CHWs wrote the script for the video, filmed the video using a CHW's cell phone, and uploaded it to YouTube, for free. Project research staff strongly believe this was one of the tools that truly fulfilled the goal of motivating participants in feeling connected to the program from the beginning.

Mobile Texting As reported in "Using Health Text Messages to Improve Consumer Health Knowledge, Behaviors, and Outcomes: An Environmental Scan," in recent years, automated mobile text messaging systems have emerged as a potentially effective approach to support improved health management among underserved populations (U.S. HHS, HRSA, 2014). As noted above, the CARIÑO program used messaging and texting to support CHWs in educating and motivating participants to achieve better health outcomes. This *mobile tool* sent pre-programmed daily texts to the participants. This communication tool allowed the CHWs to track participants' answers and provided them with a log of their own responses. Part of this was having participants text their blood pressure information on a regular basis to the CHWs. The process also allowed participants and CHWs to review responses together, especially their blood pressure readings. A critical feature of this tool was an alert if a participant entered a high blood reading level. In such cases, the CHW was immediately alerted via text. In turn, the CHW contacted participants right away by phone and was able to provide advice and if need contact the study physician.

However, the study did not have a specific protocol on training patients on how to use, send, and access text messages on their phones. As the team needed to find the best way to teach patients on how to do this, they turned to the CHWs for help. One of the CHWs created a simple bilingual fact sheet, which was then used to train participants. Using the sheet, the CHW demonstrated the participant how to use this technology on his or her own using the fact sheet as a guide. The CHWs also provided input and revisions on selecting the in the text messages to be sent such as information on stroke risk factors, nutrition information, physical activity, sleep habits, mental health, and stress management and tips and reminders that the patient should take to better their health and/or lifestyles.

From Progress Notes Form to Revised Contact Log As part of the Miami Healthy Heart Initiative (Lebron et al., 2015), CHWs conducted home visits and made phone calls to participants as part of the intervention. Most visits and calls with participants started with standardized questions including the following:

(a) How have you been since the last time I saw you?
(b) How has it been taking your medication since I last saw you?
(c) Did you have any trouble taking your medication today?
(d) Do you need help with anything in particular?

This information was collected in a Progress Notes form, where the CHW also described the visit with additional details to various other questions (i.e., Where did you meet; did you go anywhere else afterwards with the patient; did any significant issue come up; and, how long did the visit last?). The phone call progress notes had information on the duration of the call, whether it was successful or not, and a summary of information that had been given to the participant regarding health and social services. Over the course of the initial implementation of this research study, it was noted that the Progress Notes data collection instrument did not collect the full range of health education services and materials that the CARIÑO Program participant received from the CHW. In addition, the way CHW's time was utilized while capturing all of the services and information provided to program participants was not felt to be optimal for subsequent analysis of these data.

In response, for HiSSPI (Carrasquillo et al., 2018) the study team created a *Participant Monthly Contact Log*. This new Contact Log was created with detailed input from one of our CHWs, Orieta Fontán, who reviewed her progress notes over

1-month period and then provided very detailed and specific information on the depth and breadth of her activities with study participants. In the new Contact Log, visits to the participant were also broken down into the duration time, site, and social services provided, all well-documented disaggregated data that captured the range of CHW activity with participants. For example, in the Visit Location category, multiple options were included (home, clinic, campus, office, and hospital). Another category that covered social services detailed information was now being collected on filling out health insurance forms, referrals to local safety net clinics, transportation, mental health, immigration status concerns, and medical equipment (blood pressure machine) provided. This Participant Monthly Contact Log was much more effective in being able to summarize and identify CHW tasks, activities, and outreach services provided during the study. Using this revised log, the research team was able to generate data having a greater level of specificity about the many facets of the health education and social services work covered with that patient. These data would then be used in scientific manuscripts on the study intervention and findings.

All of these are examples showing how CHWs have demonstrated themselves to be a valuable stakeholder group in community-based disparities research, patient-centered research, and clinical trial interventions. CHWs have provided input on intervention forms, home visit protocol for human tissue collection, and revised data collection tools to better describe relevant health and social services provided to patients or study participants and their families. This added value increases the capacity of the research team to produce findings that are useful to patients, their families, and their caregivers when making healthcare decisions.

14.3.3.3   Part 2: Creation of Standardized Research Training for CHWs

The many important contributions that CHWs made to our study team required them to have additional skill set and training beyond what more traditional CHWs need when their focus is solely on service delivery. To be effective members of the research team, our CHWs need to better understand research procedures and the basics of informed consent, protection of human subjects, and confidentiality of patient/study participant information. In fact, such training is required at most academic institutions for all research staff engaged in research involving humans. However, the existing courses on research training being offered and required at most academic institutions were not developed for CHWs and often did not meet their training needs. To meet this need, we had been developing and creating project- and study-specific trainings for CHWs, and each time a new study was initiated or when new CHWs were being hired, we needed to train CHWs using these ad hoc training programs. As our research portfolio increased, we realized that there was redundancy in such efforts. Many of the topics covered were general information and skill sets which could be applicable for CHWs involved in any research and not project-specific skills. Thus, if there was a more structured and formalized research training for CHWs, it could avoid the redundancy of our ad hoc CHW research training.

In addition, there was increased interest from collaborative work with other state-based groups conducting research interventions, in expanding CHWs' role from providing direct service delivery to participating in evaluation and research. However, there was no centralized and structured research training program for CHWs in research, and this was repeatedly raised at the numerous group meetings. We saw this as an opportunity to build evidence-based practices (Findley et al., 2012). This need was also highlighted by CHWs themselves through the course of our interventions in clinical trials and trainings across the state.

Given the large interest in CHWs as part of the research workforce, we sought to develop and implement a training module focusing on developing CHW research skills. Such an initiative aimed to build on the increasing recognition and credibility of this fast-growing workforce and contribute towards creating a culturally competent research workforce. In a state such as Florida having a formalized CHW process, this could also be counted as part of the elective modules needed towards CHW certification or recertification. The training program could also serve as a national model for training CHWs that would then be able to be more valuable stakeholder partners in research programs and initiatives. To that end, several stakeholders including the Health Council of South Florida and the Florida Community Health Worker Coalition, Inc., sought a collaborative partner who would help support the development of a statewide research training program for CHWs.

Ultimately, funding to support the development of such a CHW research training program was received from the Patient-Centered Outcomes Research Institute (PCORI) through their Eugene Washington Engagement Award program (UMIAMI #2219). Authorized by Congress in 2010 as part of the Affordable Care Act (ACA), PCORI was created as an independent, nonprofit comparative effectiveness research funding organization. PCORI's mission is to improve people's health by supporting research that will answer outstanding questions or fill current gaps about what works best for patients and their particular circumstances so that they and those who care for them can make better-informed choices about their options. PCORI focuses on answering questions most important to patients and those who care for them based on personal circumstances, values, and desired outcomes. PCORI differs from other research entities in that they aim to produce evidence that can be easily applied in real-world settings, to help patients achieve the outcomes they want, and to reduce the burdens of major health issues (Weinert, Grieser, & Hasnain-Wynia, 2015). In addition, PCORI places a major emphasis on patient and stakeholder engagement so that their research work is informed and guided by input from patients, family caregivers, scientists, healthcare providers, insurers, health plans, and other stakeholders. Many PCORI-funded studies aim to improve healthcare delivery and reduce disparities in outcomes, especially for low-income individuals, those living in rural areas, racial and ethnic minorities, children, older adults, and people with rare diseases (Hasnain-Wynia & Sheridan, 2013). Not surprisingly, many PCORI-funded studies include CHWs and other patient advocates from across the healthcare community in their study design (Promising Practices of meaningful engagement in the conduct of research, 2013). Thus, they were very supportive of a statewide training program for CHWs in comparative effectiveness research.

14.3.3.4 Part 3: CHW Competencies and Training for Research Capacity Building

National Environmental Scan Initially we assumed that there would be existing models and toolkits for CHW training in research. We employed an environmental scan to identify such existing materials (National Academy for State Health Policy, 2017). However, what we found were repeated calls for structured research training programs to develop core competencies and skills of CHWs to strengthen their understanding of the research process (O'Brien et al., 2009; Ruiz et al., 2012). Similar to our approach, other teams in San Diego have been using their own local initiatives to standardize CHW research training (Dumbauld, Kalichman, Bell, Dagnino, & Taras, 2014). In another example from New York, one academic-community partnership developed a program with research competencies in community-based participatory research, basic research design and instrument development, informed consent, computer skills, research ethics, and institutional review board compliance as well as health-specific training such as diabetes, asthma, nutrition, and mental health (Catalani et al., 2009). However, aside from a few of these local initiatives, and unlike general CHW training and certification, where there has been rapid development of statewide and federal guidelines and toolkits, there remained much less developed around CHW research training (Tucker et al., 2018). Further, even though there have been calls for educating stakeholders on their roles in research as a promising method for engagement (Mallery et al., 2012), what existed only addressed research in a broad sense. At the time, we did not find any existing, widely disseminated materials for training in CHWs specifically in patient-centered outcomes research (PCOR) nor having CHWs themselves taking part in the process in such CHW research training program development. Thus, we agreed that we would need to develop the program ourselves.

Engagement and Mobilization of CHWs on PCOR Curriculum Development (UMIAMI# 2219) Our overarching objective was to strengthen CHWs' capacity to be involved in PCOR at the state level and increase the organizational capacity of CHW representative organizations in their promotion of PCOR. We followed PCORI engagement principles as described in their Engagement Rubric. The rubric illustrates how input from patient and stakeholder partners can be incorporated throughout the entire research process (PCORI, 2014). As a roadmap, these engagement and mobilization principles helped incorporate input into key considerations for the planning, conducting, and disseminating of the engaged research capacity-building activities of this project. Conceptually, these partners were classified as follows:

1. *Impacted Stakeholders:* patients/caregivers and CHWs as patient advocates
2. *Interested Stakeholders:* regional/local community organizations, local county public health departments, insurers, payers, federally qualified health centers, free and charitable clinics, not-for-profit organizations and education centers like community colleges, and members of the Board of Directors and Advisory Group of the FL CHW Coalition (in total, over 30 organizations in 18 months)
3. *Subject Matter Experts:* CHW curriculum developers and instructors from Florida and elsewhere to ensure a diversity of opinion and national geographical spread

First, in the planning of the project, the process of how CHWs' and stakeholder partners participated in study planning and design was described. This included definition of terms and creation of project information tools designed to encourage shared understandings. Then, in conducting the project, a detailed description on how stakeholder partners would participate in the study conduct was developed. Further, plans were also drafted so that throughout the life of the project, the project team would work with stakeholders in disseminating ongoing results and training outcomes, describing and reporting back how CHW, patient, and stakeholder partners were involved in plans to disseminate project findings and to ensure that findings were communicated in understandable, usable ways. Compensation of stakeholders for their important role in this project was also clearly articulated at the start of the project.

The next step was then to begin developing the training program. An initial preliminary draft was prepared based in part on literature review and the environmental scan that were conducted. The initial draft also relied heavily on our existing homegrown protocols on CHW training which we had used in our past research studies and CHW-led intervention programs. After this, an initial table of contents and training outline was drafted. We then received feedback from a stakeholder advisory group of CHWs, patients, and patient advocates. For this process, we developed an informational sheet for local organizations, informational slide set to be used at calls and statewide seminars, a template flyer for training recruitment, a template agenda, and project feedback form.

In developing the revised training program, these stakeholders were engaged bidirectionally in all phases. An initial outline was presented to CHWs, patients, and patient advocates through emails, webinars and calls, and two workshops with stakeholders. Focus groups with CHWs and CHW trainers were also conducted for feedback on this initial version. All these groups provided considerable input with respect to content, format literacy level selected, and training schedules' planning activities. Specifically, CHWs and allied session attendees discussed their experiences of seeking and using health information, either as patients, caregivers, or both. They also discussed their own experiences in either being approached to participate, having participated, or having assisted in implementing research studies. Stakeholders also provided feedback on selected content areas of a future training module on patient-centered research, including study design, data collection methods, ethics, informed consent, study protocols, and planned dissemination of study results. Stakeholders also had an opportunity to learn more about PCORI, its priorities, and community/patient engagement versus patient-centeredness and how the training program we were developing aligned with the priorities of the funding organization.

Content of the PCOR Training for CHWs The end result was an interactive 7-hour training that includes short video snippets, lecturettes, role plays, and individual and small group exercises. The content is divided into seven domains:*

1. *Patient-Centered Outcomes Research (PCOR):* In this introductory module, concepts of research, *patient engagement*, and *stakeholder* are defined, comparative effectiveness research is explained, and standards associated with patient-centered research are discussed. Key terms of research vocabulary are defined, and particular attention is paid to emphasize the difference between service delivery and research. CHW trainees go through a small group exercise where they create their own research study plans for a disease or health condition of interest.
2. *Ethics and Protection of Human Research Participants:* This module discusses basic ethical principles and how they apply to modern human subject research, explains the historical basis for regulating human subjects research, describes the role and jurisdiction of the Institutional Research Board, describes vulnerable populations, discusses coercion and undue influence and potential risks to subjects, identifies privacy and confidentiality protections for subjects, and discusses how to recognize ethical/professional boundaries/challenges to be faced as a local CHW.
3. *Study Allocation/Randomization:* This module provides an overview of participation in clinical trials, discusses the difference between the intervention and the comparator or control group, and conveys the importance of the randomization process and how to explain this to participants.
4. *Data Collection:* This module is an introduction to qualitative and quantitative research methods, along with basic information to identify different types of data collection methods, and the CHW's role in data collection. Examples of qualitative methods (such as observations, key informant interviews, focus groups, public forums/community consultations) are provided, along with examples of quantitative methods like questionnaires/surveys, a discussion of mixed-methods approaches, and explanation on how interviewer bias can skew the data and how to avoid this, and the module ends with a discussion on how CHWs can contribute to how data is collected with examples provided.
5. *Informed Consent Process:* This module covers the process for legally effective informed consent, lists the information that should be disclosed to subjects during the consent process, describes the process for obtaining informed consent, and includes a discussion on the voluntariness of the decision about whether or not to participate in research. Role plays are to be conducted in small groups to showcase challenges CHWs have encountered in the field while recruiting and

conducting outreach for clinical studies. Templates and sample content of inform consent forms are also discussed.

6. *Study Protocol and Data Management:* This module provides a definition of what a study protocol is, discusses the importance of study protocol adherence and documenting efforts, and identifies situations that deviate from protocol. The importance of how to report and track interactions with study participants is included, and also tips are included on how to work as a collaborative member of the team.

7. *Dissemination of Study Results:* This last section of the 7-hour course discusses how to disseminate findings to study participants, describes the dissemination of study results through health research journals, describes how CHWs can contribute to research manuscripts, and identifies innovative dissemination methods to the population at large.

Please note that in the description of the content, we use terminology and language that is familiar to researchers and readers. In the actual training sessions, however, the facilitator and materials use language and terminology that is more CHW-friendly.

Table 14.2 provides more details of the training content.

Pilot Testing of the Training Program in Florida After developing the structured research training from 2015 to 2017, the program was pilot tested and implemented among 148 CHWs across Florida. Over 30 diverse stakeholder partners were engaged at various levels in coordinating the trainings across 6 Florida regions. In addition to UM and FLCHWC, other partners involved in helping us disseminate and deliver the trainings included the Florida Department of Health, several federally qualified health centers, state-designated planning health councils, patient groups, community colleges, area health education centers, and social service organizations. Many of these sent their CHWs to the trainings and/or helped host or support the training sessions in various ways. When conducted by a recognized education provider, the program would also allow CHW trainees to receive seven elective credits towards Florida certification or renewal of their credential by the FCB.

Additional Modifications to the Program Throughout this pilot testing phase, additional feedback was received during several stages of the project on content, format, and delivery. This included further input from CHWs, patients and caregivers, CHW instructors, and supervisors from Florida, California, and Texas through consultations with national CHW curriculum experts. After these stakeholder consultations and dialogue, considerable modifications based on bidirectional dialog were made. Particular attention was paid to the training session on ethics and the protection of human subjects' rights, privacy, and confidentiality. Our revised ethics training module made the course material more CHW-friendly by including interactive activities such as role plays and small group discussions around definitions of key terms (coercion vs. persuasion, vulnerable populations, respect for persons, beneficence, justice, governmental protections, personal health information, pri-

Table 14.2 Content of the CHW training modules

Module	Module objective	By the end of this session, trainees will be able to
1. Patient-centered outcomes research (PCOR)	Demonstrate understanding of basic research and standards associated with patient-centered outcomes research	• Define key research vocabulary and difference between service delivery and research • Discuss clinical trials and various stages • Describe the PCOR *engagement* and *stakeholder* concepts • Discuss standards associated with patient-centered research
2. Ethics	Identify basic ethical principles and how they apply to modern human subject research	• Discuss the historical basis for regulating human subjects research • Describe the role and jurisdiction of the Institutional Research Board • Define vulnerable populations • Understand coercion and undue influence and potential risks to subjects • Identify privacy and confidentiality protections for subjects • Recognize ethical/professional boundaries/challenges faced as a local CHW
3. Study allocation/randomization	Demonstrate understanding of the randomization process and how to discuss this with study participants	• Identify intervention vs. comparator (control) • Discuss the importance of randomization • Proficiently explain the randomization process to study participants and its implications
4. Data collection methods	Identify different types of data collection methods and the CHW's role in data collection	• Describe examples of qualitative methods: observations, key informant interviews, focus groups, public forums, and community consultations • Describe examples of quantitative methods: questionnaires/surveys • Identify mixed-methods approaches • Understand how CHWs can contribute to how data is collected • Discuss how interviewer bias can skew the data
5. Informed consent	Demonstrate understanding of the process for legally effective informed consent	• List the information that should be disclosed to subjects during the consent process • Describe the process for obtaining informed consent • Discuss the voluntariness of the decision about whether to participate in research • Identify the regulations for waiving informed consent

(continued)

Table 14.2 (continued)

Module	Module objective	By the end of this session, trainees will be able to
6. Study protocol and reporting	Demonstrate understanding of the importance of study protocol adherence and documenting efforts	• Define what a study protocol is and identify situations that deviate from protocol • Understand a CHW's role in a research study protocol • Discuss how to report and track interactions with study participants, including phone and in person • Describe how to work with research team as a collaborative member of the team
7. Dissemination of study results	Identify conventional and innovative methods of study results dissemination	• Discuss how to disseminate findings to study participants • Describe the dissemination of study results through health research journals • Describe how CHWs can contribute to research manuscripts

For more information, see the description of Florida project at: https://www.pcori.org/research-results/2015/statewide-partnership-training-floridas-community-health-workers-patient

vacy, and institutional review boards). CHWs also provided suggestions for improvement that included making the session available in Spanish, making some content available online, and integrating more real-world scenarios, sample templates, and research study forms.

Spanish Version of the PCOR for CHW Training In a recent survey of Florida CHWs, 29% of respondents stated that Spanish was their preferred language (Tucker et al., 2018). The need for Spanish language training materials was also reiterated by members of our national CHW advisory group from California and Texas, where CHWs also serve a large proportion of Hispanic/Latino groups and also preferred to be trained in their preferred language. They noted that not only would they like to have the program expanded to their states but that a Spanish version of the training would dramatically help expand opportunities available for more CHW engagement in patient-centered research in their states. Thus, a follow-up proposal was submitted to PCORI to create a Spanish language version of the CHW research curriculum and to also expand the project to these two states. One of the original stakeholder partner organizations, the Florida Community Health Worker Coalition, Inc., would help disseminate the Spanish version of the training in Florida.

National Expansion (UMIAMI#7239) The next phase of the project occurred from 2017 to 2019 and involved partnering with two stakeholder partner organizations that had provided input to the original version of the program. Both had solid CHW and *promotores* experience and leadership roles in national CHW advocacy. One was Día de la Mujer Latina (DML), a patient advocacy group in Texas that also conducts CHW trainings in several states and Puerto Rico. The other was the Chula

Vista Community Collaborative (CVCC), a community health empowerment organization in Southern California. Using a Train-the-Trainer model, we trained 14 PCOR Champions, who in turn trained 593 PCOR-trained CHWs in those states, in English and Spanish. Dissemination of these project activities occurred across different audiences and sectors via webinars, CHW networking events, public health workforce conference workshops, Latinx (gender-inclusive term to include both Latinos and Latinas) health equity roundtable discussions, academic posters, and face-to-face presentations.

The final program evaluation and data analysis are ongoing. However, qualitative data analysis of comments in the evaluation forms of the PCOR for CHW training sessions confirms what we observed in the eyes and faces of CHWs across the nation: for many, they experience a paradigm shift in how they see themselves as public health professionals, with a transfer of skills from the direct service delivery they are used to and excel at to being mobilized and engaged as stakeholders in patient-centered research, assessment, and clinical studies.

For more information, a description of the national project is availableat: https:// www.pcori.org/research-results/2017/national-partnership-training-community -health-workers-patient-centered.

Throughout the life of the project, some challenges yielded critical decisions on several topics that molded the implementation of this national effort on capacity building for research training for CHWs.

On Mobilization and Engagement For example, there were different factors that influenced how this project was implemented, such as the level of individual staffs' and organizations' readiness for collaborations and their previous experiences with academic centers, in particular, with logistical and administrative processes such as regular schedule of invoices, processing insurance paperwork, having compatible software, and access to printing resources. The different expertise levels of the various stakeholder partner organizations, their different organizational structures (paid employee vs. volunteer-based), and various degrees of access to local resources for outreach (recently founded vs. long-standing experienced organization), all had an impact on implementation of this project that required tailored approaches to bringing all partner organizations to fully participate.

Upon a recommendation from one of the Texas stakeholder partners, DML, the main team at the University of Miami had to submit an application for content and guest instructor approvals to the Texas Department of State Health Services (DSHS) for CHW and CHW Instructor credit to be provided to trainees. Having the content of the training valid for CHW certification was instrumental in increasing attendance to the PCOR training in Texas (there is no CHW state certification program in California to date, so the continued education credit availability was not part of the discussion with partner groups there). Co-branding of informational products (recruitment flyers, training day agendas, attendance certificates) was strongly encouraged, so stakeholder organizations' logos were included on the templates and could also be used to "brand" the slides of the *Welcome* introduction section of the training program (Fig. 14.3).

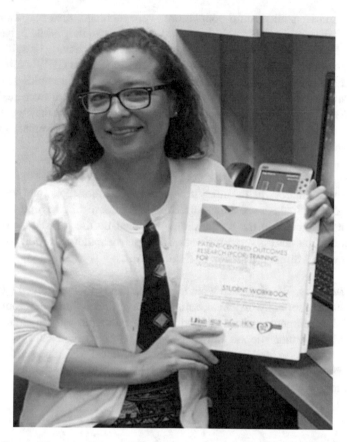

Fig. 14.3 Carmen Linarte, certified CHW candidate, with the PCOR for CHWs Training Student Manual showcasing the logos of our stakeholder partner organizations

On Content and Curriculum Development The issues related to different levels of literacy of future CHW trainees were brought up very early in creating the training materials. Upon discussions with the team, it was decided to be at twelfth grade reading level and targeting CHWs that already had some experience in the field to draw from, in other words not for new CHWs. Feedback was also elicited early in the process on a preferred training format (1 day vs. split into 2 days; sections in person/online, prescriptive vs. open) from each of the four local stakeholder partner organizations; three sites preferred one full day, and the last one requested 2 days to accommodate the working schedules of their selected CHWs. An important point of discussion in Module 1 of the training program was to spend time clarifying the distinction between service provision and research, to achieve a paradigm shift of transfer of skills from the CHWs' experiences in direct service delivery. A study research design activity for Module 1 was created as a recommendation from a CHW instructor in one of the early trainings in California for more interactivity. In Module 2, more historical examples of unethical health research with both African

American and Hispanic/Latino populations were included, also based on recommendations from early CHW trainees in evaluation forms. In Module 3, basic information on the phases of clinical studies was reinstated after having initially received feedback to delete that content. Module 6's discussion on the CHW's role as member of a research team was expanded to include specific examples from actual research studies and CHW interventions previously conducted, from real clinical studies, to which the CHW trainees responded very favorably. As they were released online throughout the life of the project, PCORI-funded project summary fact sheets per state were added in Module 7.

On Translations We discussed and sought input on how to address the diversity of literacy levels, nuances of meaning in vocabulary for concepts, and terminology variations across Spanish-speaking populations. A pilot testing session of the translation was conducted on the set of slides provided by the translator, focused on problematic terms and diverse regional Spanish vocabulary as well as avoiding terms that were a direct translation of English words.

On Sustainability We discussed what is next for newly PCOR-trained CHWs, different paths for deeper involvement, future training, professional development, and educational attainment options, including undergraduate and graduate studies. Lastly, and to further support our stakeholder partner organizations in Florida, California, Tennessee, and Texas, we provided technical assistance and individual and organizational mentorship to co-author several submissions that were accepted for presentation at recent major academic conferences.

14.3.4 Conclusion

Beyond their traditional role of direct service delivery provision, CHWs can also be an important stakeholder partner in patient-centered research. Rapid growth and utilization of CHWs has enhanced the evidence base to support CHWs in many distinct clinical areas, evaluation, community assessments, and health disparities projects. In their capacity as patients themselves, patient advocates, and healthcare professionals, CHWs can make unique and significant contributions to community-engaged disparities research projects. Our own clinical trial interventions in diabetes, stroke, HIV disease, and cancer screening demonstrate that CHWs are invaluable members of research teams.

However, there had been a national need for a structured research training program for CHWs. With PCORI support, and along with our stakeholder partners, we have now addressed this gap. The program we developed consists of seven training modules, available in English and Spanish, and is available in toolkit format including a set of slides, facilitator guide, and a CHW student workbook. The program has been pilot tested, refined, and implemented in both languages with almost 600 CHWs in Florida, California, Texas, and Tennessee. This training mechanism allows for CHWs to participate in research in multiple important ways and serves as a viable pathway to make patient-centered outcomes research more meaningful to patients and key stakeholders.

Acknowledgments Our profound thanks to PCORI, to CHWs who are training attendees in all four states for their feedback, and to CHW/CHW instructors at our stakeholder partner organizations:

- **California CHW Instructors:** Azucena Lopez de Nava, Margarita Holguin, Gabby Ruano, and Lillian Hernandez, Chula Vista Community Collaborative, San Diego
- **Florida:** Patria Alguila, CCHW and CHW Curriculum Instructor, board member of the FL CHW Coalition, and original translator of the curriculum; Lisa Hamilton, PhD, CHW Instructor and Supervisor, Co-President of FL CHW Coalition; and the CHWs who worked in our clinical interventions: Orieta Fontán at University of Miami, María Azqueta at Citrus Health, Valentine Cèsar at the Center for Haitian Studies, and Ana Rendón at Community Health of South Florida (CHI)
- **Texas CHW Instructors:** Juan Rosa, El Buen Samaritano Leadership, Austin; Mérida Escobar, South Texas Promotores Association, Edinburgh/McAllen/ Brownsville; Maria Covernali Ortiz, Familias Triunfadoras, El Paso; Mercedes Duque-Cruz, DML, Dallas/Fort Worth; and Jackie Ramos and Maria Guadalupe, DML, Houston
- **Tennessee:** Juan Canedo, Board Member, Progreso Community Center, Nashville

References

Carrasquillo, O., Lebron, C., Alonzo, Y., Li, H., Chang, A., & Kenya, S. (2017). Effect of a community health worker intervention among Latinos with poorly controlled type 2 diabetes: The Miami healthy heart Initiative randomized clinical trial. *JAMA Internal Medicine, 177*(7), 948–954. https://doi.org/10.1001/jamainternmed.2017.0926

Carrasquillo, O., McCann, S., Amofah, A., Pierre, L., Rodriguez, B., Alonzo, Y., ... Kobetz, E. (2014). Rationale and Design of the Research Project of the South Florida Center for the Reduction of Cancer Health Disparities (SUCCESS): Study protocol for a randomized controlled trial. *Trials, 15*, 299. https://doi.org/10.1186/1745-6215-15-299. PubMed PMID: 25056208; PubMed Central PMCID: PMC4127186.

Carrasquillo, O., Patberg, E., Alonzo, Y., Li, H., & Kenya, S. (2014). Rationale and design of the Miami healthy heart Initiative: A randomized controlled study of a community health worker intervention among Latino patients with poorly controlled diabetes. *International Journal of General Medicine, 7*, 115–126. https://doi.org/10.2147/IJGM.S56250. PubMed PMID: 24600243; PubMed Central PMCID: PMC3942117.

Carrasquillo, O., Seay, J., Jhaveri, V., Long, T., Kenya, S., Thomas, E., ... Kobetz, E. (2020). Increasing uptake of evidence-based screening services though a community health worker-delivered multi-modality program: Study protocol for a randomized pragmatic trial. *Trials,* *21*, 368.

Carrasquillo, O., Young, B., Dang, S., Fontan, O., Ferras, N., Romano, J. G., ... Kenya, S. (2018). Hispanic Secondary Stroke Prevention Initiative Design: Study protocol and rationale for a randomized controlled trial. *JMIR Research Protocols, 7*(10), e11083. https://doi. org/10.2196/11083

Catalani, C. E., Findley, S. E., Matos, S., & Rodriguez, R. (2009). Community health worker insights on their training and certification. *Progress in Community Health Partnerships, 3*(3), 227–235. https://doi.org/10.1353/cpr.0.0082

Chang, A., Patberg, E., Cueto, V., Li, H., Singh, B., Kenya, S., ... Carrasquillo, O. (2018). Community health workers, access to care, and service utilization among Florida Latinos: A randomized controlled trial. *American Journal of Public Health, 108*(9), 1249–1251. https:// doi.org/10.1097/MLR.0000000000000337

ClinicalTrials.gov. (2018, October 17). Miami Healthy Heart Initiative: A Behavioral Study on Cardiovascular Risk Factors (MHHI). Retrieved from https://clinicaltrials.gov/ct2/show/ NCT01152957.

Community Health Resources, LLC. (2007, October). *Building a National Research Agenda for the Community Health Worker Field: An Executive Summary of Proceedings from "Focus on the Future," an Invitational Conference.* Retrieved from http://www.chrllc.net/sitebuildercon- tent/sitebuilderfiles/chwdraftresear.chagenda.pdf.

Dumbauld, J., Kalichman, M., Bell, Y., Dagnino, C., & Taras, H. L. (2014). Case study in designing a research fundamentals curriculum for community health workers: A univer- sity-community clinic collaboration. *Health Promotion Practice, 15*(1), 79–85. https://doi. org/10.1177/1524839913504416

Findley, S., Matos, S., Hicks, A., Campbell, A., Moore, A., & Diaz, D. (2012). Building a consen- sus on CHW scope of practice: Lessons from New York. *American Journal of Public Health,* *102*(7), 1981–1987. https://doi.org/10.2105/ajph.2011.300566

Florida Center for Nursing. (2016). *2016 Annual Report.* Retrieved from https://www.hwri.org/ Portals/0/files/FHW-Emerging_Evolving_Roles_Occupations-May2016.pdf

Hasnain-Wynia, R., & Sheridan, S. (2013, August 5). *Conversations with the Latino/Hispanic com- munity.* Retrieved from https://www.pcori.org/blog/conversations-latinohispanic-community.

Ilangovan, K., Kobetz, E., Koru-Sengul, T., Marcus, E. N., Rodriguez, B., Alonzo, Y., & Carrasquillo, O. (2016). Acceptability and feasibility of human papilloma virus self-sam- pling for cervical cancer screening. *Journal of Women's Health, 25*(9), 944–951. https://doi. org/10.1089/jwh.2015.5469

Kenya, S., Jones, J., Arheart, K., Kobetz, E., Chida, N., Baer, S., & Carrasquillo, O. (2013). Using community health workers to improve clinical outcomes among people living with HIV: A randomized controlled trial. *AIDS and Behavior, 17*(9), 2927–2934. https://doi.org/10.1007/ s10461-013-0440-1

Kenya, S., Okoro, I. S., Wallace, K., Ricciardi, M., Carrasquillo, O., & Prado, G. (2016). Can home-based HIV rapid testing reduce HIV disparities among African Americans in Miami? *Health Promotion Practice, 17*(5), 722–730. https://doi.org/10.1177/1524839916629970

Kim, K., Choi, J. S., Choi, E., Nieman, C. L., Joo, J. H., Lin, F. R., & Han, H. R. (2016). Effects of community-based health worker interventions to improve chronic disease management and care among vulnerable populations: A systematic review. *American Journal of Public Health,* *106*(4), e3–e28. https://doi.org/10.2105/ajph.2015.302987

Kobetz, E., Seay, J., Koru-Sengul, T., Bispo, J., Trevil, D., Gonzalez, M., ... Carrasquillo, O. (2018). A randomized trial of mailed HPV self-sampling for cervical cancer screening among ethnic minority women in South Florida. *Cancer Causes & Control, 29*, 793. https://doi.org/10.1007/ s10552-018-1055-7

Lebron, C. N., Reyes-Arrechea, E., Castillo, A., Carrasquillo, O., & Kenya, S. (2015). Tales from the Miami healthy heart Initiative: The experiences of two community health workers.

Journal of Health Care for the Poor and Underserved, 26(2), 453–462. https://doi.org/10.1353/hpu.2015.0033

Mallery, C., Ganachari, D., Smeeding, L., Fernandez, J., Lavallee, D., Siegel, J., & Moon, M. (2012). PHP5 innovative methods for stakeholder engagement: An environmental scan. *Value in Health, 15*(4), A14. https://doi.org/10.1016/j.jval.2012.03.082

National Academy for State Health Policy. (2017, August). *State community health worker models.* Retrieved from https://nashp.org/state-community-health-worker-models/.

National Center for Chronic Disease Prevention and Health Promotion, Division for Heart Disease and Stroke Prevention. (2015, April). *Addressing chronic disease through community health workers: A policy and systems—Level approach.* Retrieved from https://www.cdc.gov/dhdsp/docs/chw_brief.pdf.

O'Brien, M. J., Squires, A. P., Bixby, R. A., & Larson, S. C. (2009). Role development of community health workers: An examination of selection and training processes in the intervention literature. *American Journal of Preventive Medicine, 37*(6 Suppl 1), S262–S269. https://doi.org/10.1016/j.amepre.2009.08.011

Patient-Centered Outcomes Research Institute. (2013, September 19). *Promising practices of meaningful engagement in the conduct of research.* Retrieved from https://www.pcori.org/events/2013/promising-practices-meaningful-engagement-conduct-research.

Patient-Centered Outcomes Research Institute. (2014, February 4). *PCORI Engagement Rubric.* Retrieved from https://www.pcori.org/sites/default/files/Engagement-Rubric.pdf

Rodriguez, B. (2019). FL CHW certification updates. In *Presentation at the 9th annual FLCHWC summit*, September 13, Orlando, FL.

Rosenthal, E. L., Brownstein, J. N., Rush, C. H., Hirsch, G. R., Willaert, A. M., Scott, J. R., … Fox, D. J. (2010). Community health workers: Part of the solution. *Health Affairs (Millwood), 29*(7), 1338–1342.2.

Ruiz, Y., Matos, S., Kapadia, S., Islam, N., Cusack, A., Kwong, S., & Trinh-Shevrin, C. (2012). Lessons learned from a community-academic initiative: The development of a core competency-based training for community-academic initiative community health workers. *American Journal of Public Health, 102*(12), 2372–2379. https://doi.org/10.2105/ajph.2011.300429

Tucker, C. M., Smith, T. M., Hogan, M. L., Banzhaf, M., Molina, N., & Rodriguez, B. (2018). Current demographics and roles of Florida community health workers: Implications for future recruitment and training. *Journal of Community Health, 43*(3), 552–559. https://doi.org/10.1007/s10900-017-0451-3

U.S. Bureau of the Census. (2016) *American Community Survey 2012–2016.* Retrieved from https://www.census.gov/acs/www/data/data-tables-and-tools/data-profiles/2016/.

U.S. Department of Health and Human Services. (2014). Health Resources and Services Administration. In *Using health text messages to improve consumer health knowledge, behaviors, and outcomes: An environmental scan.* Rockville, MD: U.S. Department of Health and Human Services. Retrieved from https://www.hrsa.gov/sites/default/files/archive/healthit/txt4tots/environmentalscan.pdf

U.S. Department of Health and Human Services, Health Resources and Services Administration, Bureau of Health Professions. (2007). *Community health worker national workforce study.* Retrieved from https://bhw.hrsa.gov/sites/default/files/bhw/nchwa/projections/community-healthworkforce.pdf.

Weinert, M., Grieser, M., & Hasnain-Wynia R. (2015). *Using community health-care workers to reduce disparities.* Retrieved from https://www.pcori.org/blog/using-community-healthcare-workers-reduce-disparities.

Welcome to CARIÑO Initiative from Dr. Carrasquillo. (2018). Retrieved from https://www.youtube.com/watch?v=OQ-jxsWGcaw.

Witmer, A., Seifer, S. D., Finocchio, L., Leslie, J., & O'Neil, E. H. (1995). Community health workers: Integral members of the health care work force. *American Journal of Public Health, 85*(8 Pt 1), 1055–1058. https://doi.org/10.2105/ajph.85.8_pt_1.1055

Part III
A Bright Future for CHWs

Chapter 15
Uniting the Workforce: Building Capacity for a National Association of Community Health Workers

Geoffrey W. Wilkinson, Ashley Wennerstrom, Naomi Cottoms, Katherine Sutkowi, and Carl H. Rush

15.1 Brief History of CHW Practice in the United States

Throughout this book, community health workers (CHWs) and their allies alike have highlighted the unique skills, roles, and competencies of CHWs working across the United States and in tribal nations. Each narrative of how individual CHWs and the programs for which they work have changed lives and even entire communities which is powerful and inspiring in its own right. However, to truly appreciate both the long-term implications of CHWs' previous efforts and their potential to revolutionize health in the future, we must examine the history of the CHW workforce, which is firmly rooted in the social justice movement.

CHWs have been working in some of the most impoverished areas in the United States and in tribal nations since the early 1950s (Hoff, 1969). The passage of two federal laws—the Federal Migrant Health Act of 1962 and the Economic

G. W. Wilkinson (✉)
Center for Innovation in Social Work and Health, Boston University School of Social Work, Boston, MA, USA
e-mail: gww@bu.edu

A. Wennerstrom
Behavioral and Community Health Sciences, Louisiana State University School of Public Health, New Orleans, LA, USA

Center for Healthcare Value and Equity, Louisiana State University School of Medicine, New Orleans, LA, USA

N. Cottoms
Tri County Rural Health Network, Inc., Helena, AR, USA

K. Sutkowi
New York City Department of Health and Mental Hygiene, New York, NY, USA

C. H. Rush
Community Resources, LLC, San Antonio, TX, USA

© Springer Nature Switzerland AG 2021
J. A. St. John et al. (eds.), *Promoting the Health of the Community*,
https://doi.org/10.1007/978-3-030-56375-2_15

Opportunity Act of 1964—promoted opportunities for CHWs to connect with under resourced areas by requiring health outreach services in migrant labor camps and impoverished neighborhoods, respectively (Perez & Martinez, 2008). Shortly thereafter, in 1968, The Indian Health Service's Community Health Representative program began with funding from the Office of Economic Opportunity (Indian Health Service, n.d.). These early programs, developed at the same time of the national community health center movement (Geiger, 2016), aimed to improve health primarily facilitating access to formal health care (Mesiter, 1990).

As CHW programs became more commonplace, several authors began to take note of CHWs' value beyond merely linking individuals to care. Specifically, they were prized for their ability to inform providers about how to address both individual and community health concerns (D'Onofrio, 1970). One 1967 description stated that CHWs could act as community organizers who would mobilize individuals and build community capacity to change social conditions (Kent & Smith, 1967). Later, in the 1990s, scholars described CHW roles as including community empowerment, advancement of social agendas, and advocacy for health system improvements (Beam & Tessaro, 1994; Eng & Young, 1992; Witmer, Siefer, Finocchio, Leslie, & O'Neil, 1995). More recently, the CHW literature has continued to stress that CHWs can promote social justice through community-level advocacy focused on changing policies related to social determinants of health (Ingram, Sabo, Rothers, Wennerstrom, & de Zapien, 2008; Perez & Martinez, 2008; Sabo, Ingram, & Wennerstrom, 2010).

CHW efforts to address social issues related to health are well documented in scientific literature in the context of specific interventions. However, an important story that has yet to be told is how CHWs have organized themselves as a workforce. In much the same manner that promoting community health requires thinking beyond merely individual clients or patients to the organizational-, community-, and policy-level factors that affect health, CHWs have realized that their livelihood and ability function as successful community advocates, rather than just liaisons to the healthcare system, which require creating higher-level infrastructure to support and organize the workforce.

This chapter aims to elucidate some of the complex history of how and why CHWs across the United States and tribal nations have organized themselves over the last two decades. A precise chronological version of the story would be difficult to convey, as multiple events and activities occurred simultaneously at local, state, and national levels. To outline the evolution of the field, the chapter begins with a description of some of the major milestones that contributed to conceptualizing CHWs, CHRs, and *promotores* a single workforce, as opposed to merely individuals who serve a single population or work on short-term health interventions. Next, there is a description of efforts to establish local and state CHW networks. Finally, there is a detailed history of over a decade of collective work that resulted in creation of the National Association of Community Health Workers (NACHW).

15.1.1   Key Milestones for the CHW Workforce

In 1970, CHWs and allies affiliated with the American Public Health Association (APHA) began organizing nationally within the Community Health Planning and Policy Development Section (American Public Health Association, 2018). The New Professionals Special Primary Interest Group (SPIG) formed with 500 CHWs and their supporters. In 2000, the New Professional SPIG changed its name to the Community Health Worker SPIG. In 2009, the SPIG reached 250 members, allowing it to become a section, a key designation that elevated CHWs into APHA governance and recognition.

An important milestone that contributed to the coalescing of the SPIG, and later section, was the release of the 1998 National Community Health Advisor Study (NCHAS) (Rosenthal et al., 1998). This was the first national study of CHW roles and activities, which helped both individuals—then working under a wide variety of titles—and their employers to recognize CHWs as a distinct workforce. The CHW SPIG passed the first APHA policy focused on CHWs in 2001 called *Recognition and Support for Community Health Workers' Contributions to Meeting Our Nation's Health Care Needs* (American Public Health Association, 2001), which articulated many CHW titles and roles outlined in the National Community Health Advisor Study.

Another seminal study was the Community Health Worker National Workforce Study published by the Health Services and Resources Administration (HRSA) in 2007 (US Department of Health and Human Services, 2007). The publication provided valuable insight into the work of an estimated 120,000 CHWs in the United States. Of equal importance, for the first time, the federal agency responsible for tracking and supporting health professionals' development had acknowledged CHWs as an important workforce.

In 2009, the CHW SPIG championed an additional development and adopted an APHA policy, *Support for Community Health Workers to Increase Health Access and to Reduce Health Inequities* (American Public Health Association, 2009). This policy outlined the first comprehensive, consensus-driven definition of CHWs:

> *Community Health Workers (CHWs) are frontline public health workers who are trusted members of and/or have an unusually close understanding of the community served. This trusting relationship enables CHWs to serve as a liaison/link/intermediary between health/ social services and the community to facilitate access to services and improve the quality and cultural competence of service delivery. CHWs also build individual and community capacity by increasing health knowledge and self-sufficiency through a range of activities such as outreach, community education, informal counseling, social support and advocacy.*

The APHA, SPIG, and other CHW leaders petitioned the US Department of Labor (DOL) in 2006 to adopt a new Standard Occupational Classification (SOC) for CHWs. The DOL adopted a new classification in 2009, SOC 21–1094, which resulted in CHWs being included as a profession in the 2010 census (US Department of Labor, Bureau of Labor Statistics, 2017). In 2010, DOL also began counting employer data on CHWs.

Additional policy success followed. In 2010, CHWs were referenced in three sections of the Patient Protection and Affordable Care Act: §5101, §5313, and §5403 (111th Congress, 2nd Session, 2010). In these sections, CHWs were defined and recognized as professionals on healthcare teams. CHWs were further referenced in the law as part of the National Health Care Workforce Commission and within grant funding to enhance the community health workforce.

Formal inclusion in the ACA fueled additional policy change in various states, which had been happening organically for several years prior. Changes to payment structures began formal recognition and reimbursement of CHWs. In 2013, the Centers for Medicare & Medicaid issued a notice in the Federal Register, 440.130—diagnostic, screening, preventative, and rehabilitative services (Centers for Medicare & Medicaid Services, 2013):

> "(c) Preventive services means services recommended by a physician or other licensed practitionerofthehealingartsactingwithinthescopeofauthorizedpracticeunderStatelawto—
>
> - Prevent disease, disability, and other health conditions or their progression
> - Prolong life
> - Promote physical and mental health and efficiency."

Per notice, states have discretion at determining who can provide such services, as long as they are recommended by a physician or other licensed provider. CHWs and their supporters advocated for states to amend their Medicaid plans to include CHWs as a provider of such services. While uptake of this approach has been limited to date, this change sparked interest from state Medicaid offices, payers, and healthcare organizations in the role of the CHW and potential for reimbursement. Though some states had already explored legislation for CHW reimbursement (Rosenthal et al., 2010), the 2013 ruling pushed additional state authorities to adopt or endorse payment mechanisms for CHWs, whether formally through reimbursement or as part of Medicaid contracts.

In 2014, the APHA CHW Section proposed a new policy statement, *Support for Community Health Worker Leadership in Determining Workforce Standards for Training and Credentialing* (American Public Health Association, 2014), outlining the need for self-determination of CHWs in CHW workforce decisions; the policy statement was approved by APHA's Governing Council. Key to this policy is a recommendation that entities—including state and local governments—seeking to draft or adopt policies about the CHW workforce should engage with the CHW workforce in development of those policies, including at least 50% self-identified CHWs.

15.1.2   Local, State, and Regional Organizing

While APHA provided one venue for organizing CHWs and their supporters, CHWs have organized into peer and professional groups since the 1960s when the Indian Health Service launched their community health representative program, leading to the National Association of Community Health Representatives or NACHR (National Association of Community Health Representatives, 2018). NACHR, founded in 1978 and governed by CHR leaders from different tribes and regions, and its tribal affiliates continue work today (US Department of Health and Human Services, Office of the Inspector General, 1993).

CHW membership organizations have taken various forms in the last half century, including as formal or informal organizations. A recent survey of current CHW membership organizations showed that over half of organizations were founded in 2010 or after (Fig. 15.1), coinciding with the passage of the ACA and recognition by the DOL (Wilkinson, Sutkowi, & Cenzon, 2018).

The same survey found that less than half of CHW membership organizations are incorporated as independent entities and that about one third have paid staff members. These organizations reported providing CHW professional development, attending conferences, training CHWs, and providing information about the workforce to employers, policymakers, and the public.

Organizing at the local, state, and regional levels has been both grassroots and grasstops. Some recent efforts have sparked stakeholders' interest in CHW organizing as funding—including funding from the Centers for Disease Control and Prevention (CDC)—has strongly encouraged engagement of CHWs in the development of workforce guidelines.

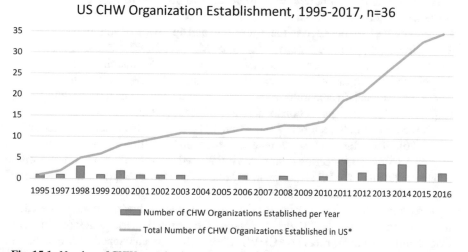

Fig. 15.1 Number of CHW organizations established by year, 1995–2017, from a survey of CHW networks conducted by NACHW

15.2   History of Developing a National CHW Organization

As CHW leaders made progress in developing an institutional base within APHA, as well as through local, state, and regional groups, they came to believe the workforce needed to have its own, independent, national voice. APHA's CHW Section was subject to the policies and procedures of the larger organization, and, since few CHWs could afford to participate in APHA, allies outnumbered CHWs in the Section's membership. The escalating national healthcare reform debate, coupled with a rising tide of research documenting CHW value in addressing healthcare and public health challenges, underscored the need for direct CHW engagement in policymaking and program development. CHWs and their allies faced a quickening stream of requests for information about core competencies, best practice models, credentialing, training, and financing. At the same time, local and state CHW organizations were emerging around the country. The time seemed right to develop a CHW organization led and controlled by workforce members.

15.2.1   American Association of CHWs (AACHW), 2006–2009

National organization building commenced in the mid-1990s, when CHW leaders convened from around the country and agreed to use "community health worker" (CHW) as a unifying umbrella term to describe a diverse workforce with over 50 documented job titles. NACHR, which had used the term "Community Health Representative," participated in the discussion and approved of adopting "CHW" as a unifying workforce title (Fox, Holderby, & Monroe, 2008). Similarly, leadership from the then-active National Association of Hispanic community health workers participated in the discussions and supported using "CHW" as a unifying term. These two national organizations represented specific components of the workforce, respectively, but no organization existed to represent all CHWs.

That changed in September 2006, when CHW leaders from across the country met in Potomac, Maryland, and agreed to form a unified national organization. They elected a 15-member steering committee comprised entirely of CHWs representing 13 states and all of the US Department of Health and Human Services regions. They organized into three subcommittees (membership/outreach, vision/bylaws, and policy), recruited an advisory council of allies, and started hosting conference calls monthly. In October 2006, they adopted the name American Association of Community Health Workers (AACHW). Their achievement capped over 6 years of meetings and discussions from 2000 through 2006 at Unity conferences, APHA annual meetings, and other venues, in which some 200 CHWs and 40 allies from 38 states participated (Fox et al., 2008). (The Unity conference provides a national forum for CHWs to gather from across the country for professional networking, learning, and leadership development. Created under the auspices of the University of Southern Mississippi, it has provided a key resource for CHW workforce identity building and organizing since 1999.)

AACHW adopted the Swahili word for self-determination, Kujichagulia, to emphasize the organization's core commitment to CHW leadership. "Community Health Workers shall determine the direction of the field," stated an AACHW presentation to the 2008 national Unity conference. "We will make the decisions concerning training and education best practices, policy development and define the field of community health workers" (Fox et al., 2008). Fidelity to this fundamental value shaped AACHW's work and direction.

AACHW was impressively productive in its short life as an organization. In 2006, AACHW leaders received a grant from the Robert Wood Johnson Foundation to support organizational infrastructure development in collaboration with the Harrison Institute at Georgetown Law Center. Work began in earnest in 2007 and resulted in a refined plan for governance structure and membership development. AACHW's bylaws committee developed vision and mission statements. AACHW's policy committee, in turn, developed a statement of core values and a CHW Code of Ethics that was disseminated nationally and used, among other purposes, to influence development of regulations for the Massachusetts program of state certification for CHWs (Wilkinson et al., 2018). The Code of Ethics was also included in 2009 in the pioneering CHW textbook, *Foundations for Community Health Workers* (Berthold, Miller, & Avila-Esparza, 2009).

Unfortunately, the demands of building and sustaining a national organization exceeded the resources AACHW was able to attract at the time. The organization depended primarily on the voluntary efforts of its leaders, who juggled AACHW-related responsibilities with the demands of their own jobs and family lives. The organization, which was never incorporated, suspended operations in 2009.

AACHW's leaders continued their national networking, using the Unity conference and APHA as structural vehicles for meeting in-person and coordinating ongoing work to promote CHW unity and workforce development. They kept the dream of a national CHW organization alive; they expanded their ranks; and they used the organizing principle of Kujichagulia to shape expectations for the behavior of allied healthcare and public health practitioners, policy makers, researchers, and advocates.

15.2.2 National Association of Community Health Workers (NACHW)

In November 2014, the CHWs who had been organizing for so many years finally received the opportunity for financial support they had been seeking for so long. A senior official with Sanofi US invited about a dozen recognized CHW leaders and allies to discuss opportunities for the company to support CHWs. Sanofi, a French-based pharmaceutical firm, had a strong interest in community-based prevention and was enthusiastic about the potential to support the CHW workforce nationally. The meeting, held in conjunction with the APHA annual meeting in New Orleans, included leaders and supporters of the former AACHW, who emphasized the value of workforce unity and self-determination. Discussions included the idea of rebuilding a national CHW organization and embraced the principle of CHW leadership. Participants in the meeting discussed lessons from the AACHW organizing experience and agreed about the importance of helping to build the capacity of state-based CHW organizations across the country. Most fundamentally, they agreed about the importance of bringing a direct CHW voice to the table in planning and policymaking with stakeholders at multiple levels about health equity and holistic health promotion.

To move the process forward, Sanofi sponsored a series of webinars in 2015 to provide technical assistance to state and local CHW associations. CHW leaders and allies planned and delivered the webinar content, featuring examples of effective CHW networks and providing information about strategic planning and organization building. Feedback was positive and underscored the need for an organization that could sustain support for the national workforce over time.

Planning for the new organization proceeded concurrently with production of the webinar series. In July 2015, an expanded group of CHW leaders and allies met at the Unity conference in Memphis, Tennessee, to discuss organizational development in more detail. By the fall, a core group of CHW leaders and allies had coalesced and were steering the process forward. This leadership group determined grant funds, for the continued effort would need to be managed by a third party. They considered several possibilities, including national philanthropies and academic centers, and chose the Center for Innovation in Social Work and Health at the Boston University School of Social Work (BU), whose leadership expressed strong support for the initiative. BU would become the fiscal sponsor for future grants to bring the new national CHW organization to life.

Planning intensified in the winter of 2016 with more frequent communication as the leadership group developed a presentation proposal for the 2016 Unity conference and started drafting its first proposal for Sanofi grant support. Several hundred CHWs from across the country attended a Unity conference presentation in Atlanta, Georgia, that July and expressed support for national organization building. Meeting between official conference sessions, planners focused on the importance of building workforce unity through an organization that could effectively represent diverse perspectives and identities, including *promotores de salud*, CHRs, and CHWs working under dozens of job titles. At this point, what to call such an organization was unclear, but participants agreed their shared values provided the basis for finding a path forward together.

Sanofi provided further funding in the fall of 2016, which enabled administrative and logistical support, and, on October 7–8, 21 CHWs and allies from 15 states met in Phoenix, Arizona, for a strategic planning retreat. The group named itself the National Coordinating Committee (NCC). They outlined a vision for the national organization, agreed on its purpose and core principles, and made formative decisions about governance and structure. They shared emerging plans during an APHA annual meeting session in Denver, Colorado, in November 2016, drawing interest and support from attendees.

The NCC continued working together into 2017 through biweekly conference calls. The NCC formed a steering committee and ad hoc work groups to maximize productivity of calls involving the entire group. At least ten NCC members were required to conduct business on any conference call, and at least half of participants had to be CHWs.

NCC members met together with the consultants in Atlanta in July 2017 for a second planning retreat, where, after careful deliberation, they chose a name for the organization: the National Association of Community Health Workers (NACHW). They approved draft vision and mission statements for NACHW, identified program priorities, worked on details of structure and governance, and agreed to refer to the leadership group as the Interim Board. Strategic planning committee members met again with the consultants in August, and strategic planning activities continued through the end of 2017.

While strategic planning was underway, organizational leaders prepared presentations for the 2017 Unity conference in Dallas, Texas, where some 400 CHWs from across the country provided input on organizational design and priorities. In addition, the NCC initiated the most comprehensive national survey of local, state, and regional CHW membership organizations ever undertaken, in cooperation with the Boston University School of Social Work. Researchers gathered data from three dozen CHW organizations across the country. After presentation of initial results at the 2017 APHA annual meeting in Atlanta, additional organizations appealed to be included in the study, and data gathering resumed from November 2017 through January 2018. The final report, presenting detailed information covering 40 distinct organizations, was distributed to respondents in June 2018 and subsequently to other interested parties.[1]

In February 2018, NACHW's leaders met in Chicago, Illinois, to address a variety of issues that had been identified but not fully considered in the consultant-led strategic planning process. The meeting provided adequate detail to proceed with hiring both an attorney to assist with NACHW's incorporation as a 501(c)(3) tax-exempt organization and a web design consultant to help implement the organization's emerging communications plan. Sanofi provided two additional grants in 2018 to support organizational launch. On October 22, 2018, the board held a Washington, DC-based event with national organizational partners to announce that NACHW would launch officially the following spring. The event was conceived as a way to catalyze support from national health organizations and was well attended, attracting some 50 participants. Presenters included a senior CDC official and the executive directors of APHA and the Trust for America's Health, along with the co-chairs of NACHW's board. Three weeks later, NACHW leaders reported on organizational development plans at the APHA annual meeting in San Diego, California.

---

[1] Plenary presentations and workshops were made at the national Unity conferences to engage CHWs from across the country in organizational planning in 2016 (Atlanta, 7/17–20) and 2017 (Dallas, 8/6–9). Scientific sessions and CHW section presentations were made, similarly, to engage CHWs and allies in organizational planning at APHA annual meetings in 2016 (Denver, 10/30–11/2) and 2017 (Atlanta, 11/5–8). In-person planning retreats were held in Phoenix (10/7–8, 2016), in Atlanta (7/21–23/17), and in Chicago (2/24–25/18). The strategic planning committee also met with consultants in Dallas on 8/6/17.

As momentum toward launch continued to build, NACHW's board maintained its intensive schedule of biweekly phone meetings. Board committees coordinated work on fundraising, outreach, and website development, policy, event planning, and developing bylaws in cooperation with NACHW's attorney. In December, 2018, the organization negotiated a Memorandum of Understanding with Health Resources in Action (HRiA), a Boston-based affiliate of the National Network of Public Health Institutes, to serve as NACHW's fiscal sponsor. In the winter of 2019, the board began recruiting 20 CHW "ambassadors" from across the country to work on membership recruitment. On March 14, 2019, NACHW was incorporated as a nonprofit organization in the state of Delaware.

NACHW launched publicly on April 15, 2019, at the Unity conference in Las Vegas, Nevada, with 850 CHWs in attendance. Board members processed into the grand ballroom of the Flamingo Hotel behind a symbolic lighted torch as the lights were dimmed, and CHWs held illuminated cell phones aloft in a scene reminiscent of a stadium concert. Board leaders inspired conferees with speeches describing the organization's mission, values, and historical promise. Participation in NACHW workshops at the conference was strong, and over 300 people paid dues to join the organization during its first 3 days.

NACHW secured approval from the US Internal Revenue Service on July 12, 2019, as a tax-exempt 501(c)(3) corporation. With funding from Care Coordination Systems and the Rx Foundation to augment Sanofi's support, NACHW began a national search for its founding executive director that summer, culminating in the hiring of Denise O. Smith on November 6, 2019. Smith, a CHW and Robert Wood Johnson Foundation Culture of Health Leader, came to NACHW from the University of Connecticut Health Disparities Institute with a strong background in healthcare administration, training, program development, and community-based service provision. Working closely with the board, she established five major priorities for the organization's first year, including updating NACHW's strategic plan; building organizational capacity in staffing, funding, and operating systems; mobilizing CHW members and allies in cooperation with NACHW's ambassadors; establishing strategic partnerships; and articulating policy and workforce development priorities. As this chapter went to press, NACHW was preparing for its first annual meeting in August, 2020, including the first election by the general membership of NACHW's board of directors.

NACHW emerged from an inclusive, deliberate planning process spanning over 4 years that depended upon the dedication of nearly two dozen CHW leaders and allies from across the country who committed themselves to hundreds of hours of voluntary cooperation to build unity and a sustainable plan to empower and support the CHW workforce. NACHW's vision, mission, and values draw upon the pioneering work of the AACHW and stand as a testament to the power of collaboration and the potential of a united, organized CHW voice:

Vision: Community health workers united nationally to support communities in achieving health, equity, and social justice.

Mission: To unify the voices of community health workers and strengthen the profession's capacity to promote healthy communities.

Values:

- *Self-empowerment.* Promoting self-actualization and self-advocacy among community health workers.
- *Self-determination.* Promoting the efforts of community health workers and the communities in which they work, to create a shared vision and direction for the future.
- *Social Justice and Equity.* Ensuring fair treatment, access, opportunity, advancement, and outcomes for individuals and communities.
- *Integrity.* Protecting and nurturing the authenticity and character of the CHW profession and promoting the contributions made by CHWs toward eliminating health disparities and advancing equity.
- *Dignity and Respect.* Building trusted relationships based on honoring the inherent value and contributions of every person irrespective of socioeconomic class, religion, race, national origin, language spoken, immigration status, abilities or disabilities, age, sex, sexual orientation, and gender identity/expression.
- *Unity.* Encouraging collaboration among community health workers to promote a common professional identity regardless of job title or work setting.

15.3 A CHW Leader's Story

15.3.1 Opportunity and Hope: Why a National Voice Matters to Me

Naomi Cottoms

Opportunity and *hope* are the two feelings experienced as I travel the roads of exploration, start-up, and capacity building. The opportunity to dream and vision while engaging with others is phenomenal. It allows for learning and understanding different perspectives. It enables one to practice the listening skills that are key to inclusion and the representation of diverse groups.

In 2012, myself and others convened a group of lay community members in the State of Arkansas working in health. We engaged with them in the thought of our work being a profession and why having a professional association could be beneficial to our efforts.

We created a steering committee to move this work forward. I was fortunate to work beside a very knowledgeable, resourceful, and caring young woman, Dr. Kate Stewart, whose commitment to social justice and equity is distinguished. Most times, I was able to follow her lead and experience her wisdom, her professional connections, and her networks. The steering committee consisted of members from the Arkansas Department of Health, the University of Arkansas for Medical Sciences at Little Rock (UAMS), and several other organizations representing community institutions and community-based organizations. This group also included several of us working in health that identified ourselves as community health workers (CHWs). It is out of this steering committee that the Arkansas Community Health Worker Association (ARCHWA) was born.

This steering committee began with monthly meetings, advancing to every other week and then weekly as needed. ARCHWA operated with the help of the steering committee and those CHWs who attended the annual conference as a support system for all CHWs in the State of Arkansas. The UAMS College of Public Health gave support through each phase of the development of ARCHWA, enabling CHWs to lead the process. In 2015, we received our IRS designation as a 501(c)(3) non-profit. I have the privilege of being a part of this wonderful organization, which is led by CHWs and provides ongoing support for the workforce. I further have had the privilege of serving as the first President of ARCHWA.

I continue to serve as a part of the leadership for CHWs in the State of Arkansas, because I believe in who we are and what we do. In our great state, we are again engaging stakeholders, this time in the conversation of whether to have certification or not. With time, individuals and organization stakeholders have changed, as well as perspectives. Therefore, we continue to inform, sharing information in an effort to ensure that the Arkansas Community understands who we are and the many valuable roles we carry out on a daily basis.

In 2016, I was afforded an opportunity to join a group of people who had been working on the development of a national CHW association. This group had observed the struggles of the state and regional groups and had participated in national studies about CHWs and their work. They were well-versed on the lay of the land, as it related to the state of CHWs, and saw the need for a national body which could aid in the empowerment of the individuals providing services as CHW throughout our nation. I was honored and excited. After accepting my invitation to this group's first meeting, I was advised of the commitment required for serving with this group. I was afraid and uncertain about adding this kind of commitment to my already overwhelming work load. Yet, I thought about our state and my fellow CHWs in Arkansas, and so I persevered. I made a commitment to participate in the meetings and to actually work with this group, providing assistance in any manner possible. I immediately began volunteering for committees and assisting wherever I could. My commitment to the call, my vision of hope, especially for those of us who believe our voices as sometimes "unheard" led me to the opportunity of serving as chairperson for the search for our new Executive Director, Mrs. Denise Smith. Working and interacting in some of the many tasks needed for the beginning of this organization has afforded me the opportunity to serve on various committees, even moving into a leadership role of being a part of the Nominations Committee and the Executive Committee. Working but enjoying my place of service with this group, I was able to be a part of the launch ceremony for the official start of this great organization, the lighting of the torch. The National Association of Community Health Workers has officially begun in due form.

Serving on this board is indeed an opportunity and a continual arousing of hope. As decisions are made and plans are envisioned, careful steps are taken to ensure inclusion, diversity, and, most of all, equity. Experiencing the process of the creation of this National Association of Community Health Workers has enabled me to learn, grow, and appreciate systems, procedures, and techniques from a variety of views including non-actuating and just plain discussion. The interactions with the other board members who hail from all over the nation enable me to interact with different value systems, different life experiences, and different levels of knowledge—a true diversity in perspectives. Yet as a group, we are all committed to this new organization and the values therein established. Our group interactions enable engagement at a level of academic proficiency yet one that allows space for human frailty. The experiences are noble and rewarding. The launch of NACHW is indeed one of opportunity and hope.

15.4   Future of CHWs in the United States

Implementation of the Patient Protection and Affordable Care Act of 2010, with its wide-ranging innovations in healthcare design and payment models, generated a veritable explosion in research about CHWs. According to a 2020 policy brief co-published by NACHW and the Association of State and Territorial Health Officials, 574 studies were published about CHWs from 2014 to 2016, compared to a total of 252 studies in the period 1994–2003. (Association of State and Territorial Health Officials and National Association of Community Health Workers, 2020). CHWs have been shown to be effective in improving health outcomes for vulnerable populations in randomized control trials and systematic reviews of interventions, and they have been shown to generate economic and social return on investment for an array of diseases, conditions, and patients, in urban and urban settings.

The prospects for CHW workforce development look bright, despite volatility in the national health policy environment. The US Bureau of Labor Statistics projects overall employment of CHWs will grow much faster than the average for all occupations from 2018 to 2028. (U.S. Department of Labor, Bureau of Labor Statistics, 2020). CHW credentialing is gaining support in red and blue states alike, and health systems are beginning to invest core budget resources for integrating CHWs into care teams because of their unique value in addressing complex patient needs. CHWs are becoming involved in behavioral health integration, and the workforce is gaining traction in an array of non-medical settings and public health disciplines.

In this context, NACHW's emergence as an organized, national voice of and for the CHW workforce is historically significant. Too many policy discussions and decisions about CHWs have happened without their active participation. Despite improving regard for the workforce, CHWs continue to struggle for professional respect. NACHW's leaders are determined to assure workforce members are "at the table, rather than on the menu" for traditionally more powerful actors to digest. Significant challenges in professional development range from workforce identity to over-medicalization of the field, from credentialing standards to access barriers, and from sustainable financing to financial exploitation. NACHW's potential to support and build CHW leadership and organizational capacity at the local, state, regional, and national levels holds enormous promise for advancing health equity and policy and system change to benefit the nation's most vulnerable members and communities.

Acknowledgments The authors thank the following NACHW leaders for participating in planning discussions about this chapter, for contributing historical information that supported its drafting, and/or for copy edits to the draft: Mae-Gilene Begay, Ramona Dillard, Durrell Fox, Lisa Renee Holderby-Fox, Gail Hirsch, and Floribella Redondo. The authors would also like to recognize all members of the founding NACHW Board of Directors:

- Mae-Gilene Begay
- Joelisa Castillo
- Naomi Cottoms
- Ramona Dillard
- Durrell Fox
- Catherine Haywood
- Wandy Hernandez
- Gail Hirsch
- Lisa Renee Holderby-Fox
- Maria Lemus
- Sergio Matos
- Susan Mayfield Johnson
- Anita McDonnell
- Floribella Redondo
- Carl Rush
- Alise Sanchez
- Julie Smithwick
- Napualani Spock
- Katherine Sutkowi
- Ashley Wennerstrom
- Geoffrey Wilkinson

Further, the authors would like to acknowledge other key leaders and supporters in the CHW field that contributed to its development and multi-decade efforts for organizing and recognition:

- J. Nell Brownstein
- Yvonne Lacey
- E. Lee Rosenthal
- Cathy Stueckemann
- Kalahn Taylor-Clark
- Noelle Wiggins

References

111th Congress, 2nd Session. (2010, May 1). *Compilation of patient protection and affordable care act.* Retrieved August 4, 2018, from https://www.hhs.gov/sites/default/files/ppacacon.pdf.

American Public Health Association. (2001, January 1). *Recognition and support for community health workers' contributions to meeting our Nation's health care needs.* American Public Health Association. Retrieved from https://www.apha.org/policies-and-advocacy/public-health-policy-statements/policy-database/2014/07/15/13/24/recognition-and-support-community-health-workers-contrib-to-meeting-our-nations-health-care-needs.

American Public Health Association. (2009, November 10). *Support for community health workers to increase health access and to reduce health inequities.* Retrieved from apha.org: https://www.apha.org/policies-and-advocacy/public-health-policy-statements/policy-database/2014/07/09/14/19/support-for-community-health-workers-to-increase-health-access-and-to-reduce-health-inequities.

American Public Health Association. (2014, November 18). *Support for community health worker leadership in determining workforce standards for training and credentialing.* Retrieved August 4, 2018, from apha.org: https://www.apha.org/policies-and-advocacy/public-health-policy-statements/policy-database/2015/01/28/14/15/support-for-community-health-worker-leadership.

American Public Health Association. (2018). *Community health workers: Who we are.* Retrieved from apha.org: https://www.apha.org/apha-communities/member-sections/community-health-workers/who-we-are.

Association of State and Territorial Health Officials and National Association of Community Health Workers (2020). *Community health workers: Evidence of their effectiveness.* Retrieved January 3, 2020, from https://www.astho.org/Programs/Clinical-to-Community-Connections/Documents/CHW-Evidence-of-Effectiveness/.

Beam, N., & Tessaro, I. (1994). The lay health advisor model in theory and practice: An example of an agency-based program. *Family & Community Health, 17*(3), 70–79.

Berthold, T., Miller, J., & Avila-Esparza, A. (Eds.). (2009). *Foundations for community health workers.* San Francisco: Jossey-Bass.

Centers for Medicare & Medicaid Services. (2013, July 15). *Medicaid and children's health insurance programs: Essential health benefits in alternative benefit plans, eligibility notices, fair hearing and appeal processes, and premiums and cost sharing; exchanges: eligibility and enrollment.* Retrieved August 4, 2018, from federalregister.gov: https://www.federalregister.gov/documents/2013/07/15/2013-16271/medicaid-and-childrens-health-insurance-programs-essential-health-benefits-in-alternative-benefit.

D'Onofrio, C. N. (1970). Aides—pain or panacea? *Public Health Reports, 85*(9), 788–801.

Eng, E., & Young, R. (1992). Lay health advisors as community change agents. *Family & Community Health, 15*(1), 24–40.

Fox, D., Holderby, L. R., & Monroe, D. (2008). Kujichagulia—Self-determination: Building AACHW, the American association of CHWs. *Unity Conference.*

Geiger, H. J. (2016). The first community health center in Mississippi: Communities empowering themselves. *American Journal of Public Health, 106*(10), 1738–1740.

Hoff, W. (1969). Role of the community health aide in public health programs. *Public Health Reports, 84*(11), 998–1002.

Indian Health Service. (n.d.). *Community health representative: About us.* Retrieved August 4, 2018, from ihs.gov: https://www.ihs.gov/chr/aboutus/.

Ingram, M., Sabo, S., Rothers, J., Wennerstrom, A., & de Zapien, J. (2008). Community health workers and community advocacy: Addressing health disparities. *Journal of Community Health, 33*(6), 417–424.

Kent, J. A., & Smith, C. H. (1967). Involving the urban poor in health services through accommodation—The employment of neighborhood representatives. *American Journal of Public Health, 57*(6), 997–1003.

Mesiter, J. S. (1990). *Un comienzo Sano: A case study of community-based prenatal intervention*. Tuscon: Southwest Border Rural Health Research Center, College of Medicine, University of Arizona.

National Association of Community Health Representatives. (2018). *NACHR*. Retrieved August 4, 2018, from nachr.net: http://www.nachr.net/.

Perez, L. M., & Martinez, J. (2008). Community health workers: Social justice and policy advocates for community health and well-being. *American Journal of Public Health, 98*(10), 11–14.

Rosenthal, E. L., Brownstein, J. N., Rush, C. H., Hirsch, G. R., Willaert, A. M., Scott, J. R., … Fox, D. J. (2010). Community health workers: Part of the solution. *Health Affairs, 29*(7), 1338–1342.

Rosenthal, E. L., Wiggins, N., Brownstein, J. N., Johnson, S., Borbon, I. A., & Rael, R. (1998). *The final report of the National Community Health Advisor Study*. Tucson: The University of Arizona.

Sabo, S., Ingram, M., & Wennerstrom, A. (2010). Social justice and health in Arizona border communities: The community health worker model. In A. J. Donelson & A. X. Esparza (Eds.), *The Colonias Reader: Economy, housing, and public health in U.S.-Mexico Border Colonias*. Tuscon: The University of Arizona Press.

U.S. Department of Health and Human Services, H. R. (2007). *Community Health Worker National Workforce Study*. Retrieved August 4, 2018, from https://bhw.hrsa.gov/sites/default/files/bhw/nchwa/projections/communityhealthworkforce.pdf.

U.S. Department of Health and Human Services, Office of the Inspector General. (1993). *Revitalizing the community health representative program*. U.S. Department of Health and Human Services. Retrieved July 30, 2018, from https://oig.hhs.gov/oei/reports/oei-05-91-01070.pdf.

U.S. Department of Labor, Bureau of Labor Statistics. (2017). *Standard occupational classification: Community health worker*. Retrieved January 3, 2020, from https://www.bls.gov/oes/2017/may/oes211094.htm.

U.S. Department of Labor, Bureau of Labor Statistics. (2020). *Health educators and community health workers. Occupational outlook handbook*. Retrieved January 3, 2020, from https://www.bls.gov/ooh/community-and-social-service/health-educators.htm.

Wilkinson, G., Sutkowi, K., & Cenzon, A. (2018). *Results of a national survey of CHW membership organizations*. National Association of Community Health Workers. Retrieved January 3, 2020, from https://nachw.org/2019/12/11/results-of-national-survey-of-chw-networks/.

Witmer, A., Siefer, D., Finocchio, L., Leslie, J., & O'Neil, E. H. (1995). Community health workers: Integral members of the health care workforce. *American Journal of Public Health, 85*(8, part 1), 1055–1058.

Chapter 16
Where Do We Go from Here? A Closing Reflection

Susan L. Mayfield-Johnson, Wandy D. Hernández-Gordon, and Julie Ann St. John

Over the years, the fact that individual health is linked to the community's health and that the health of the community is foundational to where individuals live, work, and play is increasingly evident. The collective beliefs, attitudes, and values of everyone who lives in that community profoundly affect a community's health.

Community health workers (CHWs) have been a fundamental part of the health and social services delivery systems for decades. From early accounts in history of Russian Felshers, barefoot doctors in China, and *promotores* in Latin America (Wiggins, 2009), to the landmark National Community Health Advisor Study (Rosenthal et al., 1998), and development of the National Association of Community Health Workers (NACHW) (2020), CHWs have demonstrated their resiliency in their profession and commitment to their communities.

The National Community Health Advisor Study (Rosenthal et al., 1998) first documented findings and recommendations from CHWs and practitioners on the core roles that CHWs serve as health promotion practitioners. These findings and the subsequent Community Health Worker (CHW) Core Consensus (C3) Project (2018) helped define the necessary foundation for the CHW workforce. Each of the chapters presented in this text demonstrated the meaningful contributions CHWs make to health, social, and human service delivery adaptation, and they underscore

S. L. Mayfield-Johnson
Department of Public Health, School of Health Professions, The University of Southern Mississippi, Hattiesburg, MS, USA
e-mail: susan.johnson@usm.edu

W. D. Hernández-Gordon
HealthConnect One, Chicago, IL, USA
e-mail: wandyhdz@healthconnectone.org

J. A. St. John (✉)
Department of Public Health, Texas Tech University Health Sciences Center, Abilene, TX, USA
e-mail: julie.st-john@ttuhsc.edu

© Springer Nature Switzerland AG 2021
J. A. St. John et al. (eds.), *Promoting the Health of the Community*,
https://doi.org/10.1007/978-3-030-56375-2_16

the need for more recognition on how CHWs utilize their special skills and abilities to impact and improve community health.

Recent pandemics have laid bare the deficiencies in our health and social care systems, underlining broken infrastructure, inadequate policies, and health inequalities. The demand for continued adaptations to access basic health, physiological, and social service needs takes on new meanings. Familiar barriers to care—such as cost, transportation, and language services—remains, but the new frontier requires overcoming challenges for the workforce who delivers supportive and preventative care to be responsive and creative in their solutions. CHWs are well positioned to be this workforce. Prior to the pandemic, a number of states had enacted legislation recognizing CHWs as part of a vital public health workforce (The National Academy for State Health Policy, 2019). In fact, the US Department of Homeland Security (2020, March 19) identified CHWs as "essential critical infrastructure workers" in guidance to state, local, tribal, and territorial jurisdictions and the private sector.

Despite the strong evidence of CHW effectiveness, several factors contribute to inconsistent engagement of CHWs in program management, clinical care, and research. This inconsistent engagement of CHWs contributes to ongoing inequities in the healthcare workforce, clinical and research processes in healthcare settings, and ultimately health outcomes. CHWs have long fought for respect and recognition of the CHW workforce and profession in and among other health, social, and human service professions. Integration of CHWs as members of the patient healthcare delivery team is an aim for many CHWs. Others assert their goal and work is characterized by *servicio de corazón* (service from the heart), and CHWs educate, empower, and advocate for community change in linguistically and culturally sensitive and responsive ways, sharing a desire to improve their communities so that all families may know a better way of life (Visión y Compromiso, 2019). What binds CHWs is an acknowledgment that community needs and priorities should be at the forefront when addressing the community's health. CHWs are often that voice for the community.

Community representation is vital if we want to continue to have an open dialogue and meet the needs of every individual who breathes the air, walks the sidewalks (or streets), and lives in the area, but we have to ensure that community is also represented at every table. These tables may include issues associated with local, state, or national governments; be civic in nature; have an educational emphasis; or incorporate the physical, mental, social, emotional, and spiritual well-being of its inhabitants. However, CHWs need to be present at another table, the table that includes our health, social, and human service delivery systems—the people, institutions, and resources that deliver health care and social services to meet the needs of our communities.

CHWs need to be valued and respected for the authentic voice they represent—the underserved, undervalued, and overlooked community member whose health and personhood that has been invisible to others. CHWs do not want to be another health profession that is just at the table; they want to be recognized and venerated for their unique lived experiences, their work in the trenches of the community, their exclusive knowledge of what it is like to be a member of the community being served, and the broad community connections they engage. They know which individuals, families, and elderly residents in their neighborhoods are most in need of social support and resources like food, medical supplies, and diapers. CHWs can help people apply for unemployment and disability benefits, Supplemental Nutrition Assistance Program, the Special Supplemental Nutrition Program for Women, Infants and Children, utility assistance, and prescription assistance programs. They can also offer some limited direct services through oral health and chronic disease management. CHWs want to be truly engaged in the planning, implementation, and evaluation of services and programs in which they are involved. As a CHW from rural Arkansas noted, "I want our (CHW) input and voice to be included and genuinely considered as part of the team, not as an afterthought" (N. Cottoms, personal communication, February 26, 2020).

CHWs generally come from the communities they serve and provide culturally and linguistically appropriate services. They work with diverse communities on a wide range of topics, diseases, and illnesses to provide a variety of services. They understand the system; many CHWs have walked in exactly the shoes of the community members they attend. Numerous CHWs have endured socioeconomic, racial/ethnic, and gender inequalities, but most CHWs are devoted to community health work. Often a lifetime fidelity, many CHWs feel they were called to this profession because of their experiences and struggles (Mayfield-Johnson, Rachal, & Butler, 2014). These occurrences and the subsequent proficiencies learned lend themselves to the unique contributions CHWs can offer. As such, CHWs know that such work does not have a 9 am to 5 pm schedule, requires innovative problem-solving skills, and may not be adequately compensated. In fact, CHWs often work in hourly positions that pay less than a living wage (Holgate, Albelda, & Agarwal, 2018). In the words of CHW and editor Wandy D. Hernández-Gordon:

> CHWs have to develop and wear their resilience armor. CHWs are known to have special powers. It's a combination of our life devotion and our armor of resilience. This unique profession requires being available 24 hours a day, seven days a week, to assist segregated and marginalized community members when needed with a caring, empathetic heart for service. CHW work can be stressful at times. Our kryptonite has sometimes been the need to balance advocating for community members to receive the proper resources and services they need with the dignity and respect they deserve, all while representing the protocols, required paperwork, and limited capital of our respective agencies.

These challenges can dishearten even the best CHWs.

How can we address these issues? In this text, chapter teams with CHWs as lead authors present illustrative vignettes on how CHWs can be engaged to provide these core roles: (1) cultural mediation among individuals, communities, and health and social service systems; (2) providing culturally appropriate health education and information; (3) care coordination, case management, and system navigation; (4) providing coaching and social support; (5) advocating for individuals and communities; (6) building individual and community capacity; (7) providing direct service; (8) implementing individual and community assessments; (9) conducting outreach; and (10) participating in evaluation and research. The stories, quotes, and pictures appear throughout to offer examples of what CHWs do to promote the community's health. These chapters served to demonstrate how CHWs can be uniquely positioned to improve health, community development, and access to systems of care in extensive settings, systems, and topic areas.

We know that full integration of each of the core roles has not be implemented across the country, but evidence of common and foundational CHW core roles is clear. Full acceptance and incorporation of CHWs into clinical, research, or community-based care teams has not fully actualized in all states and territories; however, each of the chapters included in this book demonstrated the need for full integration of CHWs. Full integration of CHWs include acknowledgment and trust of CHW expertise within the system. Acknowledgment includes recognizing and verbalizing CHW work as essential to other public health, social, and human service professions and to the CHWs and communities they serve. Trust incorporates respect for the unique knowledge, experiences, and contributions CHW bring to the table. Respect also includes allowances for CHWs to be noted as "community experts" in publications, presentations, and representation of respective agencies and organizations to other entities. CHWs need to represent CHWs, or as noted in the foreword, "Nothing about us without us." Finally, integration also includes adequate compensation for work. CHWs must have a living wage to ensure their ability to continue to do what they love and still afford to eat.

Our hope is that through the development of this text, we demonstrated how some teams have integrated CHWs into the care and delivery of health and social services in their communities and how other teams will ascribe to do the same with CHWs in an equitable and social justice platform—with their community's priorities and needs at the forefront. At the heart of these efforts are our communities, and CHWs will continue to fight for our communities. As a result of the work of CHWs, community members, patients, clients, our friends, and brothers and sisters learn new information and skills, increase their confidence, and enhance their abilities to advocate for themselves. Most importantly, the work of CHWs helps to reduce health inequalities among and in our communities. We hope the readers of this text will find ways to become more involved with CHWs, as a CHW, an ally, or supporter, and join the movement to advocate for equity on behalf of all of our communities.

References

Community Health Worker (CHW) Core Consensus (C3) Project. (2018). *C3 findings: Roles and competencies.* Retrieved from https://www.c3project.org/.

Holgate, B., Albelda, R., & Agarwal, V. (2018, March 15). *Community health workers: Wages, skills and roles. A report to the Massachusetts Association of Community Health Workers.* Boston, MA: The Center for Social Policy, University of Massachusetts.

Mayfield-Johnson, S., Rachal, J., & Butler, J. (2014, May). "When We Learn Better, We Do Better." Changes in Empowerment through Photovoice among Community Health Advisors in a Breast and Cervical Cancer Health Promotion Program in Mississippi and Alabama. *Adult Education Quarterly, 64*(2), 93–111. https://doi.org/10.1177/0741713614521862

National Academy for State Health Policy. (2019). *State community health worker models*. Retrieved from https://nashp.org/state-community-health-worker-models/.

National Association of Community Health Workers (NACHW). (2020). Retrieved from https://nachw.org/.

Rosenthal, E. L., Wiggins, N., Brownstein, J. N., Johnson, S., Borbon, I. A., & Rael, R. (1998). *Final report of the National Community Health Advisor Study: Weaving the future*. Tucson: The University of Arizona.

U.S. Department of Homeland Security, Cybersecurity & Infrastructure Security Agency. (2020, March 19). *Guidance on essential critical infrastructure workforce*. Retrieved from https://www.cisa.gov/publication/guidance-essential-critical-infrastructure-workforce.

Vision y Compromiso. (2019). Retrieved from http://visionycompromiso.org/who-we-are/.

Wiggins, N. (2009). CHWs throughout history and around the world. In T. Berthold, J. Miller, & A. Avila-Esparza (Eds.), *Foundations for community health workers*. San Francisco: Jossey-Bass.

Index

© Springer Nature Switzerland AG 2021
J. A. St. John et al. (eds.), *Promoting the Health of the Community*,
https://doi.org/10.1007/978-3-030-56375-2

Printed in the United States
by Baker & Taylor Publisher Services